Adolescent Gynecology

Hina J. Talib
Editor

Adolescent Gynecology

A Clinical Casebook

Springer

Editor
Hina J. Talib, M.D.
Assistant Professor, Pediatrics
Program Director, Post-doctoral Fellowship in Adolescent Medicine
Division of Adolescent Medicine
Children's Hospital at Montefiore
The Pediatric Hospital for Albert Einstein College of Medicine
Bronx, NY, USA

ISBN 978-3-319-66977-9 ISBN 978-3-319-66978-6 (eBook)
https://doi.org/10.1007/978-3-319-66978-6

Library of Congress Control Number: 2017959188

Printed on acid-free paper

This Springer imprint is published by Springer Nature
The registered company is Springer International Publishing AG
The registered company address is: Gewerbestrasse 11, 6330 Cham, Switzerland

For my mother, a physician and educator in the specialty of Pediatrics, whose footsteps I follow with confidence that comes from her unwavering support.

Foreword

The gynecologic and reproductive health care of female infants, children, and adolescents has often been fragmented without well-accepted guidelines and bodies of evidence. However, fortunately for girls and young women, a multidisciplinary medical/surgical subspecialty is now emerging into the mainstream of medical practice in the USA and to a lesser extent in other countries. This subspecialty is called pediatric and adolescent gynecology (PAG), and its practitioners include adolescent medicine specialists, endocrinologists, gynecologists, nurse practitioners, pediatricians, urologists, and psychologists/psychiatrists, all of whom have training and expertise in PAG. The case discussions in *Adolescent Gynecology: A Clinical Casebook* are written by many of the foremost US and Canadian experts in PAG and will serve as a clinical guide for PAG fellowship trainees as well as for medical students and resident trainees and primary care practitioners who are the frontline caregivers for adolescents.

The clinical case discussion format is particularly useful for addressing the many intersecting and often competing considerations that must be taken into account when providing gynecologic and reproductive health care to the adolescent age group. Approaches to common problems including pain with menstruation, excessive menstrual bleeding, menstrual hygiene for girls with special needs, vaginal discharge, and contraception are thoroughly discussed with many helpful suggestions for counseling teens and parents. For example, Drs. Sieke and Rome offer insights and advice for addressing gynecological concerns of the special needs population. They comment that "Although adolescents with disabilities may not have the same level of understanding about pubertal and sexual development as their peers, clinicians must not assume that they are not sexually active or do not have a sexual drive… Education [for] adolescents with intellectual disability … should include hygiene, contraception, consent, sexually transmitted infections, and sexual abuse prevention measures." The issues of consent and confidentiality are central to the practice of adolescent gynecology but also quite difficult to manage in the clinical encounter. Drs. Scott and Alderman in their "Case of a Girl with a Secret" answer the question, "How should providers balance the rights of adolescents' privacy regarding certain elements of their health with parents' responsibility to be a part of their adolescent child's health?" Unintended teen pregnancy, while decreasing in recent years, remains a significant problem in the USA. Access to effective contraception is an important part of the solution. Drs. Northridge and Maslyanskaya in their "Case of a Girl Seeking Birth Control" provide an in-depth discussion of the use of long-acting reversible contraception in adolescents, including medical eligibility criteria, the insertion procedure, and counseling.

In addition to cases that discuss common adolescent gynecological issues, *Adolescent Gynecology: A Clinical Casebook* also provides valuable information about some highly specialized or rare gynecological conditions affecting adolescent girls such as fertility preservation in girls undergoing cancer treatment as well as diagnosis and management of rare causes of primary amenorrhea including uterine and vaginal agenesis [Mayer-Rokitansky-Kuster-Hauser (MRKH)] and primary ovarian insufficiency (POI). Surgical and nonsurgical techniques for creation of a neovagina in adolescents with MRKH are thoroughly reviewed by Drs. Adeyemi-Fowode and Dietrich in the "Case of a Girl with Primary Amenorrhea, Cyclic Pelvic Pain, and Absent Vagina." Drs. Kanj and Gordon in their comprehensive case discussion of POI, "Case of a Girl with Delayed Puberty and High Gonadotropin Levels," not only point out the appropriate diagnostic testing for this condition but also remind us that "However, even after a thorough evaluation, approximately 90% of cases of spontaneous POI—i.e., those not secondary to cytotoxic therapy such as chemotherapy or radiation—will remain without an identifiable cause." And they further advise us that "In all cases of POI, the various components of this chronic condition must be considered, including effects on physical, emotional, and mental health…," excellent advice that applies to most adolescent gynecological problems. In the "Case of the Girl with Vulvar Swelling," Dr. Simms-Cendan clearly addresses the current controversy over cosmetic labiaplasty in teenagers and the lack of an accepted definition of labia minora hypertrophy as well as the large increase in the number of teens requesting this surgical procedure.

This excellent casebook provides an overview of many of the most common and important gynecological conditions affecting adolescent girls and distills the clinical insights of experienced PAG practitioners to help guide diagnosis and management. Its format makes it an accessible, easy-to-use resource for trainees and primary care clinicians. I believe, and sincerely hope, that it will contribute to improved gynecologic care for adolescent girls.

Susan M. Coupey, M.D.
Professor of Pediatrics
Chief, Division of Adolescent Medicine
Children's Hospital at Montefiore
The Pediatric Hospital for Albert Einstein College of Medicine
Bronx, NY USA

Preface

Pediatric and adolescent gynecology is a multidisciplinary medical/surgical subspecialty that I am passionate about, as it centers on caring for girls and young women, with and without chronic illnesses, as they navigate their changing bodies and developing sexuality, a process that can be rife with physical and emotional challenges. These challenges are often undiscovered by health professionals, as adolescent girls may not be forthcoming unless asked directly about symptoms or emotions in a sensitive manner ensuring confidentiality. This book aims to raise awareness of common and not-so-common adolescent gynecologic issues; to empower student, physician, and nursing trainees, as well as practicing providers in caring for young girls; and to update readers with advances in adolescent gynecology.

Although education in the subspecialty of pediatric and adolescent gynecology is a core element of medical training, especially in the disciplines of pediatrics and obstetrics and gynecology, it faces many barriers in training programs including lack of faculty with expertise in the field, lack of a formalized curriculum, and limited opportunities for trainees to evaluate and treat young girls with gynecologic concerns. In planning and editing this book, I have been fortunate to draw from my experience as program director of the Adolescent Medicine Fellowship Training Program at the Children's Hospital at Montefiore and as associate editor of the *Journal of Pediatric and Adolescent Gynecology*.

Puberty is a hallmark event in the development of adolescent girls, and it is a time of great physical, emotional, and social change. With this in mind, this book is organized in four sections, starting with Part I, "General and Developmental Approach to Adolescents," which includes chapters addressing adolescent confidentiality, puberty, and well care. Part II, "Menstrual Disorders," recognizes that menstrual complaints are a leading reason for physician office visits by adolescent girls in the USA. Chapters here discuss the varied concerns girls often have with their menses ranging from too heavy, to too painful, to too irregular. Part III, "Sexually Active Adolescents," highlights issues in reproductive health care including sexually transmitted infection and adolescent pregnancy both of which cause significant morbidity in adolescent girls. Finally, Part IV, "Special

Populations of Adolescents," includes chapters on girls who have sex with girls, girls who are victims of abuse, and girls with special health-care needs and chronic health conditions. Here, common gynecologic health issues are discussed in the context of these special populations to increase sensitivity to and comprehensive care of these girls.

This book uses clinical cases, a preferred method of learning by trainees, to provide a concise and clinically relevant survey of adolescent gynecology.

Teaching highlights unique to this text include the case-based format, clinical pearls and pitfalls, and suggested further reading that focuses on clinical references informed by professional society guidelines, up-to-date reviews, and the Centers for Disease Control and Prevention and other large health organizations. It is my hope that readers will enjoy learning from these clinical cases just as much as I have and that they will gain knowledge and clinical skills in the care of adolescent girls and young women.

Hina J. Talib, M.D.

Acknowledgments

This book would not be possible without the support and mentorship of Susan M. Coupey, MD, Chief, Division of Adolescent Medicine at Children's Hospital at Montefiore. Her assistance in conception and organization of the book as well as her review of the chapters was invaluable. I would also like to thank the contributing authors, who took time from their clinical practices to share their experiences and educational discussions, which I believe will be an asset to learners looking to increase their knowledge base in adolescent gynecology. I also thank Elise M. Paxson, our developmental editor at Springer for her assistance, patience, and gentle guidance in the lengthy process of completing this book. Lastly, I must credit the love and support of my husband, Nilam Patel, and the smiles and snuggles from our infant son, Isa, for carrying me through this endeavor and so much more.

Hina J. Talib, M.D.

Abbreviations

ACIP	Advisory Committee on Immunization Practices
ACS	Administration for Child Services
ADHD	Attention-deficit hyperactivity disorder
AFP	Alpha-fetoprotein
ACOG	American College of Obstetricians and Gynecologists
AUB	Abnormal uterine bleeding
BDNF	Brain-derived neurotrophic factor
β-hCG	Beta human chorionic gonadotropin
BMD	Bone mineral density
BMI	Body mass index
BV	Bacterial vaginosis
CA-125	Cancer antigen 125
CACIS	Complete androgen insensitivity syndrome
CAH	Congenital adrenal hyperplasia
CBT	Cognitive behavior therapy
CDC	Centers for Disease Control and Prevention
CLIA	Clinical Laboratory Improvement Amendments
CMT	Cervical motion tenderness
CNS	Central nervous system
COC	Combined oral contraceptive
COCP	Combined oral contraceptive pill
CPP	Chronic pelvic pain
CSEC	Commercial sexual exploitation of children
CYP3A	Cytochrome P4503A
DMPA	Depot medroxyprogesterone acetate
DMST	Domestic minor sex trafficking
DRSP	Daily Record of Severity of Problems
DSD	Disorder of sex development
DSM-5	Diagnostic and Statistical Manual of Mental Disorders, Fifth Edition
DXA	Dual-energy X-ray absorptiometry
ED	Emergency Department

EE	Ethinyl estradiol
EMR	Electronic medical record
EPT	Expedited partner therapy
FDA	US Food and Drug Administration
FHR	Fetal heart rate
FSH	Follicle-stimulating hormone
GI	Gastrointestinal
GISP	Gonococcal Isolate Surveillance Project
GnRH	Gonadotropin-releasing hormone
Hb	Hemoglobin
HFI	Hormone-free interval
HIV	Human immunodeficiency virus
HPG	Hypothalamic-pituitary-gonad
HPO	Hypothalamic-pituitary-ovarian
IBD	Inflammatory bowel disease
IEP	Individualized educational plan
IHH	Idiopathic hypogonadotropic hypogonadism
INR	International normalized ratio
IPV	Intimate partner violence
IUD	Intrauterine device
IUFD	Intrauterine fetal death
IUGR	Intrauterine growth restriction
IVF	In vitro fertilization
LARC	Long-acting reversible contraception
LBW	Low birth weight
LDHC	Lactate dehydrogenase
LGBTQ	Lesbian gay bisexual transgender queer
LH	Luteinizing hormone
MBSR	Mindfulness-based stress reduction
MGD	Mixed gonadal dysgenesis
MRKH	Mayer-Rokitansky-Kuster-Hauser
MRI	Magnetic resonance imaging
MSK	Musculoskeletal
MSM	Men who have sex with men
NAAT	Nucleic acid amplification test
NAS	Neonatal abstinence syndrome
NHTSC	National Human Trafficking Resource Center
NSAID	Nonsteroidal anti-inflammatory drug
OR	Odds ratio
PAIS	Partial androgen insensitivity syndrome
PCOS	Polycystic ovary syndrome
PID	Pelvic inflammatory disease
PMD	Premenstrual disorder
PMDD	Premenstrual dysphoric disorder
PMS	Premenstrual syndrome

POI	Primary ovarian insufficiency
POP	Progestin-only pill
PPROM	Premature preterm rupture of membranes
PRL	Prolactin
PROM	Premature rupture of membranes
PSST-A	Premenstrual Symptoms Screening Tool for Adolescents
PT	Prothrombin time
PTB	Preterm birth
PTL	Preterm labor
PTT	Partial thromboplastin time
PTSD	Post-traumatic stress disorder
RCT	Randomized controlled trial
REI	Reproductive endocrinology and infertility
SA	Spontaneous abortion
SGA	Small for gestational age
SNRI	Serotonin-norepinephrine reuptake inhibitor
SSRI	Selective serotonin reuptake inhibitor
SRI	Serotonin reuptake inhibitors
STI	Sexually transmitted infection
TRH	Thyrotropin-releasing hormone
TSH	Thyroid-stimulating hormone
US	Ultrasound
VTE	Venous thromboembolism
VVC	Vulvovaginal candidiasis
WHO	World Health Organization
WSW	Women who have sex with women
WSWM	Women who have sex with women and men

Contents

Contributors

Oluyemisi A. Adeyemi-Fowode, M.D. Division of Pediatric and Adolescent Gynecology, Department of Obstetrics and Gynecology, Baylor College of Medicine, Houston, TX, USA

Elizabeth M. Alderman, M.D. Pediatric Residency Program, The Childern's Hospital at Montefiore, The Pediatric Hospital for Albert Einstein College of Medicine, Bronx, NY, USA

Catherine Benedict, Ph.D. Department of Medicine, Zucker School of Medicine at Hofstra/ Northwell, Hempstead, NY, USA

Elizabeth Bonagura, M.S., M.D. Kosair Children's Hospital Gynecology Specialists, Louisville, KY, USA

Paula K. Braverman, M.D. Baystate Adolescent Medicine, Baystate Health, Baystate Children's Specialty Center, Springfield, MA, USA

Division of Adolescent and Transition Medicine, Department of Pediatrics, University of Cincinnati College of Medicine, Cincinnati Children's Hospital Medical Center, Cincinnati, OH, USA

Karen Browner-Elhanan, M.D. Pediatrics-Adolescent Medicine, Renown Children's Hospital, Reno, NV, USA

Gale R. Burstein, M.D., M.P.H. Erie County Department of Health, Buffalo, NY, USA

Marina Catallozzi, M.D., M.S.C.E. Division of Child and Adolescent Health, Department of Pediatrics, Heilbrunn Department of Population and Family Health, Columbia University Medical Center, Morgan Stanley Children's Hospital at New York Presbyterian, New York, NY, USA

Chanelle Coble, M.D. Department of Pediatrics, NYU School of Medicine/ Bellevue Hospital, New York, NY, USA

Ellen L. Connor, M.D. University of Wisconsin, Adolescent PCOS Clinic, American Family Children's Hospital, Madison, WI, USA

Susan M. Coupey, M.D. Professor of Pediatrics, Chief, Division of Adolescent Medicine, Children's Hospital at Montefiore, The Pediatric Hospital for Albert Einstein College of Medicine, Bronx, NY, USA

Kristina Derrick, M.D., Sc.M. Department of Pediatric Endocrinology, Children's Hospital at Montefiore/Albert Einstein College of Medicine, Bronx, NY, USA

Jennifer E. Dietrich, M.D., M.Sc. Obstetrics and Gynecology and Pediatrics, Texas Children's Hospital, Baylor College of Medicine, Houston, TX, USA

Nancy A. Dodson, M.D., M.P.H. Division of Adolescent Medicine, Department of Pediatrics, Children's Hospital at Montefiore, Bronx, NY, USA

Allison Eliscu, M.D., F.A.A.P. Division Chief of Adolescent Medicine, Department of Pediatrics, Stony Brook Children's Hospital, Stony Brook, NY, USA

Jonathan D. Fish, M.D. Pediatric Hematology/Oncology and Stem Cell Transplantation, Steven and Alexandra Cohen Children's Medical Center of New, New York, NY, USA

Zucker School of Medicine at Hofstra/Northwell, Hempstead, NY, USA

Nathalie Fleming, M.D., F.R.C.S.C. Division of Gynecology, Department of Surgery, Children's Hospital of Eastern Ontario, Ottawa, ON, Canada

Department of Obstetrics, Gynecology and Newborn Care, The Ottawa Hospital, Ottawa, ON, Canada

Faculty of Medicine, University of Ottawa, Ottawa, ON, Canada

Risa L. Fridy, M.D. Mount Sinai Hospital, Icahn School of Medicine, New York, NY, USA

Donna Futterman, M.D. Adolescent AIDS Program, Einstein College of Medicine, Children's Hospital at Montefiore, Bronx, NY, USA

Hanna R. Goldberg, M.S. Faculty of Medicine, University of Toronto, Toronto, ON, Canada

Catherine M. Gordon, M.D., M.Sc. Division of Adolescent and Transition Medicine, Department of Pediatrics, University of Cincinnati College of Medicine, Cincinnati Children's Hospital Medical Center, Cincinnati, OH, USA

Elissa Gross, D.O., M.P.H. Division of Hospital Medicine, The Pediatric Hospital for Albert Einstein College of Medicine, Children's Hospital at Montefiore, Bronx, NY, USA

S. Paige Hertweck, M.D. University of Louisville School of Medicine, Kosair Children's Hospital, Louisville, KY, USA

Amanda M. Jacobs, M.D. Division of Adolescent Medicine, Department of Pediatrics, Children's Hospital at Montefiore, Albert Einstein College of Medicine, Bronx, NY, USA

Megan Jacobs, M.D., F.A.A.P. Section of Adolescent Medicine, Department of Pediatrics, University of Colorado – School of Medicine, Children's Hospital Colorado, Aurora, CO, USA

Rula V. Kanj, M.D. Division of Pediatric and Adolescent Gynecology, Department of Obstetrics and Gynecology, University of Cincinnati College of Medicine, Cincinnati Children's Hospital Medical Center, Cincinnati, OH, USA

Lauren A. Kanner, M.D. Division of Pediatric Endocrinology, Department of Pediatrics, University of Wisconsin School of Medicine and Public Health, Madison, Madison, WI, USA

Paritosh Kaul, M.D. Section of Adolescent Medicine, Department of Pediatrics, University of Colorado – School of Medicine, Children's Hospital Colorado, Aurora, CO, USA

Sari Kives, M.D. Section of Gynecology, Hospital for Sick Children, Toronto, ON, Canada

Sofya Maslyanskaya, M.D. Division of Adolescent Medicine, Children's Hospital at Montefiore, The Pediatric Hospital for Albert Einstein College of Medicine, Bronx, NY, USA

Jasmine Multani, H.B.Sc. Faculty of Medicine, University of Toronto, Toronto, ON, Canada

Alexandra C. Nevin Lam, M.D. Department of Obstetrics and Gynecology, North York General, Toronto, ON, Canada

Jennifer L. Northridge, M.D. Division of Adolescent Medicine, Joseph M Sanzari Children's Hospital, The Pediatric Hospital for Hackensack University Medical Center, Hackensack, NJ, USA

Rollyn M. Ornstein, M.D. Division of Adolescent Medicine and Eating Disorders, Penn State Hershey Children's Hospital, Hershey, PA, USA

Aristotle Panayiotopoulos, M.D. Department of Pediatric Endocrinology, Northwell Health, Staten Island, NY, USA

Priscilla Rahmer, F.N.P. Pediatric Hematology/Oncology and Stem Cell Transplantation, Steven and Alexandra Cohen Children's Medical Center of New York, New York, NY, USA

Maria H. Rahmandar, M.D. Division of Adolescent Medicine, Ann & Robert H. Lurie Children's Hospital of Chicago, Hempstead, NY, USA

Division of Pediatric and Adolescent Gynecology, Cincinnati Children's Hospital Medical Center, Chicago, IL, USA

Jessica Rieder, M.D., M.S. Division of Adolescent Medicine, The Pediatric Hospital for Albert Einstein College of Medicine, Children's Hospital at Montefiore, Bronx, NY, USA

Ellen S. Rome, M.D., M.P.H. Cleveland Clinic Lerner College of Medicine at Case, Cleveland, OH, USA

Center for Adolescent Medicine, Cleveland Clinic Children's Hospital, Cleveland, OH, USA

Susan L. Rosenthal, Ph.D., A.B.P.P. Division of Child and Adolescent Health, Department of Pediatrics, Columbia University Medical Center, Morgan Stanley Children's Hospital at New York Presbyterian, New York, NY, USA

Xiomara Santos, M.D. Department of Obstetrics and Gynecology, Orlando Health Physicians Group, Orlando, FL, USA

Nadia L. Scott, M.D., M.H.S. Division of Adolescent Medicine, Department of Pediatrics, The Children's Hospital at Montefiore, Bronx, NY, USA

Erin H. Sieke, B.A. Cleveland Clinic Lerner College of Medicine at Case, Cleveland, OH, USA

Courtney Sims, M.D. Department of Pediatrics, The Pediatric Hospital for Albert Einstein College of Medicine, Children's Hospital at Montefiore, Bronx, NY, USA

Judith Simms-Cendan, M.D. Department of Clinical Sciences, University of Central Florida College of Medicine, Orlando, FL, USA

Jean Someshwar, M.D. Division of Adolescent and Young Adult Medicine, Children's National Health System, George Washington University, Washington, DC, USA

Lawrence R. Stanberry, M.D., Ph.D. Department of Pediatrics, Columbia University Medical Center, Morgan Stanley Children's Hospital at New York Presbyterian, New York, NY, USA

Bianca Stortini, M.D. Division of Gynecology, Department of Surgery, Children's Hospital of Eastern Ontario, Ottawa, Canada

Department of Obstetrics, Gynecology and Newborn Care, The Ottawa Hospital, Ottawa, Canada

Faculty of Medicine, University of Ottawa, Ottawa, ON, Canada

Hina J. Talib, M.D. Assistant Professor, Pediatrics, Program Director, Post-doctoral Fellowship in Adolescent Medicine, Division of Adolescent Medicine, Children's Hospital at Montefiore, The Pediatric Hospital for Albert Einstein College of Medicine, Bronx, NY, USA

Kanani E. Titchen, M.D. Division of Adolescent Medicine, Children's Hospital at Montefiore, the Pediatric Hospital for Albert Einstein College of Medicine, Bronx, NY, USA

Simone Vigod, M.D., M.Sc., F.R.C.P.C. Psychiatry, Reproductive Life Stages Program, Women's Mental Health Program, Women's College Hospital, Toronto, Ontario, Canada

Part I
General and Developmental Approach to Adolescents

Chapter 1
Case of a Girl with a Secret

Nadia L. Scott and Elizabeth M. Alderman

The assurance of confidentiality in sexual, reproductive, and mental health is an essential element of the therapeutic relationship between adolescents and their health-care providers. Research has shown that adolescents may forgo needed health care for these sensitive concerns if they believe this information will be shared with their parents. To address this issue, laws have been enacted to protect confidentiality when an adolescent seeks care in areas such as sexually transmitted infection testing, contraception, and outpatient mental health services. Confidentiality laws can vary by state and may depend on a practitioner's assessment of the minor's ability to make informed decisions regarding his or her health. In some circumstances, however, confidentiality cannot be assured, such as when the adolescent's safety is at stake. There are also other challenges to preserving confidentiality such as billing for services, the electronic medical record, and patient portals. For this reason, providers should familiarize themselves with the laws regarding adolescent confidentiality in their state and include discussions of confidentiality in each adolescent patient encounter.

E.H. is a 15-year-old girl with no significant past medical history who presents to your office for her annual physical prior to starting her sophomore year in high school. You have been her physician since she was an infant. Her mother has accompanied her to your office. She is weighed, her vital signs are recorded, and she and her mother are placed in an exam room. The patient and her mother state that she has been well since her last visit. She was an honor roll student last year and is planning on taking several Advanced Placement courses in the fall. You are ready to

N.L. Scott, M.D., M.H.S. (✉)
Division of Adolescent Medicine, Department of Pediatrics,
The Children's Hospital at Montefiore, Bronx, NY, USA
e-mail: nascott@montefiore.org; scott.nadia@gmail.com

E.M. Alderman, M.D.
Pediatric Residency Program, The Children's Hospital at Montefiore,
The Pediatric Hospital for Albert Einstein College of Medicine, Bronx, NY, USA

H.J. Talib (ed.), *Adolescent Gynecology*,
https://doi.org/10.1007/978-3-319-66978-6_1

commence the physical exam, and you ask E.H.'s mother to sit in the waiting room while you exam E.H. You explain to E.H. and her mother that in addition to the exam, you will be asking E.H. a series of additional questions. You also explain that anything discussed with E.H. during this time will be kept between yourself and E.H. except if E.H. discloses information that demonstrates she wishes to harm herself or others or is in danger in some other way. You further explain that this confidential interview is a component of every health-care maintenance visit you conduct with an adolescent patient.

Once E.H.'s mother has left the room, you begin to ask questions related to sexual and behavioral health. E.H. states that she and her boyfriend of 1 year have recently started having sexual intercourse, and she is interested in obtaining contraception. E.H. states that she has not told her mother she is sexually active and begs you not to tell her mother. She states that some of her classmates have told her about the oral contraceptive pill, and though she thinks she may like to try it, she is worried about her parents finding out when they receive a bill for your services.

Questions

1. How should providers begin a discussion on confidentiality with patients and parents?
2. How should providers balance the rights of adolescents' privacy regarding certain elements of their health with parents' responsibility to be a part of their adolescent child's health?
3. What limitations exist to the confidential relationship between health-care provider and adolescent patient?
4. How are confidential health-care services that are provided to adolescent patients paid for without informing their parents whose insurance is billed?
5. In an era of electronic medical records and electronic patient portals, what new challenges have arisen to ensuring confidential health-care services for adolescents?

Discussion

Background

Adolescents exist in a unique place physically, socially, and psychologically. As they grow physically into adults, they also begin to separate emotionally from their parents and begin to develop a distinct set of behaviors, opinions, and values.

The practice of adolescent medicine is also distinct in that it encompasses aspects of health and the human experience that are considered very private such as romantic and sexual relationships, reproductive choices, and mental and emotional health. As adolescents begin to assert their independence from their parents, they often want to keep the aforementioned aspects of their life and health private. An adolescent's fear that his or her parents will discover health information that one wishes to keep confidential is sometimes so strong that some adolescents will defer needed health care to prevent an intentional or unintentional breach of their confidentiality. Therefore, to be an effective adolescent health-care provider, one must examine issues of privacy, confidentiality, consent, and the provider-patient relationship with a different lens than that used for patients of other ages. Because of these unique aspects of adolescence, confidentiality and consent are integral parts of an effective therapeutic relationship with an adolescent patient. In order to ensure the integrity of this relationship, confidential care may be provided to adolescents for selected services, including sexually transmitted infection screening and treatment, mental health services, contraception, and pregnancy, depending on the state of medical practice.

The power of consent and the protection of confidentiality are closely connected in the provision of adolescent health care. Consent in the context of health services is informed permission given without coercion or duress by an individual for medical services or interventions. Minors (defined as anyone below the age of 18 years old) are not legally considered competent to evaluate the significance of medical diagnoses or to assess the potential risks and benefits of recommended medical treatments. Parents or legal guardians, therefore, are in most cases tasked with the right and the responsibility of giving consent for medical care for their minor children. Anyone 18 years or older, on the other hand, is no longer a minor and considered legally capable of giving consent if they have the mental capacity to understand the risks and benefits of medical care.

These general guidelines of consent become more complicated for adolescents. Every state has its laws related to the ability of minors to consent. These decisions encompass reproductive and sexual health such as diagnosis and treatment of sexually transmitted infections, contraception, pregnancy-related care, outpatient mental health and substance abuse services, and sexual assault treatment. In addition to the ability to consent to these services, adolescents may have the right to receive these services confidentially without parental notification except in the case where an adolescent gives explicit permission for confidential diagnoses and interventions to be shared with parents by the provider.

In general, areas outside these protected services still remain in the purview of the parent or guardian. This means that parents have the right to be informed of any test results or medical diagnoses and to give or withhold consent for medical testing or procedures outside of the realm of the confidential areas described above.

Mature and Emancipated Minors

Some minors are entitled to consent for all of their own health care. *Emancipated minors* are those who are married, are parents, are enrolled in the armed forces, or are financially independent [1]. Minors who are parents may not only have the right to consent to all of their own health care, but also that of their children depending on state law. Pregnant minors also have expanded rights. Pregnant adolescents have the right to confidentiality for all health care related to prenatal care including non-gynecologic issues that could potentially adversely affect a pregnancy [1].

A *mature minor* may also have extended consent and confidentiality protections. A mature minor is defined as an individual below the age of 18 years of age who demonstrates a level of intellectual and psychosocial development that renders them able to understand the import of medical decisions and their consequences [1]. This definition can vary from state to state and among providers as health-care providers must use their judgment in individual cases to determine if an adolescent patient can be considered a mature minor. Individual characteristics that might help to define an adolescent as a mature minor are age, level of education, intelligence, life experience, and previous involvement with their own health-care decision making. An additional consideration is the service for which consent is sought. Generally, if a service is minimally risky and within established medical protocols, a mature minor could consent to that service without parental input. The mature minor doctrine is typically applied on a case-by-case basis and varies in its extent of practice from state to state [2].

Policy and Legislation Supporting Adolescent Confidential Care

Since the 1980s, confidential care for adolescents has been supported by health policy and legislation. Multiple professional organizations dedicated to the health of children and adolescents have created policy statements recognizing the central necessity of confidential health care for adolescents. The American Academy of Pediatrics (AAP), the Society for Adolescent Health and Medicine (SAHM), the American Medical Association (AMA), and the American College of Obstetrics and Gynecology (ACOG) have all issued policy statements that emphasize the importance of confidentiality between the adolescent patient and health-care provider in the areas of sexual and mental health [2].

Federal and state legislation has also sought to address the provision of confidential health care for adolescent patients. These are typically extensions of the common law privacy protections which ensure confidentiality in the provision of reproductive health care and family planning such as those outlined in cases such as Griswold v. Connecticut [3].

Title X, passed in 1970 as a part of the Public Health Service Act, provides federal financial support for the provision of affordable family planning and sexual health care. In 1978, Title X was expanded to include a mandate stating that clinics must provide confidential sexual and reproductive health services to adolescents. As approximately 20% of the 4.5 million patients served in Title X clinics annually are below the age of 19, protections allotted to Title X recipients also affect the large number of adolescents that seek care in those facilities [4].

Another piece of federal legislation which helps to dictate the provision of confidential health care to adolescents is the Health Insurance Portability and Accountability Act or HIPAA. HIPAA, passed in 1996, outlines strict regulations for how protected health information is utilized, disseminated, and secured. HIPAA also includes a provision that makes confidential the records of any adolescent over the age of 18 years, emancipated or mature minors, and minors accessing services that they are able to consent to by individual state law such as sexual health-care services, mental health care, and substance abuse therapy [5]. On the other hand, HIPAA also states that minors' health records that fall outside of these categories may be accessed by parents and guardians as they are considered the "personal representatives" of their minor children [6].

Federal legislation, though strong in its endorsement of confidential health services for adolescents, is put into practice slightly differently in each state. For example, all 50 states and the District of Columbia allow minors to consent to sexually transmitted infection testing and treatment without parental notification [7]. On the other end of the spectrum of services lies abortion. 26 of the 50 states require the consent of one or both parents before an abortion can be performed, and 12 states require one or both parents to be notified of a minor's intention to obtain an abortion before it can be performed. It should be noted that all 38 of these states have provisions for minors to obtain abortion without parental consent or notification by appealing to a judge (judicial bypass) or in the case of a medical emergency and imminent harm to the mother [7]. Because of the variation among state laws and policies and the propensity for these regulations to change with new state legislation, health-care providers who serve adolescents should familiarize themselves with the confidentiality and consent laws of the state in which they practice.

There are certain situations where confidentiality cannot be assured. If an adolescent patient discloses suicidal or homicidal intent, confidentiality must be broken and the parent informed of this situation for the safety of the child. Parents must also be informed if a child discloses abuse as well as the appropriate child protection authorities. Complete confidentiality also cannot be assured if an adolescent has a reportable communicable infection such as chlamydia, gonorrhea, syphilis, or HIV. Health-care providers are required to report positive test results to the local department of health who then reports them to the Centers for Disease Control. Patients who test positive for these infections may be contacted by the Department of Health in order to determine sexual contacts so that they may be treated. Typically, however, a health-care provider would not be required or permitted to report these results to the parent of an adolescent patient.

What Impact Does Confidentiality Have on How Adolescents Utilize Health Care?

The importance of confidentiality in providing effective clinical health care for adolescent patients has also been supported by research. A study of 562 California high school students showed that when adolescents were assured of conditional confidentiality, they were significantly more likely to disclose health information such as sexual practices, substance abuse, and mental health status [8]. Similarly, in a study of teenagers utilizing contraceptive services at Wisconsin family clinics, 50% stated they would not return to these clinics if parental notification of oral contraceptive use was required. Only 1% of those surveyed said that they would stop having sex if this occurred. Those surveyed would simply stop using contraception or use a less effective method [9].

Provision of Confidential Care for Adolescent in Practice

Despite the proven importance of confidentiality protections in adolescent health care, in practice, there is a wide variation between states as well as individual practitioners that serve adolescents.

In a 2014 study which audiotaped the visits of 49 primary care providers in North Carolina, only 51% of visits included a portion of the visit where the adolescent patient was interviewed without a parent, and only 31% of visits included an assurance of confidentiality [10]. A study of 372 primary care practices in the Washington, D.C., area showed a discordance between what services office staff believed were available to adolescent patients confidentially (and presumably what they might be relaying to patients) as compared to the doctors in the same practice [11]. Overall, pediatrics practices were also much less likely to provide health-care services defined as "medically emancipated conditions" such as pelvic exams, contraceptive counseling, and STI testing that should be provided to adolescents confidentially. The authors hypothesized that this discrepancy may be due to pediatricians' unfamiliarity with sexual health-care services, discomfort with "keeping" portions of adolescent visits secret from parents with whom they may have a long-standing relationship or misinformation about confidentiality laws, and what services fall under their purview [11].

Paying for Confidential Care

One challenging aspect of providing confidential care to adolescents is payment for confidential services. Most adolescents are insured as dependents under their parents' health insurance plans, and this can inadvertently endanger the provision of confidential care if charges are sent to parents or guardians regarding services provided to their adolescent children. These breaches can occur inadvertently in the setting of Explanation of Benefits (EOBs), reviews sent to the policyholder of services when any member of the plan accesses care. These occurrences or even the fear of these occurrences by adolescents on their parents' plans may cause some teens to forgo needed care [12]. Some states have enacted laws to remedy this problem and those that exist vary by state. 12 of 50 states have provisions in place to help protect from breaches of confidentiality on EOBs [7]. These include regulations that state that if a written request is submitted by an adolescent, all communications regarding that minor's health-care claims for confidential services must be sent directly to the adolescent patient or that insurance companies must seek the adolescent patient's permission before sending EOBs with sensitive health information. At the federal level, the Affordable Care Act passed in 2010 extends health-care coverage to young adults up to age 26 on their parents' plans. While this policy provides health insurance to many young people who were previously uninsured, it also leaves open the possibility of an increased number of accidental breaches of confidentiality when adolescents or young adults seek to have their parents' insurance pay for confidential services. The ACA also requires the complete cost coverage of preventative health services including STI testing and contraception. To counteract the risk of inadvertent breaches, the Society of Adolescent Medicine, the American Academy of Pediatrics, and the American College of Obstetricians and Gynecologists have released a policy statement that states because these services are paid in full leaving no residual financial liability, they should not be included on EOB forms [13].

Adolescent Confidential Care in the Electronic Medical Record Age

Another potential area for breaches of confidentiality in the provision of adolescent health care is through patient accessible electronic medical records. Professional organizations have made recommendations for institutions that help protect adolescent confidentiality when setting up their electronic medical records [14, 15]. Many medical practices and health-care systems have patient portals to facilitate patient access to their own medical records. In the case of minors, their guardians also have access to their health records which clearly could pose an issue if an adolescent patient's records contain sensitive information such as results of STI testing or contraceptive prescriptions. Solutions to this problem are still in their infancy and vary from institution to institution. Some institutions create two portals: one that is accessible by the parents and one that is accessible by the adolescent that contains sensitive aspects of the medical chart such as sexual or mental health [16]. Other electronic medical record systems have a separate section where providers enter confidential information about adolescent patients which is not visible in any after visit summaries accessible to parents.

Conclusions

Providing the highest level of health care to adolescents requires health-care providers to call on a diverse set of skills in order to provide effective care. One of the most difficult aspects is honoring the adolescent's newly developing physiological and social autonomy by allowing them to consent to and receive confidential health-care services for sexual and reproductive health, outpatient mental health, and substance abuse services.

Though it has been repeatedly shown that adolescents may forgo essential health-care needs if they fear a breach in confidentiality, the question of how to ensure consistent confidential care for them is more challenging. Between the myriad and frequently changing state laws dictating which services are confidential and under which circumstances, reimbursement notifications, and the increasing presence of patient and parent accessible electronic medical information, confidential care can be challenging to effectively provide.

Health-care providers should familiarize themselves and their staff with the confidentiality provisions of their state and health-care system. They should also develop a comfort with the treatment of adolescent patients including sexual and mental health care and familiarize their adolescent patients and their parents with the most effective adolescent medical visit. This visit consists of a portion with the adolescent alone and the parent and teen being aware that whatever is discussed during this private time will remain confidential.

Clinical Pearls and Pitfalls

- Adolescents may be entitled to confidential health care for health care related to sexuality, mental health, illicit substance use, and sexual assault.
- State laws dictate the ability for adolescents to receive confidential care.
- Practitioners must take the developmental stage of the adolescent into consideration when determining if an adolescent may consent to confidential services.
- Whenever possible, parents and guardians should be encouraged to participate in the health care of their adolescent child.
- Confidential health care cannot be assured for an adolescent if the adolescent is a danger to herself or others, discloses abuse that state law mandates medical provider to report, or tests positive for an infection that must be reported to the local department of health.

References

1. Feierman J, Lieberman D, Schissel A, et al. Teenagers, health care and the law. New York Civil Liberties Union; 2009. http://www.nyclu.org/files/thl.pdf. Accessed 12 Sept 2016.
2. Berlan E, Bravender T. Confidentiality, consent, and caring for the adolescent patient. Curr Opin Pediatr. 2009;21:450–6.
3. American Civil Liberties Union. Timeline of important reproductive freedom cases decided by the Supreme Court; 2015. https://www.aclu.org/timeline-important-reproductive-freedom-cases-decided-supreme-court#comment-0. Accessed 12 Sept 2016.
4. Health and Human Services. Title X: the national family planning program; 2014. http://www.hhs.gov/opa/pdfs/title-x-national-family-planning-overview.pdf. Accessed 12 Sept 2016.
5. American College of Gynecologists. Committee opinion: adolescent confidentiality and electronic health records; 2014. http://www.acog.org/Resources-And-Publications/Committee-Opinions/Committee-on-Adolescent-Health-Care/Adolescent-Confidentiality-and-Electronic-Health-Records. Accessed 12 Sept 2016.
6. English A, Ford C. The HIPAA privacy rule and adolescents. Perspect Sex Reprod Health. 2004;36(2):80–6.
7. Guttmacher Institute. 2016. www.guttmacher.org. Accessed 12 Sept 2016.
8. Ford C, Millstein S, et al. Influence of physician confidentiality assurances on adolescents' willingness to disclose information and seek future health care. JAMA. 1997;278(12):1029–34.
9. Reddy D, Fleming R, Swain C. Effect of mandatory parental notification on adolescent girls' use of sexual health care services. JAMA. 2002;288(6):710–4.
10. Bravender T, Lyna P, et al. Physicians' assurances of confidentiality and time spent alone with adolescents during primary care visits. Clin Pediatr. 2014;53(11):1094–7.
11. Akimbami L, Gandhi H, Cheng T. Availability of adolescent health services and confidentiality in primary care practices. Pediatrics. 2003;111(2):394–401.
12. Frerich E, Garcia C, Long S, et al. Health care reform and young adults' access to sexual health care: an exploration of potential confidentiality implications of the affordable care act. Am J Public Health. 2012;102(10):1818–21.
13. Burstein G, Blythe M, Santelli J, et al. Confidentiality protections for adolescents and young adults in the health care billing and insurance claims process. J Adolesc Health. 2016;58(3):374–7.
14. Anoshiravani A, Gaskin GL, Groshek MR, et al. Special requirements for electronic medical records in adolescent medicine. J Adolesc Health. 2012;51(5):409–14.
15. American Academy of Pediatrics, Committee on Adolescence and Council on Clinical and Information Technology. Standards for health information technology to ensure adolescent privacy. Pediatrics. 2012;130(5):987–90.
16. Bayer R, Santelli J, Klitzman R. New challenges for electronic health records; confidentiality and access to sensitive health information about parents and adolescents. JAMA. 2015;313(1):29–30.

Chapter 2
Case of a Girl Due for Human Papillomavirus Immunization

Maria H. Rahmandar and Paula K. Braverman

Case

JH is a healthy 12-year-old female with an unremarkable past medical history who presents for a sports pre-participation physical for soccer. When discussing her gynecologic history, JH reports menarche 6 months ago around her 12th birthday. She has monthly periods without excessive bleeding or cramping. Family history is only notable for celiac disease in her mother and rheumatoid arthritis in her paternal grandmother.

During a confidential social history, JH shares that she lives with her parents and older brother. Her family is health conscious: her father is a salesman for a nutritional supplement company, and her mother only buys organic fruits and vegetables. The family is also very religious, and JH is active in her church youth group. JH is about to start seventh grade and typically receives As and Bs. She has a lot of friends on the soccer team and wants to be a teacher and coach. She feels safe at home and denies any mood concerns and abuse history or that she or any of her teammates have tried tobacco, alcohol, and other drugs. She identifies as female and has crushes

M.H. Rahmandar, M.D. (✉)
Division of Adolescent Medicine, Ann & Robert H. Lurie Children's Hospital of Chicago, Chicago, IL, USA

Division of Pediatric and Adolescent Gynecology, Cincinnati Children's Hospital Medical Center, Cincinnati, OH, USA
e-mail: MRahmandar@luriechildrens.org

P.K. Braverman, M.D.
Baystate Adolescent Medicine, Baystate Health, Baystate Children's Specialty Center, Springfield, MA, USA

Division of Adolescent and Transition Medicine, Department of Pediatrics, University of Cincinnati College of Medicine, Cincinnati Children's Hospital Medical Center, Cincinnati, OH, USA

H.J. Talib (ed.), *Adolescent Gynecology*,
https://doi.org/10.1007/978-3-319-66978-6_2

on boys but is not allowed to have a boyfriend now and reports that she does not plan to even kiss a boy until she gets married.

On physical examination, vital signs and body mass index are within normal limits. JH appears healthy, athletic, and cooperative with tanner IV breast and pubic hair and no abnormalities on comprehensive examination.

JH is cleared for sports and developmentally appropriate anticipatory guidance is offered. However, when routine immunizations are discussed, her mother consents to the meningococcal, tetanus, diphtheria, and acellular pertussis vaccines but hesitates with the human papillomavirus (HPV) vaccine. She wants to avoid "unnecessary" vaccines and has several questions:

1. Does my daughter really need the HPV vaccine if she is not going to have sex until marriage?
2. My son never got the vaccine; should he get it?

Discussion

Messages for patient and family: *You welcome the family's questions and strongly recommend the vaccine for both the patient and her brother. You discuss with both the patient and her family that HPV is a common infection that can lead to cancer and genital warts. HPV is well known to cause cervical cancer in females and is associated with oropharyngeal, penile, anal, and other genital cancers. Her older brother should also be immunized to decrease both the acquisition and spread of HPV between himself and his future partner(s).*

Background discussion: HPV is the most common sexually transmitted infection in the USA with 20–24-year-old females having among the highest prevalence [1]. Certain HPV types can lead to cutaneous manifestations (common skin warts), while others are associated with genital or oropharyngeal lesions (precancer and cancers) [2]. Genital HPV infections are generally acquired via skin-to-skin contact, most often sexual intercourse [2]. Though HPV infections can cause clinical manifestations, most HPV infections are asymptomatic and clear spontaneously in 2 years [3]. In addition, cervical cancer is very rare in females under age 20, and it takes years for cancer to develop after exposure to the virus leading to the recommendation to delay Pap smears until age 21 [3]. It is the persistence of infection with high-risk HPV types (such as HPV 16, 18, 31, 33, 45, 52, 58) which leads to cancers in women and men, many of which could be prevented by the HPV vaccine [2]. Low-risk HPV types 6 and 11 cause about 90% of genital warts (condylomata acuminata) and are associated with recurrent respiratory papillomatosis and conjunctival papillomas [2]. Genital warts are not precancerous lesions but still can be bothersome, as well as difficult to treat [2].

Each year in the USA, around 30,000 cases of HPV-related cancers are diagnosed [2]. HPV infections are responsible for nearly all cervical and anal cancers and most oropharyngeal, vaginal, and vulvar cancers [4]. The incidence of anal and

Table 2.1 HPV-associated cancers

Site	Average annual #	% Attributable HPV	% Caused by HPV 16 or 18	% Additional caused by HPV 31, 33, 45, 52, 58
Cervix	11,967	96%	66%	15%
Vulva	3136	51%	49%	14%
Vagina	729	64%	55%	18%
Penis	1046	36%	48%	9%
Anus: F	3089	93%	79%	11%
Anus: M	1678	93%	79%	4%
Oropharynx: F	2370	63%	51%	10%
Oropharynx: M	9356	63%	63%	4%

Data from [6, 14]

oropharyngeal cancers have been increasing in the USA [5]. These cancers are most commonly caused by the HPV types found in the licensed HPV vaccines [6] (Table 2.1).

Messages for patient and family: *You can let the family know that HPV vaccines have been in use for over a decade and studied in clinical trials for even longer. Further, HPV vaccine is strongly recommended by the major medical groups. The most recently released 9-valent vaccine protects against even more high-risk HPV types.*

Background discussion: Several vaccines have been developed to help decrease risks and subsequent sequelae related to acquisition of HPV infection. The US Food and Drug Administration (FDA) has approved the use of three HPV vaccines, which protect against two, four, or nine types of HPV. After FDA licensing and review of available studies, recent Advisory Committee on Immunization Practices' (ACIP) vaccination guidelines (March 2015) reaffirmed the recommendations for vaccination of all males and females at ages 11–12 with catch-up for females aged 13–26 and males aged 13–21 [7]. The recommendations permit use in males and females as young as age 9 and males ages 22–26. However, it is important to note that the vaccine is specifically recommended in several special populations including cases of sexual abuse or assault (starting at age 9), catch-up vaccination through age 26 for men who have sex with men, and in both males and females who are immunocompromised [7, 8] (Table 2.2). All guidelines from major medical organizations agree with ACIP regarding the age group for routine immunization. In December 2016, the Centers for Disease Control and Prevention (CDC) approved the use of a two-dose series for boys and girls initiating HPV vaccination prior to age 15; the three-dose series is still recommended for those who start HPV immunization between ages 15 through 26 [9].

Messages for patient and family: *For maximum protection, the patient should complete the entire series of shots. You can also emphasize the recommendation of universal vaccination at ages 11–12, since, even if the patient is not exposed to HPV prior to marriage, younger adolescents achieve a better antibody response to the vaccine than older teens. It is important to emphasize that this is a cancer prevention*

Table 2.2 Characteristics of HPV vaccines and ACIP recommendations

Characteristic or recommendation	Bivalent (2vHPV)	Quadrivalent (4vHPV)	9-valent (9vHPV)
Brand name	Ceravix	Gardasil	Gardasil 9
Viruslike particles contained	16, 18	6, 11, 16, 18	6, 11, 16, 18, 31, 33, 45, 52, 58
Manufacturer	GlaxoSmithKline	Merck	Merck
Recommendations	• Females only • Routine at age 11 or 12 • Can be started at age 9 • Catch-up for females ages 13–26	• Females and males • Routine at age 11 or 12 • Can be started at age 9 • Catch-up for females ages 13–26 (including immunocompromised) • Catch-up for males ages 13–21 • Catch-up for MSM and immunocompromised males ages 22–26	• Females and males • Routine at age 11 or 12 • Can be started at age 9 • Catch-up for females ages 13–26 (including immunocompromised) • Catch-up for males ages 13–21 • Catch-up for MSM and immunocompromised males ages 22–26 • Two doses for females and males under age 15
Proven protection against	• Cervical cancer precursors in females	• Cervical, vulvar, and vaginal cancer precursors in females • Genital warts in females and males • Anal precancers in males	• Protection over the 4vHPV from five additional HPV types for cervical, vulvar, and vaginal cancer precursors in females

MSM men who have sex with men; recommendations from [7]

vaccine against a virus that the vast majority of individuals will be exposed to from future sexual partners.

Background discussion: HPV vaccines were initially recommended as a three-dose series, with the minimum time between doses 1 and 2 being 4 weeks and between doses 2 and 3 being 12 weeks [2]. There must be a minimum of 24 weeks between doses 1 and 3. A two-dose series has been approved by the CDC for males and females beginning HPV vaccination before the age of 15, with doses given 6–12 months apart [9]. Completion of a vaccine series with the same type of HPV vaccine is ideal in order to be consistent with the vaccine research studies. However, in cases where the previous vaccine type is unknown or unavailable, ACIP recommends completing the series, with the available HPV vaccine, rather than restarting the entire three-dose series [7].

Completion of the vaccine series results in production of vaccine-type HPV antibodies, or seropositivity, in over 99% of healthy individuals, and the antibody response produced by the two-dose series is non-inferior to that of the three-dose series [9]. Antibody titers decrease in the first 2 years after vaccination but then tend to stabilize at levels which are significantly higher than those resulting from natural HPV infection [2]. Furthermore, HPV antibody responses are significantly higher in

9–15-year-olds compared to older adolescents and young adults, contributing to the recommendation to vaccinate all 11–12-year-olds [2, 7]. The antibody titers for the 9-valent vaccine are non-inferior to the quadrivalent vaccine [2].

In the HPV vaccine research studies, there was no identified lower threshold of antibody level below which an individual would not be protected from vaccine-related HPV types [2]. In practical terms, HPV antibody titers are not commercially available nor used in the clinical setting. We do know, however, that these vaccines are incredibly effective at preventing HPV-related disease [2] (Table 2.2). The protection from the bivalent and quadrivalent vaccines does not decrease even a decade after vaccination, as evidenced by the lack of breakthrough disease in 8–10-year follow-up studies [2]. Though HPV vaccines are most effective if given before a patient's sexual debut, the vaccines can be used in patients who have been sexually active or even have evidence of current or past HPV infection. Individuals are unlikely to be infected with all vaccine-preventable types of HPV and will receive protection from the types to which they have not been exposed. It should also be noted that the vaccine is not therapeutic [2]. In other words, HPV vaccines do not treat disease but only can prevent disease.

Messages for patient and family: *You can reassure the family that the HPV vaccine's safety is monitored closely and patients usually only have minor side effects with the injection, similar to all vaccines given to children and adolescents. The vaccine is even safe and recommended in patients with a family history of autoimmune diseases, such as celiac disease and rheumatoid arthritis.*

Background discussion: HPV vaccines are generally well tolerated and safe. The vaccines cannot cause infection since they are not live viruses but consist of bioengineered viruslike particles from the capsid proteins of the HPV types contained in the vaccine [2, 7]. HPV vaccination can be given to patients who are immunocompromised although the immunologic response may not be as robust as in immunocompetent individuals. It is also can be used by those who are breastfeeding (note: quadrivalent and 9-valent vaccines are considered safe in lactating women, but the bivalent vaccine has not been studied in breastfeeding patients) [2, 4]. Although there is no evidence of adverse pregnancy outcomes (pregnancy category B) and a pregnancy test is not required before vaccination, there have been no specific HPV vaccine studies in pregnant women. As such, HPV vaccines are not recommended in pregnant women and should be postponed until the pregnancy is completed (providers can notify the pregnancy registry for pregnant women who inadvertently receive the 9-valent vaccine at 1-800-672-6372; other HPV vaccine pregnancy registries have been closed with concurrence from the FDA) [2]. HPV vaccines have also not been shown to increase the risk of autoimmune diseases. Though some case reports have associated vaccination with development of multiple sclerosis, larger studies have shown no causal relationship [10].

It is common for parents to state concerns that consenting to the HPV vaccine will give their son or daughter license to become sexually active. Immunization with the HPV vaccine has not been shown to increase risky sexual activity [11]. In one recent study, researchers utilized a retrospective medical chart review, over a 3-year period, in order to prevent self-reporting bias and documented clinical outcome

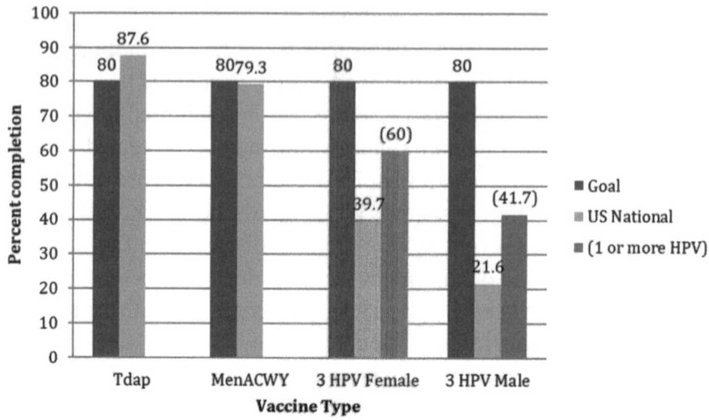

Fig. 2.1 2014 National Immunization Survey: adolescent vaccines (ages 13–17). Data from the US Department of Health and Human Services and National Center for Health Statistics, 2014; US Department of Health and Human Services and Office of Disease Prevention and Health Promotion, 2016

markers of sexual activity. The study found that females who received the HPV vaccine were no more likely than those who never received the vaccine to seek contraception and testing for pregnancy or STIs or be diagnosed with a pregnancy or STI. This study also showed that HPV vaccination was not associated with earlier age of initiation of sexual activity. As with all STIs, it is important to provide counseling that HPV transmission can also be reduced by abstinence, consistent condom use, and circumcision in males [1].

All three vaccine types have a similar side effect profile [7]. The most common adverse event is injection site pain, swelling, or redness [2]. Less commonly, systemic symptoms, such as headache, dizziness, fever, nausea, or fatigue, can be seen [2]. Syncope has been noted in adolescents following any vaccine, including the HPV vaccine [2]. To prevent syncopal episodes, patients should be observed sitting or lying for 15 minutes after injection [2]. The only HPV-specific serious adverse event reported has been rare anaphylaxis in patients allergic to vaccine components [1]. Therefore, the vaccine is contraindicated in individuals with an allergy to any vaccine components, including yeast in the quadrivalent and 9-valent or latex in the syringe stopper of the bivalent vaccine. The Vaccine Adverse Event Reporting System, among other vaccine surveillance programs, continuously collects and reviews potential adverse events [4]. No deaths have been caused by the vaccine [12]. As with all vaccines, the HPV vaccine can be given during mild illness but should be deferred during moderate-to-severe acute illness [2]. HPV vaccination does not change cervical cancer screening recommendations, because there are other HPV types that can cause cervical cancer that are not covered by the vaccine [7].

Despite what is known about the impressive immunogenicity, efficacy, and safety profiles of these vaccines, HPV vaccine uptake in the USA has been poor (Fig. 2.1).

Although HPV vaccine uptake is much lower than the healthy children 2020 goal of 80%, it is also notable that uptake is lower than other vaccines on the adolescent platform [13]. As of 2014, in the USA, only 39.7% of females and 21.6% of males had completed three doses of the HPV series, and 60% of females and 41.7% of males had received at least one dose of the HPV series [14]. The promising news is that even with the poor immunization rate, vaccine-type HPV prevalence in the US population has decreased which suggests herd immunity, and there are fewer cases of genital warts in the adolescent age group [15, 16]. Other countries have been successful in achieving high rates of vaccination by including the HPV vaccine in their national vaccine program [3]. Some countries have also found decrease in genital warts and cervical dysplasia [16]. After just 3 years of the HPV vaccine program, Australia noted a decrease in cervical dysplasia [3].

Studies have evaluated various strategies to help increase vaccination rates, and one study showed high rates of series completion when families could choose the method by which they were reminded, whether via text, email, phone call and multiple methods or also by reminding the adolescent themselves [17]. More importantly, families are more likely to vaccinate against HPV if their physician strongly recommends the vaccine [12]. It is considered best practice to update vaccines at all patient visits and not miss opportunities by only reserving immunizations for the annual well visit.

Clinical Pearls and Pitfalls

1. HPV is the most common sexually transmitted virus in the USA. Genital warts result from low-risk HPV types and cancers can result from persistent infection with high-risk types.
2. HPV is responsible for most cervical, anal, oropharyngeal, vaginal, and vulvar cancers, along with some penile cancers.
3. HPV vaccines are safe and effective at protecting against HPV-related cancers and genital warts.
4. HPV vaccination should be routinely recommended to females and males ages 11 and 12. Vaccination can start at age 9 and recommended at this age with a history of sexual abuse. Catch-up vaccination is recommended for females ages 13–26 (bivalent, quadrivalent, or 9-valent) and males ages 13–21 (quadrivalent or 9-valent). Vaccination is also recommended for MSM and all immunocompromised individuals including males ages 22–26.
5. HPV antibody response is more robust when given at younger ages.
6. HPV vaccines are most effective if given before a patient becomes sexually active and is exposed to the virus, but neither sexual activity nor evidence of current or past HPV infection is a contraindication to vaccination.
7. Though the HPV vaccine is not approved in pregnant females, no safety concerns have been identified during pregnancy, and a pregnancy test is not required prior to vaccination.

8. HPV vaccines are generally well tolerated. The most common side effect is injection site discomfort. The most common adverse event is syncope, as is seen with other adolescent vaccines. No deaths have been caused by the vaccine.
9. HPV series completion rates are low in the USA, but a strong recommendation from a physician is one of the most important factors in increasing vaccination rates.

References

1. Committee on Infectious Diseases. HPV vaccine recommendations. Pediatrics. 2012;129:602–5.
2. American Academy of Pediatrics. Human papillomaviruses. In: Kimberlin DD, Brady MT, Jackson MA, Long SS, editors. Red Book®: 2015 Report of the Committee on Infectious Diseases; 2015.
3. American College of Obstetricians and Gynecologists. Practice Bulletin No. 157: cervical cancer screening and prevention. Obstet Gynecol. 2016;127:e1–e20.
4. Centers for Disease Control and Prevention. Human papillomavirus-associated cancers—United States, 2004-2008. MMWR Morb Mortal Wkly Rep. 2012;61:258–61.
5. Jemal A, Simard EP, Dorell C, Noone AM, Markowitz LE, Kohler B, Eheman C, Saraiya M, Bandi P, Saslow D, Cronin KA, Watson M, Schiffman M, Henley SJ, Schymura MJ, Anderson RN, Yankey D, Edwards BK. Annual Report to the Nation on the Status of Cancer, 1975-2009, featuring the burden and trends in human papillomavirus(HPV)-associated cancers and HPV vaccination coverage levels. J Natl Cancer Inst. 2013;105:175–201.
6. Saraiya M, Unger ER, Thompson TD, Lynch CF, Hernandez BY, Lyu CW, Steinau M, Watson M, Wilkinson EJ, Hopenhayn C, Copeland G, Cozen W, Peters ES, Huang Y, Saber MS, Altekruse S, Goodman MT. US assessment of HPV types in cancers: implications for current and 9-valent HPV vaccines. J Natl Cancer Inst. 2015;107:djv086.
7. Petrosky E, Bocchini JA Jr, Hariri S, Chesson H, Curtis CR, Saraiya M, Unger ER, Markowitz LE. Use of 9-valent human papillomavirus (HPV) vaccine: updated HPV vaccination recommendations of the advisory committee on immunization practices. MMWR Morb Mortal Wkly Rep. 2015;64:300–4.
8. Markowitz LE, Dunne EF, Saraiya M, Chesson HW, Curtis CR, Gee J, Bocchini JA Jr, Unger ER. Human papillomavirus vaccination: recommendations of the Advisory Committee on Immunization Practices (ACIP). MMWR Recomm Rep. 2014;63:1–30.
9. Meites E, Kempe A, Markowitz LE. Use of a 2-dose schedule for human papillomavirus vaccination—updated recommendations of the advisory committee on immunization practices. MMWR Morb Mortal Wkly Rep. 2016;65:1405–8.
10. Scheller NM, Svanstrom H, Pasternak B, Arnheim-Dahlstrom L, Sundstrom K, Fink K, Hviid A. Quadrivalent HPV vaccination and risk of multiple sclerosis and other demyelinating diseases of the central nervous system. JAMA. 2015;313:54–61.
11. Bednarczyk RA, Davis R, Ault K, Orenstein W, Omer SB. Sexual activity-related outcomes after human papillomavirus vaccination of 11- to 12-year-olds. Pediatrics. 2012;130:798–805.
12. Brady MT. Pediatricians can lay out evidence to allay fears over HPV vaccine. AAP News. 2014.
13. U.S. Department of Health and Human Services & Office of Disease Prevention and Health Promotion. Healthy People 2020: immunization and infectious diseases [online]. 2016. https://www.healthypeople.gov/2020/topics-objectives/topic/immunization-and-infectious-diseases/objectives. Accessed 29 Mar 2016.

14. U.S. Department of Health and Human Services & National Center for Health Statistics. National immunization survey-teen. In: Prevention, C. F. D. C. A, editor. 2014. Hyattsville, MD.
15. Markowitz LE, Liu G, Hariri S, Steinau M, Dunne EF, Unger ER. Prevalence of HPV after introduction of the vaccination program in the United States. Pediatrics. 2016;137:1–9.
16. National Center for Immunization and Respiratory Diseases. HPV vaccine information for clinicians [online]. Centers for Disease Control and Prevention; 2015. http://www.cdc.gov/hpv/hcp/need-to-know.pdf
17. Kempe A, O'Leary ST, Shoup JA, Stokley S, Lockhart S, Furniss A, Dickinson LM, Barnard J, Daley MF. Parental choice of recall method for HPV vaccination: a pragmatic trial. Pediatrics. 2016;137:1–10.

Suggested Educational Reading, References, and Policies

Tips and Toolkits

American Academy of Pediatrics. HPV champion toolkit [online]. https://www.aap.org/en-us/advocacy-and-policy/aap-health-initiatives/Pages/HPV-Champion-Toolkit.aspx
Brady MT. Pediatricians can lay out evidence to allay fears over HPV vaccine. AAP News. 2014.
Centers for Disease Control and Prevention. HPV vaccine for preteens and teens [online]. 2015. http://www.cdc.gov/vaccines/who/teens/vaccines/hpv.html

Chapters, Policy Statements, and Guidelines

American Academy of Pediatrics. Human papillomaviruses. In: Kimberlin DD, Brady MT, Jackson MA, Long SS, editors. Red Book®: 2015 Report of the Committee on Infectious Diseases; 2015.
Meites E, Kempe A, Markowitz LE. Use of a 2-dose schedule for human papillomavirus vaccination—updated recommendations of the Advisory Committee on Immunization Practices. MMWR Morb Mortal Wkly Rep. 2016;65:1405–8.
Petrosky E, Bocchini JA Jr, Hariri S, Chesson H, Curtis CR, Saraiya M, Unger ER, Markowitz LE. Use of 9-valent human papillomavirus (HPV) vaccine: updated HPV vaccination recommendations of the advisory committee on immunization practices. MMWR Morb Mortal Wkly Rep. 2015;64:300–4.

Chapter 3
Case of a Girl with Delayed Puberty and Inflammatory Bowel Disease

Kristina Derrick and Aristotle Panayiotopoulos

Case

A 13-year and 8-month-old girl presented with concern of no breast or pubic hair development. Over the previous 2 years, her height percentile declined from 75th to 10th%, and weight declined from 25th to 5th%. Her midparental height was 5′7.5″ (171.5 cm). Her mother had menarche at 13 years of age, her sister had menarche at 12 years of age, and her father had a growth spurt after high school.

At age 11 years and 5 months, she started having abdominal pain, bloody diarrhea, and weight loss. She was diagnosed with inflammatory bowel disease (IBD). Over the next 2 years, she had frequent exacerbations of the IBD. At age 13 years and 8 months, she was evaluated for her delayed puberty. Exam showed a thin girl with no dysmorphic features, acanthosis, hirsutism, goiter, abdominal tenderness, or abnormal neurologic exam. Pubertal staging was Tanner 1 breast tissue and Tanner 1 pubic hair, with normal external female genitalia. Labs showed LH 0.1 mIU/ml, FSH 0.9 mIU/ml, estradiol <2 pg/ml, prolactin 9.6 ng/ml, serum hCG <2 mIU/ml, TSH 1.30 μU/ml, total testosterone 22 ng/dl, free testosterone 2.8 pg/ml, DHEAS 37 μg/dl, androstenedione 42 ng/dl, 17-hydroxyprogesterone 32 ng/dl, anti-Mullerian hormone 6.53 ng/ml, and karyotype 46,XX. Bone age x-ray showed a skeletal maturity age of 11 years at chronological age of 13 years and 8 months, consistent with delayed bone age. Pelvic ultrasound showed a uterus with prepubertal shape and ovaries that were small for age with a few follicles. She had a DXA scan that showed bone density *z* scores of −2.1 in the lumbar spine, −0.4 in the hip, and −0.5 in the forearm. However, since her bone age was 12 years old, *z* scores

K. Derrick, M.D., Sc.M. (✉)
Department of Pediatric Endocrinology, Children's Hospital at Montefiore/Albert Einstein College of Medicine, Bronx, NY, USA
e-mail: kderrick@montefiore.org

A. Panayiotopoulos, M.D.
Department of Pediatric Endocrinology, Northwell Health, Staten Island, NY, USA

H.J. Talib (ed.), *Adolescent Gynecology*,
https://doi.org/10.1007/978-3-319-66978-6_3

were adjusted and showed −0.8 in the lumbar spine, 0.3 in the hip, and 0.5 in the forearm, which are all within normal range (z score above −2.0).

Etiologies of delayed puberty, including Turner syndrome, gonadal dysgenesis, polycystic ovarian syndrome (PCOS), nonclassic congenital adrenal hyperplasia (CAH), thyroid disorder, hyperprolactinemia, primary ovarian insufficiency, hypothalamic amenorrhea, and hypogonadotropic hypogonadism, were ruled out. Her low levels of LH, FSH, and estradiol showed that she was not yet in puberty. The suspected cause was functional delayed onset of hypothalamic-pituitary-gonadal activity due to her IBD, which resulted in active inflammation and malnutrition. It was expected that as her IBD was under better control and she gained weight, she would spontaneously start puberty. Thus, no intervention was required for pubertal development.

Follow-up evaluation at 14 years and 5 months showed that her IBD was well controlled, and she had improved to 15th% in weight and 30th% in height. She had Tanner 2 breast tissue and Tanner 3 pubic hair. Her LH was 1.4 mIU/ml, FSH 2.9 mIU/ml, and estradiol 13 pg/ml. At 15 years and 11 months, approximately 1 year and 8 months after the first signs of breast development, she had menarche. An exam 2 weeks later showed Tanner stage 5 breasts and Tanner stage 4 pubic hair. Her height and weight were at 80th% (Fig. 3.1), and her height of 5′6.5″ (169 cm) was within range of her midparental height. Her bone age x-ray showed skeletal maturity age of 15 years, showing catch-up growth and skeletal maturation due to pubertal hormones. She had not had any fractures but was advised to optimize calcium and vitamin D intake and to repeat DXA scan in 1 year.

The patient and her parents want to know if there is any future health risk due to her delayed puberty, such as osteoporosis or infertility.

Discussion

Normal Puberty and Delayed Puberty

Puberty is a period of growth and development between childhood and adulthood that results in attainment of secondary sex characteristics, adult height, and reproductive capacity. The normal progression of pubertal stages was defined by Tanner through cross-sectional and longitudinal studies of healthy children [1–3]. Puberty in girls starts with breast development to Tanner stage 2. Most girls have breast development at age 8–13 years, with peak height velocity at Tanner 3 breasts, and menarche occurring 2–3 years after breast development begins. The appearance of pubic hair, axillary hair, and body odor are called adrenarche and occur in parallel to the breast changes but may start before or after breast development begins. Adrenarche is controlled by hormones produced in the adrenal gland, in contrast to breast development (puberty) that is controlled by hormones produced by the ovaries. At the time of puberty, the hypothalamus secretes gonadotropin-releasing hormone (GnRH) at increasing frequency and amplitude. GnRH stimulates the pituitary to release luteinizing hormone (LH) and follicle-stimulating hormone (FSH), which

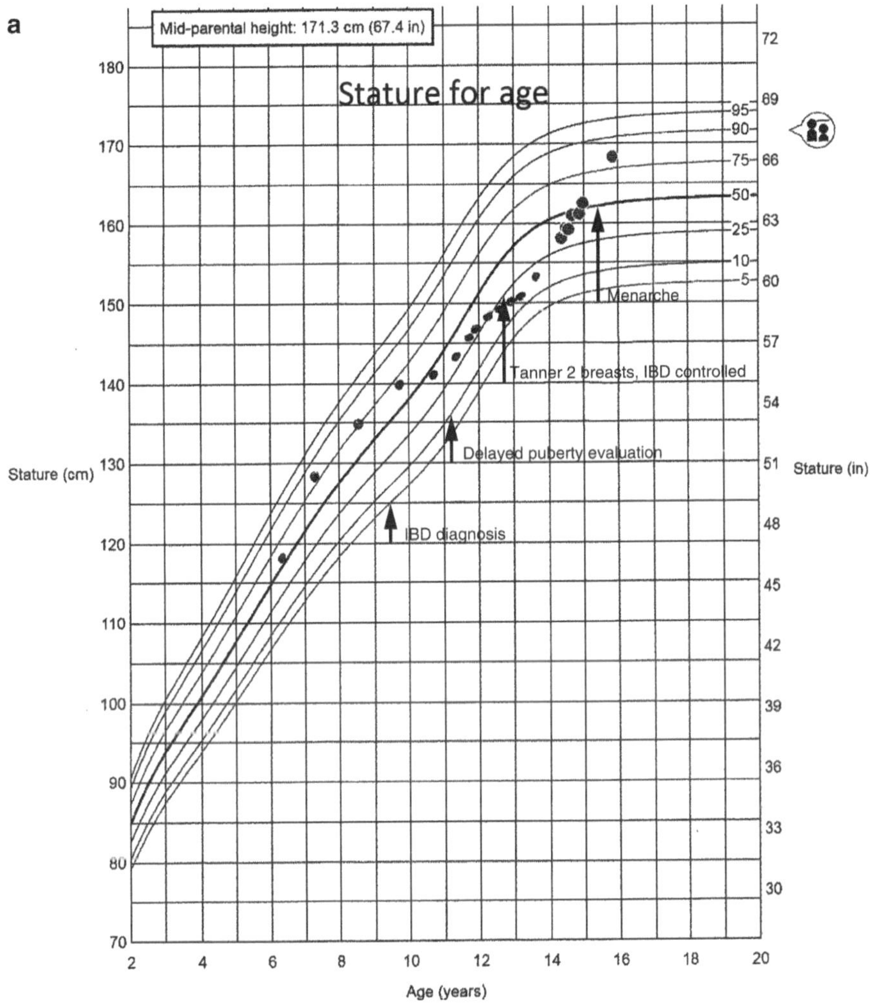

Fig. 3.1 Growth chart [(**a**) stature for age and (**b**) weight for age]

act on the ovary to make estrogens. Estrogens promote the development of secondary sex characteristics such as breast development and widening of the hips. Estrogens also promote linear growth and, ultimately, cause the epiphyses (growth plates) of the long bones to fuse and prevent further increase in height.

Delayed puberty is defined as puberty occurring two standard deviations beyond the mean age. Girls should be evaluated for delayed puberty in the following situations: (1) no breast development by age 13, (2) no menarche within 3 years of thelarche, (3) no menarche by age 14 with signs of hirsutism, (4) no menarche by age 14 with history or exam suggestive of excessive exercise or eating disorder, and (5) no menarche by age 15 [4]. Patients with delayed puberty will not have achieved the pubertal growth spurt, so they may appear to have dropped percentiles on the growth

b

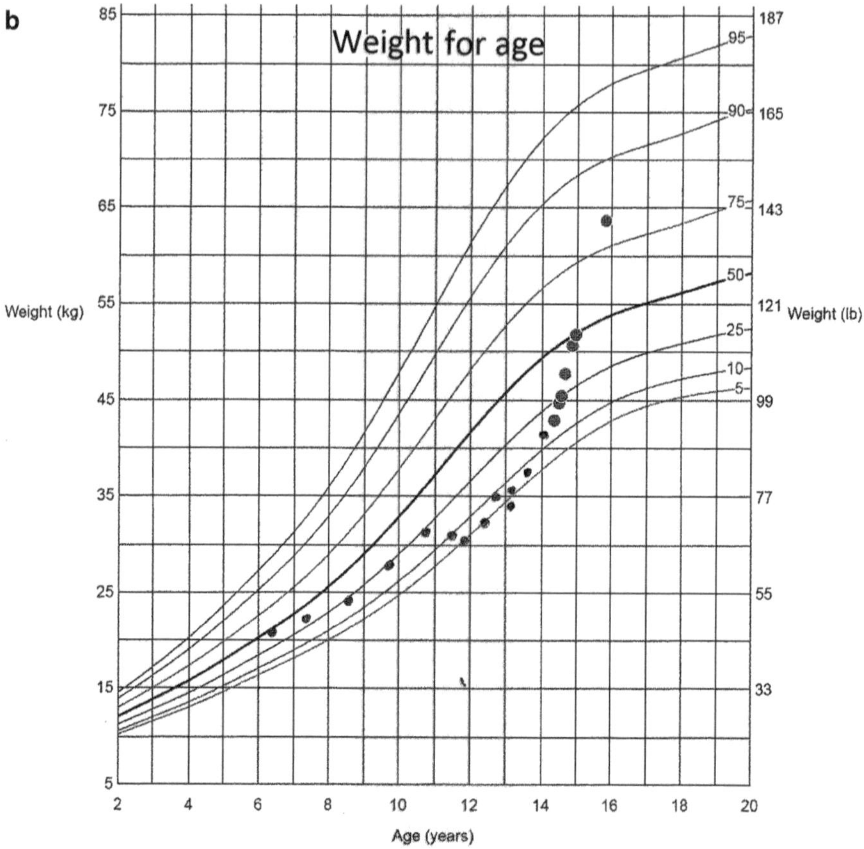

Fig. 3.1 (continued)

curve. An x-ray of their left hand (bone age x-ray) will show the maturity of the patient's epiphyses that can be compared to a standard (such as the atlas of Greulich and Pyle) and used to predict height based on current height and bone age.

Causes of Delayed Puberty and Evaluation

The differential diagnosis of delayed puberty includes many causes of endocrine and non-endocrine nature. The causes may be separated into three categories: (1) functional delayed onset of hypothalamic-pituitary-gonadal (HPG) activity (low LH/FSH, reversible or resolves with time), (2) hypogonadotropic hypogonadism (low LH/FSH), and (3) hypergonadotropic hypogonadism (high LH/FSH – primary gonad problem) (Table 3.1) [5]. There are some additional conditions that do not clearly fit into these categories and may have normal or abnormal LH and FSH levels. A careful history and examination may help to focus the differential diagnosis and subsequent workup (Table 3.2). An LH level under 0.2–0.6 mIU/ml or FSH

Table 3.1 Causes of delayed puberty and specific laboratory and imaging tests (in addition to LH and FSH)

Causes of delayed puberty	Tests to consider
Functional delayed onset of hypothalamic-pituitary-gonadal activity (low LH/FSH, reversible or resolves with time) – Constitutional delay (diagnosis of exclusion) – Uncontrolled illness: Inflammatory bowel disease, celiac disease, systemic lupus erythematosus, cystic fibrosis, chronic kidney disease, hypothyroidism, hyperthyroidism, sickle cell disease – Malnutrition, including anorexia – Excessive exercise, including female athlete triad (primary amenorrhea, disordered eating/low energy, low bone mineral density) – High prolactin	– Bone age x-ray – ESR, CBC, celiac serology, BMP, TSH, free T4, DXA – DXA – Prolactin
Permanent hypogonadotropic hypogonadism (low LH/FSH) – Kallmann syndrome – Congenital GnRH deficiency – Multiple pituitary hormone deficiencies (optic nerve hypoplasia, genetic, trauma, surgery) – Intracranial disorders or injury (surgery, irradiation, trauma, infarction – Sheehan syndrome) – Idiopathic hypogonadotropic hypogonadism (IHH) – Prader-Willi, Laurence-moon, Bardet-Biedl syndromes	– MRI brain/olfactory bulbs – Free T4, IGF-1, morning cortisol, prolactin for any suspected pituitary problem – Specific genetic testing
Hypergonadotropic hypogonadism (high LH/FSH – Primary gonad problem) – Turner syndrome (45,XO or 46,XX/45,XO mosaic or other variants without two full X chromosomes) – Damage to gonads (trauma, chemotherapy, irradiation, autoimmune, mumps infection) – Other genetic causes (e.g., FMR1 premutation)	– Karyotype – Ovarian antibodies, adrenal antibodies – FMR1 premutation testing
Other conditions with variable LH/FSH – Disorder of sex development/gonadal dysgenesis (e.g., 46XY DSD) – Androgen insensitivity syndrome – Polycystic ovarian syndrome – Nonclassic congenital adrenal hyperplasia	– Karyotype, testosterone, DHEAS – Karyotype, testosterone, estradiol, DHEAS – Testosterone, DHEAS – 17-hydroxyprogresterone
Anatomic conditions causing delayed menarche in the setting of normal puberty (normal LH/FSH) – Mayer-Rokitansky-Kuster-Hauser syndrome (MRKH) – Imperforate hymen – Transverse vaginal septum	Pelvic ultrasound hCG

Table 3.2 History and physical exam evaluation of delayed puberty

History
– Age of breast or pubic hair development
– Growth chart trend in height and weight (recent crossing of percentiles)
– Excessive exercise or restrictive eating behaviors
– Chronic illnesses (including inflammatory bowel disease, celiac disease, systemic lupus erythematosus, cystic fibrosis, chronic kidney disease, hypothyroidism, sickle cell disease)
– Medications (including glucocorticoids)
– Family history of pubertal timing
– Mother's and father's height to calculate midparental height for girls
Midparental height for girls = $\frac{(\text{father's height in inches} - 5) + (\text{mother's height in inches})}{2}$
Exam
– Height and weight percentile
– Tanner staging of breasts
– Tanner staging of pubic hair
– Normal external female genitalia
– Presence and amount of axillary hair
– Signs of hyperandrogenism: Hirsutism on the face, chest, and abdomen; severity of acne
– Acanthosis nigricans

level under 0.2–1.0 mIU/ml, depending on the assay, may be considered low [6]. An LH or FSH level above the normal range for a menstruating female is considered high, though it should be repeated as normal girls may have sporadic high levels.

Functional delayed onset of HPG activity is most commonly due to constitutional delay of growth and puberty, which is a diagnosis of exclusion [6]. Constitutional delay occurs more often in males than in females and is seen in families with a history of delayed puberty (and associated pubertal growth spurt). Asking the parents' age at puberty can help establish this as a possibility; most mothers remember their age at menarche, and fathers may recall when they first started shaving or if they continued growing after high school. LH and FSH will be low, but they will rise appropriately when the child's puberty starts at a later age. The child may have a lower height percentile that will improve after the delayed pubertal growth spurt.

Functional delayed onset of HPG activity may be due to poor nutrition or energy balance, inflammatory disease, or states of chronic disease. Women with anorexia, malnutrition, and the female athlete triad (primary amenorrhea, disordered eating or low energy, low bone mineral density) may present with low body mass index and decreased fat tissue composition. This is associated with low levels of the hormone leptin, which has a key role in GnRH release and stimulation of puberty. Clues in the patient's history that may suggest these conditions include food restriction, binging/purging behavior, or excessive exercise. Some patients with uncontrolled or undiagnosed illnesses such as inflammatory bowel disease (IBD), celiac disease, or systemic lupus erythematosus may have pubertal delay related to both malnutrition and inflammation. Pro-inflammatory cytokines, including IL-1 and TNFα, may impair both GnRH and gonadal steroid production [7]. Growth failure may be an early sign of IBD or celiac disease, related to both poor nutrition and inflammation affecting the growth plate and growth hormone pathway. Other warning signs of gastrointestinal disease may include abdominal pain, constipation, diarrhea, or bloody stools. In this setting, helpful tests may include a celiac panel testing for antibodies, specifically tissue transglutaminase IgA and IgG and total IgA level, as well as ESR to look for inflammation. Hypothyroidism or hyperthyroidism may affect pubertal development if the condition is uncontrolled or undiagnosed. Hypothyroidism may present as weight gain, fatigue, depression, concentration difficulty, constipation, or cold intolerance. Hyperthyroidism may present as weight loss, fatigue, anxiety, tremor, diarrhea, or heat intolerance. Evaluation includes a thyroid-stimulating hormone (TSH) level, with or without a paired free thyroxine (free T4) level. Other medical conditions such as cystic fibrosis, chronic kidney disease, or sickle cell disease may need to be brought into better control in order for puberty to progress. Some genetic causes of obesity such as Prader-Willi syndrome and Bardet-Biedl syndrome are associated with functional hypogonadism as well.

Rarely, patients may have high prolactin levels interfering with GnRH secretion. Elevated prolactin may be due to pituitary tumor, medication (antipsychotics that are dopamine antagonists, such as Risperdal), or severe hypothyroidism causing elevation of thyrotropin-releasing hormone (TRH). Patients may present with galactorrhea, and if there is a pituitary tumor, they may have headaches or visual changes (particularly bitemporal hemianopsia). If a high prolactin level is found, further investigation should be done to determine the source, as treatment may normalize LH and FSH.

Permanent hypogonadotropic hypogonadism is LH/FSH deficiency in the absence of a known or suspected disease or malnutrition state affecting the whole body. In the absence of conditions such as IBD or other chronic illnesses, anorexia, and female athlete triad, one may consider disorders that affect the hypothalamus or pituitary and cause LH/FSH deficiency. Among patients with a known history of pituitary hormone deficiencies or those at risk, due to optic nerve hypoplasia, intracranial surgery, trauma, or genetic etiologies, a deficiency of LH and FSH would be a likely cause of delayed puberty. Patients may have congenital GnRH deficiency, either as an isolated hormone deficiency or combined with other pituitary deficiencies. Some genes associated with multiple pituitary hormone deficiencies include *POU1F1*, *PROP1*, *LHX3*, *LHX4*, and *HESX1* [8]. Isolated GnRH deficiency may be related to mutations in genes encoding GnRH (*GNRH1*), the GnRH receptor (*GNRHR*), or the kisspeptin receptor (*KISS1R*) [8]. In Kallmann syndrome, commonly associated with reduced or absent sense of smell, the GnRH neurons and the olfactory bulb fail to migrate into their proper position. Patients have low LH and FSH levels, and MRI of the brain may show abnormal olfactory bulb position. Numerous genes are linked to Kallmann syndrome, including *KAL1*, *FGFR1*, *FGF8*, *PROK2*, and *PROKR2* [8].

Finally, some patients have low LH and FSH levels with no clear cause, which is called idiopathic hypogonadotropic hypogonadism (IHH). It can be difficult to differentiate this group from those with constitutional delay of puberty, but those with constitutional delay will eventually start puberty and progress at a normal tempo, while those with IHH will not start puberty spontaneously.

Patients with a high LH and FSH level fall into the category of hypergonadotropic hypogonadism that is concerning for a problem with the gonads (ovaries). Premature ovarian insufficiency is the most common cause in this group, with Turner syndrome being the leading diagnosis. In Turner syndrome, part or all of the second X chromosome is missing, resulting in dysgenetic "streak" gonads. These gonads cannot respond appropriately to LH and FSH to make estrogen, resulting in ovarian insufficiency. Many girls with Turner syndrome are not diagnosed until they have delayed puberty, even though they may have been short for some time. Additional phenotypic features of Turner syndrome can include a high-arched palate, webbed neck, large carrying angle (with arms held at the side and palms facing forward, the angle between the hand and the body), widely spaced nipples, and shield chest. Some patients may have mild or none of the classic features of Turner syndrome if they have a mosaic karyotype (45,XO/46,XX). While a few patients with Turner syndrome enter puberty spontaneously and even achieve menarche, most patients need treatment to start and maintain pubertal development and regular menses. All girls with delayed puberty should be evaluated for Turner syndrome with a karyotype.

Other causes of premature ovarian insufficiency include idiopathic ovarian failure, autoimmune ovarian failure with documented ovarian antibodies (or adrenal antibodies that cross-react with similar tissue), and fragile X with an FMR1 premutation. In addition there are iatrogenic causes, such as chemotherapy (particularly cyclophosphamide) or irradiation to the pelvic area.

Undiagnosed disorder of sex development (DSD) should also be considered, particularly in cases where karyotype and phenotype (including internal genitalia) or in contradiction. These patients may have absent ovaries and dysgenetic gonads or have some testicular tissue (ovotestes). LH and FSH may be high if the gonads are not functional; otherwise, they may be low or normal. A karyotype to evaluate for 46,XY DSD and testing androgen levels (testosterone, DHEAS) may be helpful. One rare condition is androgen insensitivity syndrome, where the androgen receptor has a mutation preventing it from responding to testosterone in fetal development and at puberty. These patients will appear as normal females but have a 46,XY karyotype, high androgen levels, and low estrogen levels.

Other conditions with variable LH and FSH values include polycystic ovarian syndrome and nonclassic congenital adrenal hyperplasia (CAH). Polycystic ovarian syndrome is diagnosed in adolescents with irregular or absent periods with clinical or laboratory signs of hyperandrogenism. Girls may have excess hair on the face, chin, chest, or abdomen as well as significant acne. High testosterone levels are common, and DHEAS levels may be elevated as well. Girls with insulin resistance due to obesity may be more likely to have PCOS, but there is a growing subset of girls recognized to have PCOS with a lean physique. Another consideration in girls with delayed puberty is nonclassic CAH, where there is a milder defect in the 21-hydroxylase enzyme that causes classic CAH diagnosed in the newborn period. These patients may have signs of hyperandrogenism including hirsutism, excess acne, and clitoral enlargement. DHEAS and testosterone may be elevated. The diagnostic test for nonclassic CAH is a 17-hydroxyprogesterone level which, if high, should prompt a referral to endocrinology.

Mayer-Rokitansky-Kuster-Hauser (MRKH) syndrome is a condition where the fallopian tubes, uterus, and top part of the vagina fail to form. In this case the ovaries function properly, and there is no delay in breast development, but the patient may need a procedure to have a period or may never have a period (MRKH).

In determining the diagnostic approach to a female with delayed puberty, one appropriate stepwise method starts with determining the LH and FSH [9]. If the LH and FSH are high, then causes of hypergonadotropic hypogonadism (particularly Turner syndrome) should be investigated. If the LH and FSH are low, then the clinician should consider and evaluate for any likely systemic condition that could be causing the delayed puberty (such as IBD, thyroid disease, female athlete triad) or diseases with known delayed puberty (such as Prader-Willi syndrome). If this evaluation is negative, the patient may benefit from endocrine referral and close monitoring (at least every 6–12 months). A bone age x-ray may show a bone age that is delayed (defined as more than two standard deviations below the chronologic age) in patients with constitutional delay as well as potentially any of the other conditions. This is due to the lack of estrogen to stimulate bone growth and maturation; thus, a bone age x-ray should be interpreted in the context of history, examination, and laboratory results.

Treatment

In patients with constitutional delay of puberty, the initial approach is watchful waiting. Discussion with the patient involves reassurance and emphasis on the variance in the age when puberty begins and the rate at which it develops. Low-dose estrogen (oral or transdermal) may be considered as an option, in particular when there is psychosocial distress secondary to poor self-esteem or difficult peer interactions [6]. If estrogen therapy is initiated, puberty should be monitored with both clinical and biochemical parameters, along with linear growth and bone age evaluation. Therapy is continued until appropriate pubertal staging is achieved for age.

In girls with permanent hypogonadism due to hypogonadotropic hypogonadism or hypergonadotropic hypogonadism, long-term estrogen therapy will be required. As in girls with constitutional delay, low-dose estrogen is started with gradual increase until adult replacement doses are achieved. Conjugated estrogens at 0.3 mg daily have been a suggested dose to start with, but even lower doses have become more commonly used (oral micronized estradiol 0.25 mg/day or transdermal estradiol 14 μg/day). Cutting a transdermal patch and wearing it for less time are options to provide lower doses, and have been used in girls with Turner syndrome. These doses are significantly lower than what is required to initiate menstrual flow.

Estrogen doses are increased gradually over a period of 2–3 years. The slow increase of estrogen without the presence of progestin is crucial in the appropriate breast development and growth. After 15–24 months of estrogen therapy, or when vaginal breakthrough bleeding occurs, progestin is added to induce endometrial cycling. Two hundred milligram of oral micronized progesterone or 5 mg of oral medroxyprogesterone is given for 12 days of the month [10]. The adult dose of estradiol is 100 μg/day (transdermal).

In patients with functional delayed onset of HPG, it is important to correct or improve underlying pathology to achieve normal progression of puberty. Correcting any nutritional or energy expenditure imbalances is necessary by providing lifestyle modification options or cognitive behavioral therapy as needed. Once the underlying cause is resolved, pubertal progression is usually achieved within 1 year.

Long-Term Considerations

The psychosocial distress which is experienced by girls with delayed puberty is acknowledged but not well studied. The period in which this is experienced is primarily during the early years in which delay is noticed but may have long-term negative effects. Furthermore, less is known on how estrogen therapy may interfere with any psychosocial distress patient may be having. When considering estrogen therapy for delayed puberty, the clinician should consider the permanence of the condition, how the child is coping with this disorder, and how any intervention will affect her in both positive and negative ways.

Women with reversible hypogonadotropic hypogonadism should not have diminished fertility provided their menses are normal. Fertility may require specific treatment options in other patients. Women with permanent hypogonadotropic hypogonadism require treatment with exogenous LH and FSH to induce ovulation and fertility. Women with ovarian failure may have the option of donor oocytes if their uterus is normal with estrogen treatment, but a fertility specialist will need to consider whether pregnancy is safe.

Although adult height may be compromised in patients with delayed puberty due to causes other than constitutional delay, growth hormone therapy has not been shown to be of benefit. In addition, it is uncertain how delayed puberty and its management may affect adult bone health. Patients with underlying illnesses such as IBD may have negative effects on their bone density due to the disease process, nutrition, and inflammation as well as due to delayed puberty. There may be disease-specific risks to bone density that persist after gonadal function is normalized [11]. Careful monitoring of bone density with regular DXA scans and optimizing calcium, vitamin D, and weight-bearing physical activity are important to help the child achieve optimal bone density.

Clinical Pearls and Pitfalls

- Patients with chronic illnesses, especially those that affect gastrointestinal tract or cause chronic inflammation, can have delayed puberty.

- Health care providers taking care of children and adolescents with chronic illnesses such as IBD, SLE, and sickle cell disease should monitor for delayed puberty and refer to endocrinology as needed.
- Lack of breast development by 13 years, lack of menarche by 15 years, or lack of menarche within 3 years of breast development warrants evaluation.
- Causes of delayed puberty can be separated based on low or high puberty hormones (LH, estradiol) and history or exam findings suggestive of causes of functional delay of hypothalamic-pituitary-gonadal (HPG) axis maturation (chronic illness, excessive exercise, constitutional delay).
- Constitutional delay of puberty is a diagnosis of exclusion.

References

1. August GP, Grumbach MM, Kaplan SL. J Clin Endocrinol Metab. 1972;34(2):319–6.
2. Marshall WA, Tanner JM. Variations in pattern of pubertal changes in girls. Arch Dis Child. 1969;44(235):291–303.
3. Marshall WA, Tanner JM. Variations in pattern of pubertal changes in boys. Arch Dis Child. 1970;45(239):13–23.
4. ACOG committee opinion No. 651: menstruation in girls and adolescents: using the menstrual cycle as a vital sign. Obstet Gynecol. 2015;126(6):e143–6.
5. Wei C, Crowne EC. Recent advances in the understanding and management of delayed puberty. Arch Dis Child. 2016;101:481–8.
6. Palmert MR, Dunkel L. Clinical practice. Delayed puberty. N Engl J Med. 2012;366(5):443–53.
7. Ezri J, Marques-Vidal P, Nydegger A. Impact of disease and treatments on growth and puberty of pediatric patients with inflammatory bowel disease. Digestion. 2012;85(4):308–19.
8. Larson A, Nokoff NJ, Meeks NJ. Genetic causes of pituitary hormone deficiencies. Discov Med. 2015;19(104):175–83.
9. Abitbol L, Zborovski S, Palmert MR. Evaluation of delayed puberty: what diagnostic tests should be performed in the seemingly otherwise well adolescent? Arch Dis Child. 2016;101:767–71.
10. Crowley WF, Pitteloud N. Diagnosis and treatment of delayed puberty. In: Snyder PJ, Middleman AB, Geffner M, editors. UpToDate. Waltham, MA. Accessed 8 Apr 2016.
11. Williams KM. Update on bone health in pediatric chronic disease. Endocrinol Metab Clin North Am. 2016;45(2):433–41.

Suggested Educational Reading, References, and Policies

Abitbol L, Zborovski S, Palmert MR. Evaluation of delayed puberty: what diagnostic tests should be performed in the seemingly otherwise well adolescent? Arch Dis Child. 2016;101:767–71.

Crowley WF, Pitteloud N. Diagnosis and treatment of delayed puberty. In: Snyder PJ, Middleman AB, Geffner M, editors. UpToDate. Waltham, MA. Accessed 8 Apr 2016.

Kaplowitz PB. Delayed puberty. Pediatr Rev. 2010;31(5):189–95.

Palmert MR, Dunkel L. Clinical practice. Delayed puberty. N Engl J Med. 2012;366(5):443–53.

Wei C, Crowne EC. Recent advances in the understanding and management of delayed puberty. Arch Dis Child. 2016;101:481–8.

Chapter 4
Case of a Girl with Vulvar Swelling

Judith Simms-Cendan and Xiomara Santos

A 13-year-old girl presents with her mother to the clinic. She complains that she has noticed a bulge in her "private area." She is very competitive in gymnastics that at times the area becomes irritated after practice. Her mother examined her and was concerned that she has abnormal, swollen growth of the skin and has scheduled an appointment for evaluation.

On further questioning, the patient reports that she has become self-conscious about her genital appearance. She has done Internet searches and is concerned she has abnormal genitalia that are not attractive. She reports tenderness, especially after balance beam work, but it is minimal and resolves after her shower. She has not noticed any burning on urination. She began menses 18 months ago and is using tampons without difficulty but at times feels that hygiene can be difficult during her menses due to the "extra skin." She has no other medical or surgical history. She is in the eighth grade, doing well in school and active in sports. She has no history of eating disorders. She has never been sexually active and denies a history of sexual abuse. She denies drug or alcohol use. Most days she is happy but has been stressed balancing school and gymnastics.

On physical examination she is a healthy-appearing 13-year-old with a normal body mass index. She has Tanner IV breast development. On pelvic exam, she has completely removed her pubic hair by shaving. Her labia majora, clitoris, and urethral meatus are normal. Her labia minora are visible without retraction of the labia

J. Simms-Cendan, M.D. (✉)
Department of Clinical Sciences, University of Central Florida College of Medicine, Orlando, FL, USA
e-mail: judith.simms-cendan@ucf.edu

X. Santos, M.D.
Department of Obstetrics and Gynecology, Orlando Health Physicians Group, Orlando, FL, USA
e-mail: xiomara.santos@orlandohealth.com

H.J. Talib (ed.), *Adolescent Gynecology*,
https://doi.org/10.1007/978-3-319-66978-6_4

majora and measure 3 cm in width from introitus to lateral edge. No lesions nor erythema are noted.

Her mother looks worried and asks, “Is my daughter normal? Does she need surgery?” The patient states, “I don’t like the way I look. Can you fix this?”

Discussion

In the age of widely available images of vulvar anatomy through web searches, and unfortunately easily accessible Internet pornography, adolescent girls are increasingly presenting with concerns about their genital appearance and requesting surgical correction. Between 2014 and 2015, there was an 80% increase in girls aged 18 and younger undergoing cosmetic labiaplasty [1]. This increase reported by the American Society for Aesthetic Plastic Surgery reflects data from survey by the society of physicians used for national projections and probably underestimates the number of labiaplasties performed as some physicians performing labiaplasty on adolescents may not classify it as cosmetic. Approach to care of adolescent girls presenting with concerns about their genital appearance requires an understanding of the wide variety of normal appearance, time, and resources to educate the patient and her family and a cautious, conservative approach to management prior to considering any surgical intervention.

Adolescents undergo several changes as part of normal pubertal development, including growth of their labia minora [1]. There has been increased awareness and focus on the appearance of the external genitalia, leaving many adolescents wondering if their body is normal [2]. It is not uncommon for an adolescent to report these concerns to a health-care provider. While most cases can be managed with education and reassurance, some might require further intervention [3]. Knowledge of normal genital anatomy and pubertal changes is important to be able to manage adolescents presenting with concerns about their labia.

The labia minora are very sensitive to stimulation, and their stimulation may be a component of the normal sexual response. Recent research has demonstrated the presence of free endings and other sensory structures in the labia minora from biopsy specimens of labia minora considered waste tissue in 10 girls under the age of 10 undergoing surgery by a pediatric urologist [4]. Schober et al. surveyed 62 healthy adult women about the appearance and sexual sensitivity of the labia. In 11% of women reporting self-perceived larger labia minora, there was a higher rating of sexual pleasure [5]. That same study showed women’s assessment of their anatomy is highly variable in what is considered to be normal.

There is no standard definition of labia minora hypertrophy in the literature (Fig. 4.1) [2, 6]. Review of the literature of studies that measured labia minora size in adult women demonstrated a wide variety of labia minora width, with measurements ranging from 3 to 50 mm [7]. There are no such studies in adolescent girls. In adult women, there is no statistical association with labial size and ethnicity, age, hormone use, or history of sexual activity [5]. While patients may consider it

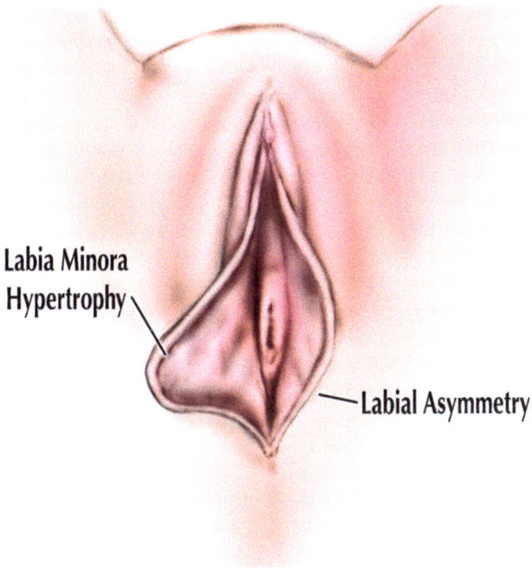

Fig. 4.1 Labia minora hypertrophy

abnormal to have the labia minora protrude beyond the labia majora, caution should be taken before diagnosing the appearance as that of labial hypertrophy, especially in those with a labia measuring 4 cm or less [8].

Common symptoms of adolescents presenting with labial hypertrophy include irritation, pain, and interference with personal hygiene (especially during menses) [1, 3, 9]. In many cases adolescents report interference with sports, like running, cycling, horseback riding, and swimming, and interference with sexual activity [3]. Concerns about the appearance of the labia minora can affect their self-esteem and result in significant psychological distress for the adolescent particularly when wearing specific clothing, like a bathing suit or formfitting clothing [3, 9]. In addition, many parents are unaware of the normal variation of the labia minora and might express their concerns about their daughter's appearance when comparing it to their own [1, 3]. This can add to the psychological and emotional distress of the adolescent.

After obtaining a detailed history about the adolescent's concerns and symptoms, the provider should proceed with a physical examination [3]. In most cases, especially in the nonsexually active adolescent, an internal pelvic exam with the use of speculum can be avoided, and an external pelvic exam would be sufficient to evaluate her concerns. Other conditions that can present with similar symptoms and need to be excluded on exam are vulvitis, vaginitis, lichen sclerosus, cysts, lipomas, abscesses, and childhood asymmetric labium majus enlargement [3]. Areas to be inspected include the hair distribution, skin, labia majora and minora, clitoris, urethra meatus, introitus, and perineal body. The labia minora can be measured from the midline to the lateral free edge while holding it fully extended.

Table 4.1 Conservative measures for management of labia hypertrophy

Conservative measures
Reassurance about normal vulvar anatomy Referral to resources to show the variations of normal
Proper genital hygiene to avoid irritation Use simple soaps, use of emollients, avoid scented gels
Use comfortable underwear Avoidance of formfitting clothing

Patient Education Is Key

Once other conditions have been excluded, the provider should provide reassurance and education to the adolescent about their normal anatomy and pubertal development [1, 3, 7]. The external genitalia continue to grow and change throughout puberty, including enlargement of the labia majora, which may significantly reduce the prominence of the labia minora.

There are excellent resources, such as *Petals* by Nick Karras and the Labia Library (web based out of Australia) that can be used to educate girls and their families about the wide variety of genital anatomy. In addition, the patient should be educated about how the labia might appear more prominent if the pubic hair is removed.

Conservative Management of Symptoms

The first approach to discomfort with sports or clothing should be conservative. The use of protective emollients, especially those that are silicon based, can provide relief. Some girls find they have less chafing with looser underwear, where others find they do well with tighter underclothes, and experimentation of these options should be encouraged. Improved hygiene and sitz baths are also important measures that can relieve symptoms (Table 4.1) [1, 7].

Surgical correction of labial hypertrophy in adolescence remains very controversial. There are some who view cosmetic surgery akin to female genital mutation, and some countries such as Great Britain have restricted its use under the age of 18 years.

Labioplasty: A Controversial Intervention in Adolescents

If significant bothersome symptoms persist, such as labia becoming entrapped in clothing or intractable inflammation, then surgical correction can be considered [1, 3]. Some authors recommend avoiding surgery in those younger than 15 years old in order to avoid need for second procedure in the future (if the labia continues to grow) [3]. Proceeding with surgery at an older age also allows the adolescent to be more mature and participate in informed consent.

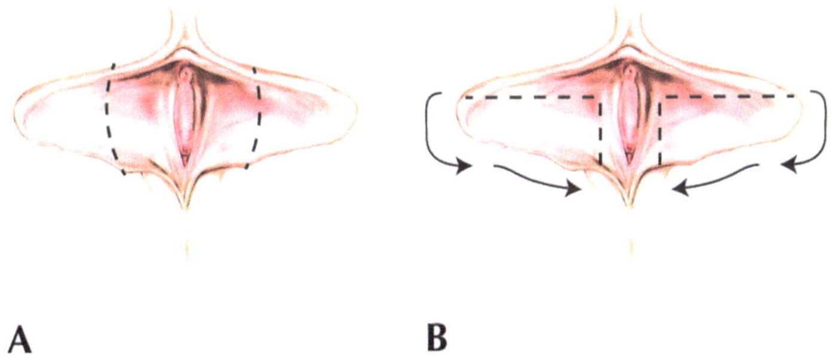

Fig. 4.2 (**a**) Straight resection of excess tissue. (**b**) Wedge resection of excess tissue

When considering surgical correction of labia hypertrophy, commonly referred as labiaplasty, it is important to review the motivation and goals of the surgery. The provider should assess whether or not the adolescent has realistic goals of the surgical outcomes and benefits [1]. The adolescent should be screened for body dysmorphic disorder and referred to a mental health professional if there is suspicion of it [1, 10]. Labial cosmetic surgery in adolescence in general is discouraged.

Several labiaplasty techniques have been described in the literature including straight amputation, wedge resection, and de-epithelization, among others [3, 8–10]. See Fig. 4.2.

Goals of the wedge resection technique include decreased exposed scar and maintenance of nerve innervation at the periphery; however, there is a higher rate of wound breakdown with this technique. Most studies in adult women report high satisfaction rates and low rate of complications [8, 10]. The most common complications reported are wound dehiscence, hematoma, and postoperative bleeding [10]. One small study in adult women of sexual functioning after labiaplasty showed improved satisfaction in genital appearance but no long-term improvements in sexual function [11]. However, there is a lack of prospective studies, and some authors discourage performing labiaplasty on adolescents given the lack of valid research on long-term outcomes with the possibility of loss of labial sensation being one of the major concerns [7]. The adolescent and her parents or guardian should be fully informed of the potential risks of surgery prior to proceeding.

Clinical Pearls and Pitfalls

1. Many patients and their families require only education. Using books like *Petals* by Nick Karras can teach girls that there is a wide variety of normal vulvar anatomy and provide reassurance.
2. Consider psychological evaluation for body dysmorphic disorder. Cosmetic surgery of the genitals is discouraged in minors.
3. Surgical correction should be reserved for very symptomatic individuals. Genital surgery may affect subsequent sexual response and function.

Resources for Patient Education

- Petals, by Nick Karras. A book with black and white photos depicting the wide range of normal vulvar anatomy. Nickkarras.com.
- The Great Wall of Vagina. Art exhibition of plaster casts of vulvas showing the wide range of normal. Greatwallofvagina.co.uk.
- 101 Vagina. One Hundred and One Women: One Hundred and One Stories, by Philip Werner. A book with black and white photos with stories designed to break down perceptions about what is normal and combat body image shame. 101vagina.com
- The Labia Library. Excellent website with information on normal size, symmetry, color and symptom management and color photos in lithotomy and standing. Labialibrary.org.au.

Resource for Physicians

- ACOG Committee Opinion on Breast and Labial Surgery in Adolescents Number 662. http://www.acog.org/Resources-And-Publications/Committee-Opinions/Committee-on-Adolescent-Health-Care/Breast-and-Labial-Surgery-in-Adolescents

References

1. American College of Obstetricians and Gynecologists. Breast and labial surgery in adolescents. Committee Opinion No. 662. Obstet Gynecol. 2016;127:e138–40.
2. Bercaw-Pratt JL, Santos XM, Sanchez J, Ayensu-Coker L, Nebgen DR, Dietrich JE. The incidence, attitudes and practices of the removal of pubic hair as a body modification. J Pediatr Adolesc Gynecol. 2012;25:12–4.
3. Reddy J, Laufer MR. Hypertrophic labia minora. J Pediatr Adolesc Gynecol. 2010;23:3–6.
4. Schober J, Aardsma N, Mayoglou L, Pfaff D, Martin-Alguacil N. Clin Anat. 2015;28:392–8.
5. Schober J, Martin Alguacil N, Cooper R, Pfaff D, Meyer-Bahlburg H. Self assessment of anatomy, sexual sensitivity, and function of the labia and vagina. Clin Anat. 2015;28:355–62.
6. The American Society for Aesthetic Plastic Surgery. 2015 Cosmetic Surgery National Data Bank Statistics. http://www.surgery.org/sites/default/files/ASAPS-Stats2015.pdf
7. Runacres SA, Wood PL. Cosmetic labiaplasty in an adolescent population. J Pediatr Adolesc Gynecol. 2016;29(3):218–22.
8. Rouzier R, Louis-Sylvestre C, Paniel BJ, Haddad B. Hypertrophy of labia minora: experience with 163 reductions. Am J Obstet Gynecol. 2000;182(1):35–40.
9. Lynch A, Marulaiah M, Samarakkody U. Reduction labiaplasty in adolescents. J Pediatr Adolesc Gynecol. 2008;21(3):147–9.
10. Oranges CM, Sisti A, Sisti G. Labia minora reduction techniques: a comprehensive literature review. Aesthet Surg J. 2015;35(4):419–31.
11. Veale D, Naismith I, Eshkevari E, Ellison N, Costa A, Robinson D, Abeywickrama L, Kavouni A, Cardoza L. Psychosexual outcome after labiaplasty: a prospective case-comparison study. Int Urogynecol. 2014;25:831–9.

Chapter 5
Case of the Girl with Abdominal Pain

Hanna R. Goldberg, Jasmine Multani, and Sari Kives

Case

A 14-year-old female presented to the emergency room with an 8-day history of right lower quadrant abdominal pain. She also complained of nausea, vomiting, sweating, and headache. The patient described the severity of the pain as fluctuating between a 4 and 7 out of 10. She characterized the pain as a constant ache with occasional stinging sensations lasting up to 5 min. She had no dysuria and her bowel movements had been soft and somewhat loose.

On gynecological history, the patient had regular menstrual cycles with no associated dysmenorrhea. Her last menstrual period was 26 days prior to presentation. The patient's past medical, surgical, and family histories were unremarkable. She was not taking any medication and had no allergies.

On physical exam, vital signs were normal. Her abdomen was soft, but tender in the right lower quadrant to both palpation and percussion. An ultrasound was ordered.

H.R. Goldberg, M.S. (✉) • J. Multani, H.B.Sc.
Faculty of Medicine, University of Toronto, Toronto, ON, Canada
e-mail: hanna.goldberg@mail.utoronto.ca; jasmine.multani@mail.utoronto.ca

S. Kives, M.D., M.Sc.
Section of Gynecology, Hospital for Sick Children, Toronto, ON, Canada
e-mail: kivess@smh.ca

H.J. Talib (ed.), *Adolescent Gynecology*,
https://doi.org/10.1007/978-3-319-66978-6_5

Discussion

What Features on this Patient's History Are Worrisome and Why?

Regardless of age, any female presenting with lower quadrant abdominal pain, nausea, and vomiting, with or without fever, should be investigated for adnexal torsion. Adnexal torsion is the twisting of the adnexa around its vascular pedicle. It can lead to compromised ovarian venous and arterial flow and consequently ischemia and necrosis. It is commonly associated with the presence of an ovarian cyst. Adnexal torsion is worrisome as failure to recognize this diagnosis can lead to permanent loss of ovarian function. Characteristic findings of adnexal torsion on ultrasound include an enlarged ovary and absence of flow on Doppler. Ultrasound may also show a solid mass with multiple peripheral cysts as a result of ovarian congestion and transudation of fluid into follicles. While absent flow is suggestive of torsion, ultrasound may also demonstrate adequate flow in a transiently torsed adnexa. Optimal management of adnexal torsion involves immediate laparoscopic detorsion.

Back to the Case

The reported ultrasound showed a right ovarian complex cyst that measured $4.0 \times 5.1 \times 4.5$ cm. The cyst had features suggestive of a hemorrhagic cyst. Surrounding ovarian parenchyma showed arterial and venous Doppler flow. There was no evidence of appendicitis.

What Features on History and Ultrasound Help to Differentiate the Etiology of Adnexal Masses?

Adnexal Masses

Adnexal masses include functional cysts, benign neoplasms, and malignant neoplasms. The probability of each histologic type of adnexal mass varies according to the age and menarchal status of the patient. Ultrasound is the best diagnostic investigation for evaluation of adnexal pathology in all age groups. On ultrasound, ovarian masses may appear as cystic, solid, or complex (encompassing both cystic and solid characteristics). In non-virginal patients, transvaginal pelvic ultrasound allows for resolution and differentiation of cystic components. Virginal patients, however, typically undergo an abdominal ultrasound with a full bladder, which has limited positive predictive value. Color flow Doppler is helpful for assessing torsion as well as ectopic pregnancy.

Functional Cysts

Functional cysts are among the most common type of adnexal mass found in the adolescent population. They arise as a result of dysfunctional ovulation or failure of mature follicles to involute. The incidence of functional cysts peaks in the postnatal and postmenarcheal periods as a result of prenatal exposure to maternal hormones and hormonal changes during puberty, respectively. Functional cysts encompass simple or follicular, corpus luteal, and hemorrhagic cysts.

The typical presentation of functional cysts is chronic aching abdominal pain. This can be periumbilical or localized to the lower quadrant. Torsion, perforation, infarction, or hemorrhage of a functional cyst can result in an acute pain. Large cysts can also lead to a sense of abdominal fullness or bloating and can impact urination, leading to frequency or retention.

Functional cysts are identified on ultrasound as simple, anechoic, thin-walled masses. However, hemorrhagic functional cysts may appear complex on ultrasound and may have variety of different appearances depending on the stage of evolution of the clot. Lacelike reticular echoes or an intracystic solid clot is the most typical appearance of a hemorrhagic cyst seen on ultrasound.

Benign Neoplasms

Along with functional cysts, benign neoplasms are among the most common type of adnexal mass found in the adolescent population. Ovarian mature cystic teratomas, also known as dermoid cysts, are benign germ cell tumors. They are the most common type of benign neoplasm diagnosed in adolescents.

The presentation of benign neoplasms can vary widely. Patients may present with abdominal pain or increased abdominal girth, with or without associated nausea and vomiting. Some patients may be completely asymptomatic with the mass discovered as an incidental finding on routine examination.

Benign neoplasms are seen on ultrasound as complex, hypoechoic masses. Complexity of a mass, however, does not necessarily point to a benign neoplasm since tubo-ovarian abscesses, hemorrhagic cysts, and rarely endometriomas are all cysts that have complex attributes on imaging.

Malignant Neoplasms

While the majority of adnexal masses in the pediatric and adolescent population are benign, approximately 10–20% are malignant. Malignant ovarian neoplasms occur more often in premenarchal patients in comparison to postmenarchal patients.

Similar to functional cysts and benign neoplasms, patients with malignant tumors commonly present with lower abdominal pain. They may also present with an abdominal mass or increased abdominal girth. Tumor markers, such as alpha-fetoprotein (AFP), cancer antigen 125 (CA-125), lactate dehydrogenase (LDH), and beta human chorionic gonadotropin (ß-hCG), are often elevated; however, they may be normal as well.

Malignant ovarian masses are found to be complex on ultrasound with ill-defined, irregular borders and central necrosis and may include thick septations of papillary projections. They may also appear as completely solid lesions. Size of the mass on ultrasound is a predictor of malignancy. Masses that are identified as complex and greater than 8 cm or solid of any size should raise suspicion of malignancy.

Given the Diagnosis of a Hemorrhagic Cyst, How Would You Manage the Patient? What Are Important Reasons for Earlier Return?

Management

The goal of management of functional ovarian cysts in the pediatric and adolescent population is conservative management with observation, as functional cysts should resolve spontaneously. Serial ultrasounds often demonstrate resolution of functional cysts in the absence of treatment. Thus, it is recommended that functional cysts be managed expectantly, with follow-up ultrasound. There is not sufficient data in the literature to support recommendations of specific time intervals for follow-up of a functional ovarian cyst. However, since most functional cysts resolve after 2–3 months, follow-up over this time period is appropriate. If serial ultrasounds demonstrate that the cyst has recurred, combined hormonal contraceptives can be used to prevent further recurrence. The patient should return earlier if she experiences any symptoms of adnexal torsion. If the cyst persists and is greater than 4 cm, diagnostic laparoscopy is recommended to rule out other adnexal pathologies (Fig. 5.1).

Back to the Case

It was recommended that the patient follow up with gynecology in 8 weeks to confirm resolution of the cyst. The patient was counseled to return to the emergency department if she had symptoms of adnexal torsion, including acute lower abdominal pain, associated with nausea, vomiting, or fever.

At the follow-up visit, the patient described minimal abdominal pain. She denied any associated symptoms, such as nausea or vomiting. On exam, the abdomen was

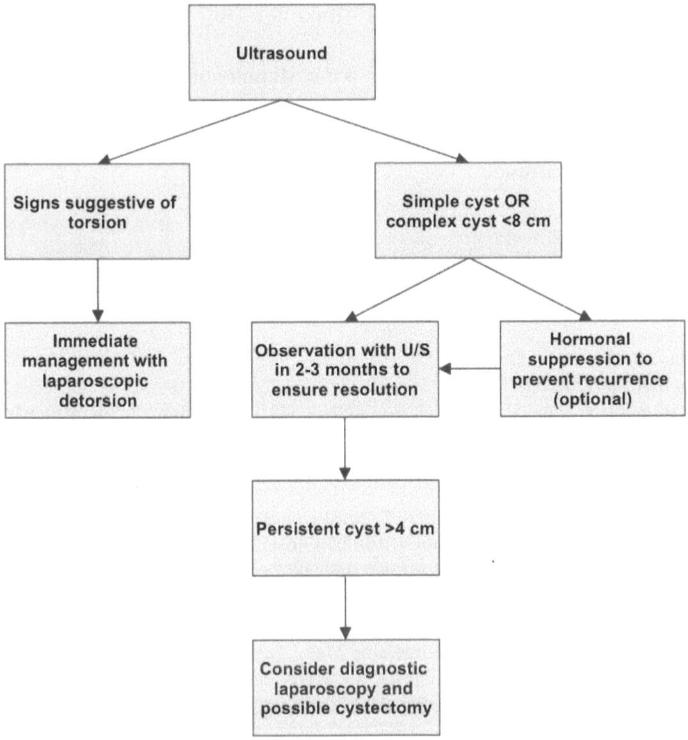

Fig. 5.1 Management of postmenarchal patient presenting with abdominal pain

soft and mildly tender in the right lower quadrant. Ultrasound showed a normal uterus and normal ovaries with complete resolution of the hemorrhagic cyst.

Clinical Pearls and Pitfalls

- Ultrasound is the best diagnostic tool for evaluation of adnexal pathology.
- Adnexal torsion should be ruled out in cases of patients presenting with lower abdominal pain, especially those with associated nausea and vomiting.
- Patients with functional cysts typically present with chronic, aching lower abdominal pain.
- On ultrasound, functional cysts may appear simple or complex, such as in cases of hemorrhagic cysts.
- Goal of management is preservation of structure and function of the ovary with conservative management.
- Functional cysts resolve spontaneously, without any treatment.

- Follow-up ultrasound should be performed to ensure resolution of a functional cyst.
- If the cyst persists and is greater than 4 cm, diagnostic laparoscopy and possible cystectomy is recommended.
- If a functional cyst recurs, combined hormonal contraceptives can be used to prevent further recurrence.

Bibliography

1. Kirkham YA, Kives S. Ovarian cysts in adolescents: medical and surgical management. Adolesc Med. 2012a;23:178–91.
2. Kives S, Gascon S, Dubuc E, Van Eyk N et al. No. 341-Diagnosis and management of adnexal torsion in children, adolescents and adults. J Obstet Gynaecol Can. 2017;39(2):82–90.
3. Kokoska ER, Keller MS, Weber TR. Acute ovarian torsion in children. Am J Surg. 2001;180(6):462–5.
4. Graif M, Shalev J, Strauss S, Engelberg S, Mashiach S, Itzchak Y. Torsion of the ovary: sonographic features. AJR Am J Roentgenol. 1984;143(6):1331–4.
5. White M, Stella J. Ovarian torsion: 10-year perspective. Emerg Med Australas. 2005;17(3):231–7.
6. Shadinger LL, Andreotti RF, Kurian RL. Preoperative sonographic and clinical characteristics as predictors of ovarian torsion. J Ultrasound Med. 2008;27:7–13.
7. Rogers EM, Cubides GC, Lacy J, Gerstle JT, Kives S, Allen L. Preoperative risk stratification of adnexal masses: can we predict the optimal surgical management? J Pediatr Adolesc Gynecol. 2014;27:125–8.
8. Templeman CL, Fallat ME. Benign ovarian masses. Semin Pediatr Surg. 2005;14(2):93–9.
9. Kirkham YA, Lacy JA, Kives S, Allen L. Characteristics and management of adnexal masses in a Canadian pediatric and adolescent population. J Obstet Gynaecol Can. 2011;33:935–43.
10. Okai T. Transvaginal sonographic appearance of hemorrhagic functional ovarian cysts and their spontaneous regression. Int J Gynecol Obstet. 1994;44:47–52.
11. Zhang M, Jiang W, Li G, Xu C. Ovarian masses in children and adolescents - an analysis of 521 clinical cases. J Pediatr Adolesc Gynecol. 2014;27(3):e73–7.
12. Laufer MR. Adnexal masses. In: Emans JE, Laufer MR, editors. Emans, Laufer, & Goldstein's pediatric and adolescent gynecology. 6th ed. Philadelphia: Lippincott Williams & Wilkins; 2012. p. 381.
13. Surratt JT, Siegel MJ. Imaging of pediatric ovarian masses. Radiographics. 2001;11:533–48.
14. Fisher M, Lara-Torre E. Update on key topics in adolescent gynecology. J Pediatr Adolesc Gynecol. 2013;26:51–7.

Recommended Reading

Kirkham YA, Kives S. Ovarian cysts in adolescents: medical and surgical management. Adolesc Med. 2012b;23:178–91.

Kives S, Gascon S, Dubuc E, Van Eyk N et al. No. 341-Diagnosis and management of adnexal torsion in children, adolescents and adults. J Obstet Gynaecol Can. 2017;39(2):82–90.

Part II
Menstrual Disorders

Chapter 6
Case of a Girl with Irregular Periods, Acne, and Hirsutism

Lauren A. Kanner and Ellen L. Connor

Case

CC is a 17-year-old female of Irish and German American descent, with a past medical history of premature adrenarche and obesity presenting with oligomenorrhea. She had menarche at age 11 years after adrenarche at age 7 and thelarche at age 9. Her menses were irregular after menarche and continued to occur every 2–3 months with amenorrhea for the past 6 months. Menses tended to last 5 days with heavier flow in the first 2 days and some mild cramping. She also describes moderate acne since age 9, partially responsive to topical acne treatments. Family history is positive for her mother with obesity and type 2 diabetes and a healthy sister and father. Her mother achieved pregnancy with CC using clomiphene.

On physical examination, her vital signs were within normal range for age; BMI is at the 97th percentile. CC has generalized obesity. Skin exam reveals open and closed comedones on face, chest, and back. She has acanthosis nigricans around her posterior neck and in the axillae with notable skin tags present. Evidence of stubble from shaving of sideburns and chin is notable. Coarse, black hair is noted midline on abdomen and back, as well as some terminal hair between the breasts. She is noted to have shaved legs but coarse hair on her lower arms. She has Tanner V breasts and Tanner V pubic hair. GU exam is consistent with normal-appearing, estrogenized external female genitalia with no clitoromegaly.

Laboratory results are as follows: TSH of 2.2 μIU/mL (0.35–4.94 μIU/mL) with Free T4 1.4 ng/dL (0.7–1.5 ng/dL). 17-OH progesterone is 105 ng/dL (9–208 ng/

L.A. Kanner, M.D.
Division of Pediatric Endocrinology, Department of Pediatrics, University of Wisconsin School of Medicine and Public Health, Madison, WI, USA

E.L. Connor, M.D. (✉)
University of Wisconsin, Adolescent PCOS Clinic, American Family Children's Hospital, Madison, WI, USA
e-mail: elconnor@pediatrics.wisc.edu

H.J. Talib (ed.), *Adolescent Gynecology*,
https://doi.org/10.1007/978-3-319-66978-6_6

dL) with DHEAS of 206 μg/dL (65–371 μg/dL) and androstenedione of 1.8 ng/mL (0.35–2.05 ng/mL). Prolactin is 14 ng/mL (4.2–23 ng/mL). Total testosterone is elevated at 64 ng/dL (11–62 ng/dL) with free testosterone 11.2 pg/mL (1.2–7.5 pg/mL). Hemoglobin A1c is 6.1%. A 2-h oral glucose tolerance test is performed with fasting glucose of 92 mg/dL and 2-h insulin glucose of 137 mg/dL. A 24-h urinary-free cortisol is normal. A transabdominal ultrasound demonstrates an endometrial stripe of 3 cm and right ovary volume of 12 cm and left ovary of 8 cm with multiple "string of pearl cysts" notable on bilateral ovaries.

Discussion of hyperandrogenism, secondary amenorrhea, and ultrasonographic findings is held with CC and her mother. Their questions are as follows:

1. How should periods be managed?
2. Can the acne and unwanted hair growth be addressed?
3. How do we know this is PCOS?

Discussion

Differential Diagnosis

The differential diagnosis of polycystic ovary syndrome (PCOS) must be carefully considered. The lack of absolute criteria for diagnosing PCOS makes ruling out all other possible causes of similar symptoms of paramount importance. Causes of irregular menses or amenorrhea, excess acne, and/or excess body hair must be carefully sought. Clinicians must be aware that a family history of PCOS, premature adrenarche, or a personal history of insulin resistance can occur in young women with other pathologies causing amenorrhea, acne, or hirsutism. Thus, every girl presenting with these symptoms should be thoroughly evaluated.

Multiple causes should be considered for irregular menses or secondary amenorrhea. A logical evaluation begins with determining whether the cause is associated with normal, low, or high gonadotropin levels. If LH and FSH levels are elevated, primary ovarian failure is likely, and the evaluation should be directed toward determining etiology. Genetic causes such as Turner syndrome, gonadal dysgenesis, fragile X, and galactosemia can lead to primary ovarian failure. Primary gonadal failure may also be autoimmune with antiovarian antibodies or idiopathic. Low LH and FSH levels may indicate hypothalamic or pituitary dysfunction, which can be the result of CNS disease or lesion, eating disorder or malnutrition, or the female athlete triad. Normal LH and FSH levels with irregular menses or secondary amenorrhea can be seen in patients recovering from eating disorders or the female athlete triad, as well as in patients with PCOS, who may sometimes but not always have an LH/FSH ratio > 2. Hypothyroidism, pregnancy, Cushing syndrome, and hyperprolactinemia should be ruled out as causes of oligomenorrhea or amenorrhea.

Signs of true virilization should be sought out. If virilization is present, it can manifest as excess muscle mass, deepening voice, severe early acne, early and

Table 6.1 Diagnostic criteria for PCOS [1, 4–6]

Androgen Excess-Polycystic Ovary Syndrome Society (AE-PCOS Society)	National Institute of Health/National Institute of Child Health and Human Development Criteria (NIH/NICHD)	Rotterdam criteria
Includes: • Biochemical and/or clinical hyperandrogenism	**Includes:** • Biochemical and/or clinical hyperandrogenism	**Two of the three criteria:** • Biochemical and/or clinical hyperandrogenism
Plus at least one of the following: • Oligomenorrhea/ oligo-ovulation [4] • Ultrasound findings consistent with polycystic ovaries	• Oligomenorrhea/ oligo-ovulation [4]	• Oligomenorrhea/ oligo-ovulation [4] • Ultrasound findings consistent with polycystic ovaries

All criteria require exclusion of other causes of findings, see section on differential diagnoses

severe hirsutism, and/or clitoromegaly. In these cases, testosterone levels may be more elevated than seen in PCOS. Virilization should alert the clinician to the need to rule out adrenal or ovarian tumors, congenital adrenal hyperplasia, and disorders of sexual differentiation.

Excess acne can be familial without serious pathology, particularly in the peripubertal period. Adolescent PCOS diagnosis should therefore not be diagnosed on the basis of mild acne without hyperandrogenemia. Evaluation of hirsutism should be made to rule out familial hypertrichosis and should be ethnic specific when using the Ferriman-Gallwey scale, noting that some ethnicities have much less body hair and are therefore virilized at a lower score. For Caucasian or African American patients such as CC described above, using the modified Ferriman-Gallwey scale of nine areas, a score of at least 8 would be consistent with hirsutism, while a lower score would be needed to define hirsutism in an Asian girl. Evaluation of hair must determine whether the hair is vellus (not androgen dependent) or terminal (androgen responsive).

Evaluation

Diagnosis of adolescent PCOS remains an area of discussion among clinicians and researchers, even more of a conundrum than sorting out the various criteria for diagnosis of PCOS in adult women (Table 6.1).

Evaluation of an adolescent for polycystic ovary syndrome requires both clinical and laboratory evaluations and consideration of ultrasound investigation as well (Table 6.2). A detailed menstrual history should be obtained to confirm oligomenorrhea and/or polymenorrhea and that the patient is 2 years postmenarche.

Table 6.2 Diagnosis of PCOS in an adolescent [2, 8]

Presentation of androgen excess	Oligomenorrhea, oligo-ovulation, polymenorrhea	Ultrasound evidence of polycystic ovarian morphology[a,b]
• Hirsutism including mild or focal hirsutism • Moderate to severe inflammatory acne • Elevated serum total and free testosterone • A single androgen level > 2 SD above the mean for specific assay should not be considered evidence of hyperandrogenism if otherwise asymptomatic adolescent girl	• Interval < 20 days or >45 days more than 2 years after menarche • Interval > 90 days in consecutive menses • Lack of menses by age 15 years • Lack of menses >2–3 years after thelarche	• No specific criteria to define polycystic ovarian morphology in adolescents but may consider: • Ovarian volume > 12 cm^3 [a]Do not use follicle count. Multifollicular pattern does not have a relationship with hyperandrogenism and is more common in adolescents [b]Enlarged ovaries but otherwise regular menses and without hyperandrogenism does not indicate the diagnosis of PCOS

Oligomenorrhea is defined as menses occurring less than every 3 months with cycles >35 days in adults and >45 days in adolescents. Polymenorrhea is defined as menses with <25 day intervals for adults and <20 day interval cycles in adolescents [1, 2]. Primary amenorrhea in a small subset of girls may delay diagnosis of PCOS, but lack of menarche by age 15 or 2–3 years after true thelarche raises suspicion for PCOS.

Transabdominal or transvaginal ultrasound can be obtained to screen for polycystic ovarian morphology with transvaginal imaging preferred but not possible or tolerated in many adolescent patients. To meet criteria for PCOS, an adult ultrasound would demonstrate ≥12 antral follicles in at least one ovary measuring 2–9 mm in diameter or ovarian volume ≥ 10 cm^3. However, in an adolescent, an ovarian volume ≥ 12 cm^3 has been recommended by some authorities, and multifollicular morphology should not be used as this morphology may be difficult to distinguish from adolescent patterns. String of pearl morphology is sometimes but not necessarily found in adolescent evaluation of the ovaries by ultrasonography.

Hyperandrogenism in PCOS can be defined as either biochemical, with mild elevation of free and/or total testosterone, with free testosterone elevation more common, or clinical, based on physical exam features of androgen excess, mainly hirsutism, severe acne, or alopecia. Alopecia is uncommon in adolescence. The Ferriman-Gallwey score can be used for documenting hirsutism with a score of 8 or more consistent with hirsutism in Caucasian or African American girls. However, there can be ethnic variation in hirsutism affecting sensitivity of the scores, and some adolescents will have focal hirsutism but not elicit a high Ferriman-Gallwey score. Hirsutism refers specifically to excessive coarse sexual hair (terminal hair developing in a male pattern distribution) and must be distinguished from hypertrichosis which is generalized vellus hair growth distributed in a nonsexual pattern.

To meet the diagnostic criteria for hyperandrogenemia for PCOS and rule out other differential diagnoses, laboratory work is recommended (Table 6.3).

Table 6.3 Laboratory work recommended to diagnose hyperandrogenemia for PCOS

Consistent with (but not diagnostic of) PCOS
• ↑ Free and total testosterone • LH/FSH ratio > 2, ↓ sex hormone binding globulin
Consistent with other differential diagnoses
• Adrenal pathology: significant ↑ DHEAS, androstenedione, 17-OH progesterone, or 24 h urinary-free cortisol (or 11 pm salivary cortisol) • Thyroid pathology: abnormal TSH, free T4, or free T3 • Pituitary pathology: significantly ↑prolactin or FSH • Androgen secreting tumor (ovary or adrenal gland): ↑↑↑free and total testosterone
Additional evaluation to consider for metabolic conditions associated with PCOS
• Oral glucose tolerance test • Fasting insulin and glucose for glucose to insulin ratio • Hemoglobin A1c • Fasting lipid panel • Liver function tests

Treatment

Goals: The goals for treatment of PCOS are multiple. Restoration of menstrual function is a primary goal of treatment, both for fertility and for uterine health. Since menstrual cycles with PCOS can be anovulatory and irregular, routine shedding of the endometrial lining may not occur despite estrogen effect, increasing endometrial thickening. Without proper shedding of the lining, the risk for uterine cancer increases. Therefore, regulation of menses with shedding of the endometrial lining (if not undergoing pharmacologic menstrual suppression) of at least every 3 months is needed for uterine cancer prevention. Additionally, restoring menstrual function with menstrual regularity might improve a girl's knowledge of her cycles, potentially decreasing the risk of unintended and undetected pregnancy for sexually active adolescents. Another goal for PCOS treatment is to control the effects of hyperandrogenism, namely, hirsutism, alopecia, and acne, which can cause psychological distress for an affected adolescent. Some methods of treatment will prevent or ameliorate hyperandrogenism, while others diminish the end organ effects of hyperandrogenism. Because insulin resistance is associated with the excess ovarian androgen production in both lean and obese girls with PCOS, an important goal for treatment in PCOS is to address insulin resistance associated with the diagnosis both through lifestyle modifications and medication management [2].

Lifestyle Changes: Changes in nutrition and increase in physical activity aid in decreasing insulin resistance through decreased adipose tissue and improving cellular insulin sensitivity, especially with exercise. Often meeting with a nutritionist and/or exercise physiologist can aid in making realistic lifestyle changes as adolescents with PCOS may have struggled to lose weight or improve fitness in the past, and an in-depth assessment of their energy balance can provide specific goals for areas of change. Mediterranean diet may benefit insulin-resistant girls by decreasing insulin excursions.

Hormonal Therapy: The use of hormonal contraceptives can aid in both restoration of menstrual function and decrease of androgen effect. Most often therapy is provided as an estrogen-progesterone combination oral contraceptive. Such therapy should not be used in those with open epiphyses and significant potential remaining growth or in girls with a personal history of thromboembolic events or chronic disease predisposing to such events. Strong family histories of thromboembolic events necessitate hematologic evaluation before a girl is placed on estrogen-containing hormonal therapy.

Androgen Blockers: Many adolescents with hyperandrogenism employ topical treatments for the physical findings associated with hyperandrogenism. Such therapies include depilatory products, waxing or laser treatments for hirsutism, and topical or oral antibiotics or retinoids for acne. Other oral medications can be used to decrease the effects of hyperandrogenism. Spironolactone is an aldosterone antagonist, potassium-sparing diuretic with secondary antiandrogenic effects via peripheral androgen antagonism, and decreased testosterone biosynthesis [3]. It is contraindicated during pregnancy as a teratogen for male fetuses and should not be used in patients with hyperkalemia or renal insufficiency. Other antiandrogenic agents occasionally employed in adolescents with PCOS include finasteride, a 5 α-reductase inhibitor, and flutamide, a selective antagonist of the androgen receptor. The hepatotoxicity of flutamide and potential side effects of finasteride have made them less desirable as choices in adolescents. Topical eflornithine, which blocks ornithine transcarboxylase in the hair follicle, can prevent hair growth but requires twice daily administration without interruption and is generally not covered by insurance, with cost being prohibitive for most teens needing to use it over several areas of the body simultaneously and continuously.

Metformin: Metformin is an antihyperglycemic medication in the biguanide family for improving insulin sensitivity and has been used in management of PCOS in adult women. It improves insulin sensitivity by increasing peripheral glucose uptake and utilization along with decreasing hepatic glucose production and decreasing intestinal absorption of glucose to lower overall blood glucose levels. Although metformin has been associated with weight loss, it should not be given to patients for the purpose of weight loss itself since the associated weight loss is modest and primarily occurs with concurrent lifestyle modifications. It is not FDA approved for PCOS or weight loss in adolescents.

Clinical Pearls and Pitfalls

PCOS Pearls

1. PCOS diagnosis in adolescents should not be made until a girl is at least 2 years postmenarchal.
2. Before a diagnosis of PCOS can be made in a girl, adrenal or ovarian secreting tumors, congenital adrenal hyperplasia, hypothyroidism, pregnancy,

prolactinoma, Cushing syndrome, ovarian failure, and other causes of symptoms must be excluded.

3. The diagnosis of PCOS requires hyperandrogenism and oligo-anovulation or polycystic ovaries according to the Androgen Excess-PCOS Society criteria. The diagnosis of PCOS requires hyperandrogenism and oligo-anovulation according to the NIH criteria. The diagnosis of PCOS requires two of the three criteria of hyperandrogenism, oligo-anovulation, and/or polycystic ovaries according to the Rotterdam criteria.
4. Hyperandrogenism in PCOS can be clinical in the form of severe acne or hirsutism and/or biochemical in the form of mild elevations in free testosterone and/or total testosterone.
5. Oligo-ovulation may cause irregular, frequent, or heavy menses due to anovulatory bleeding.
6. Although not part of any diagnostic criteria, many girls with PCOS are insulin resistant, regardless of BMI. Acanthosis nigricans, hypertriglyceridemia, and decreased HDL may be signs of insulin resistance.
7. In selected patients, weight loss or improved fitness, through dietary modification and increased moderate physical activity, can improve menstrual regularity and hyperandrogenism.
8. Combined estrogen and progesterone therapy, usually in the form of an oral contraceptive pill, is a mainstay of menstrual regulation and amelioration of hyperandrogenism signs.
9. Spironolactone may be used to treat physical signs of hyperandrogenism by blocking the androgen receptor but will take 3–6 months to demonstrate full effect.
10. Decreasing insulin resistance through dietary change, fitness, and +/− medication may improve symptoms in PCOS.

Suggested Educational Reading, References, and Policies

- Rotterdam, NIH, and Androgen Excess-PCOS Society Task Force Guidelines [1, 4–7]
- Criteria for adolescent PCOS diagnosis [2, 8]

References

1. Revised 2003 consensus on diagnostic criteria and long-term health risks related to polycystic ovary syndrome. Fertil Steril. 2004;81:19–25.
2. Witchel SF, Oberfield S, Rosenfield RL, et al. The diagnosis of polycystic ovary syndrome during adolescence. Horm Res Paediatr. 2015.
3. Corvol P, Michaud A, Menard J, Freifeld M, Mahoudeau J. Antiandrogenic effect of spirolactones: mechanism of action. Endocrinology. 1975;97:52–8.

4. Azziz R, Carmina E, Dewailly D, et al. The Androgen Excess and PCOS Society criteria for the polycystic ovary syndrome: the complete task force report. Fertil Steril. 2009;91:456–88.
5. Carmina E, Oberfield SE, Lobo RA. The diagnosis of polycystic ovary syndrome in adolescents. Am J Obstet Gynecol. 2010;203:201.e1–5.
6. Fauser BC, Tarlatzis BC, Rebar RW, et al. Consensus on women's health aspects of polycystic ovary syndrome (PCOS): the Amsterdam ESHRE/ASRM-Sponsored 3rd PCOS Consensus Workshop Group. Fertil Steril. 2012;97:28–38.e25.
7. Zawadzki J, Dunaif A. Diagnostic criteria for polycystic ovary syndrome: towards a rational approach. In: Dunaif A, Givens JR, Haseltine FP, Merriam GR, editors. Polycystic ovary syndrome, vol. 4. Boston: Blackwell Scientific Publications; 1992. p. 377–84.
8. Witchel SF, Roumimper H, Oberfield S. Polycystic ovary syndrome in adolescents. Endocrinol Metab Clin N Am. 2016;45:329–44.

Chapter 7
Case of a Girl with Painful Periods, Pain with Bowel Movements, and Dyspareunia

Elizabeth Bonagura and S. Paige Hertweck

A 16-year-old girl presents to pediatric and adolescent gynecology office with chief complaint of persistent abdominal and pelvic pain. She reports that she has had cramping and sharp pain as long as she can remember and thinks it started with menarche at age 12. Her pain previously started a day or two prior to her menstrual cycle and lasted through the first 2–3 days of her menses, but now she endorses pain on a near daily basis. The pain is most severe however just before and during her menses, which last 5 days and occur every 28 to 30 days. The patient describes the flow as heavy, and she changes 4–5 pads per day but denies soaking through her pads at night. She also endorses intermittent constipation and pain with bowel movements but denies any pain with urination or increased frequency of urination. She denies nausea or vomiting and blood in her stool or urine. She is currently sexually active with a single partner for the last year and reports one lifetime partner. She has never been tested for sexually transmitted infections but does endorse pain with intercourse.

The patient's medical history is significant for childhood asthma, but she denies any prior surgeries, allergies, or use of tobacco, alcohol, or illicit substances. However, she reports missing multiple days of school throughout the year due to her pain and states she quit the soccer team because of pain and missed practices as well. She has never been pregnant, and her family history is significant for mother, maternal aunt, and maternal grandmother with history of endometriosis and diabetes in the same grandmother.

E. Bonagura, M.S., M.D. (✉)
Norton Children's Gynecology Specialists, Louisville, KY, USA
e-mail: ebonagura@gmail.com

S.P. Hertweck, M.D.
University of Louisville School of Medicine, Kosair Children's Hospital, Louisville, KY, USA
e-mail: Paige.Hertweck@nortonhealthcare.org

H.J. Talib (ed.), *Adolescent Gynecology*,
https://doi.org/10.1007/978-3-319-66978-6_7

She has tried use of ibuprofen to treat her pain and has seen four other doctors prior to this visit including two pediatricians, a gastroenterologist, and a general obstetrician-gynecologist who put her on an oral contraceptive pill over a year ago to help with her painful menses. She takes them as prescribed and reports they initially helped a little bit, but now she feels they are not helping at all.

A physical exam performed in the office reveals normal vital signs in a well-nourished female in no acute distress. She is easily conversing. Heart and lung exams are within normal limits although her abdominal exam is significant for mild tenderness diffusely to deep palpation but no masses, rebound, or guarding. She consents to both a speculum and bimanual exam and has no cervical motion tenderness and does have mild adnexal and uterine tenderness of a small, mobile, anteverted uterus but no adnexal masses. The vagina is patent, and there are no vulvar, vaginal, or cervical lesions identified. Her musculoskeletal and neurologic exams are within normal limits. An ultrasound is ordered which reveals a normal uterus measuring 6 cm × 3.5 cm × 2 cm, the endometrial stripe is 0.7 cm, and there are normal appearing bilateral ovaries with no evidence of mass. A sexually transmitted disease panel for gonorrhea, chlamydia, trichomonas, and mycoplasma is negative. After discussion with the patient and her family, a decision is made to proceed with diagnostic laparoscopy with possible resection of endometriosis and placement of levonorgestrel IUD.

The procedure is performed without complication, and intraoperative findings reveal several clear vesicular and red-flame-like lesions scattered along with posterior cul-de-sac and the bilateral uterosacral ligaments consistent with stage 1 endometriosis. Several contiguous lesions are resected, and the remainder is burned intraoperatively, and final pathology reveals endometrial stroma and glands confirming diagnosis of endometriosis. Postoperatively, the patient asked: "What is endometriosis?" and "What should I expect in the future, am I cured by surgery?"

Discussion

Dysmenorrhea, or pain with menses, is a very common complaint in adolescents. The pain associated with menses may be accompanied by nausea, vomiting, diarrhea, headaches, fatigue, dizziness, or, rarely, even syncope. Most of the time, dysmenorrhea is found to be primary in nature rather than secondary as a result of pelvic pathology. Some studies have shown that patients with primary dysmenorrhea have higher levels of prostaglandins (PGF2α and PGE2) than that found in women without dysmenorrhea. Exogenous administration of these compounds can, in fact, induce similar symptoms as those mentioned above [1]. Cyclooxygenase, which is critical to production of precursors of PGF2α and PGE2, is blocked by nonsteroidal anti-inflammatory drugs (NSAIDs), thus making the use of NSAIDs typically first-line therapy and very effective in treating primary dysmenorrhea. Combined hormonal therapies, such as oral contraceptive pills, are another commonly used treatment for dysmenorrhea. They are thought to work by ovulation suppression and induction of endometrial hypoplasia. When primary treatment with NSAIDs and/or hormonal suppression fails to treat painful periods, secondary causes need to be considered. Secondary dysmenorrhea is defined as pain with menses due to pelvic pathology, such as that seen in this case, where the patient was found to have endometriosis. In making a diagnosis of primary or secondary amenorrhea, history taking is critical. Assessment of acute or chronic nature of pain, quality, location, associated symptoms, medications (and dosages) tried, assessment of bowel function, sexual activity, family history, and past medical and surgical history can all be very revealing in reaching a diagnosis.

A complete physical exam is required to assess for potential etiologies of pelvic pain. Of particular concern would be the presence of an abdominal mass or an obstructive genital outflow tract anomaly that may be noted easily on an abdominal exam. Pelvic exams, however, can be challenging in young adolescents, especially those who are not sexually active. While an internal vaginal exam is felt not to be mandatory, some type of pelvic assessment is required to rule out obstructive anomalies and pelvic masses [2]. Visualization of the external genitalia with placement of a cotton swab into the vagina can assess for vaginal patency. A recto-abdominal exam and/or a pelvic ultrasound can be utilized to evaluate for anomalies and masses without a need for vaginal exam. However, in adolescents who are tampon users or are sexually active who complain of moderate to severe pain, both a speculum and bimanual exam should be strongly considered [1]. Evaluation urine and genital tract for infection with urinalysis, urine culture, screening for bacterial vaginosis, candida, gonorrhea, chlamydia, and other potentially suspected infections should be undertaken. If genital tract obstruction is suspected, MRI is the gold standard for evaluation.

Endometriosis, a commonly seen cause of secondary dysmenorrhea, is defined as presence of endometrial tissue outside of the uterus. Diagnosis of endometriosis is challenging with patients not infrequently seeing nine or more providers before being given a definitive diagnosis, and adolescents on average see four or more doctors before getting a diagnosis [2, 3]. This patient presents with nonspecific cyclic and acyclic pelvic pain, which has a broad differential. She is currently sexually active and endorses pain with intercourse as well as with her menses and also constipation. The initial differential in a patient like this should include both gynecologic and non-gynecologic etiologies of abdominal pain such as chronic pelvic inflammatory disease, constipation, pelvic floor dysfunction, musculoskeletal pain, irritable bowel syndrome, psychosocial complaints, or a mixture of these. There can be an overlap of causes of pain. It is not uncommon for patients to have both endometriosis and other disorders. One retrospective study of adolescents with musculoskeletal causes of pelvic pain revealed that 10% also had endometriosis [4].

If the patient's pain is acute, one should evaluate potentially life-threatening conditions such as ectopic pregnancy, bowel perforation, and appendicitis as well as adnexal torsion, genital tract obstruction, urinary tract infection, renal stones, mittelschmerz pain, and pelvic inflammatory disease.

A thorough history is thus critical to diagnosis given the large differential for pelvic pain. Adolescents with endometriosis commonly present with complaints of pelvic pain that may be cyclic, acyclic, or both. The most commonly documented complaint in this population is acquired or progressive dysmenorrhea (64–94%), and pain is usually described as cyclic and acyclic pain as seen in this case study. Sixty-one percent of patients with both cyclic and acyclic pain were found to have endometriosis compared to cyclic or acyclic pain alone. Patients will also present with complaints of acyclic pain (36–91%), dyspareunia (14–25%), and gastrointestinal complaints (2–46%) [3]. Another significant finding, associated with a diagnosis of endometriosis, is interference of pain with daily activities such as participation in physical and social activities and poor school attendance as seen in this patient. It is important to know that the typical presentation in adolescents is not necessarily the same as that in adults who often seek medical attention for pelvic masses and infertility as well as pain. Most adults diagnosed with endometriosis report symptoms since the teen years making early diagnosis important for treatment of symptoms, prevention of progression, and prevention of infertility.

A particularly key finding in this patient's history, which should raise suspicion for endometriosis, is chronic pelvic pain resistant to medical treatment with oral contraceptives or NSAIDs. It has been reported in studies done in the 1990s that up to 70% of these patients will be found to have visible endometriosis on diagnostic laparoscopy [5, 6]. This finding of high rates of endometriosis in those with chronic pelvic pain not responsive to treatment was confirmed in review by Janssen et al. done in 2013, with 62% of adolescents meeting this criteria having visually confirmed endometriosis [7]. An additional risk factor for endometriosis that this patient has is her extensive family history of the disease. She also experienced early menarche along with early-onset dysmenorrhea, which has been shown to be associated with a diagnosis of endometriosis as well. Obstructive-type Mullerian anomalies are also associated with increased rates of endometriosis, which is thought to be due to increased retrograde menstruation. The rate of association of obstructive anomalies with endometriosis has been quoted in the literature to range from 5% up to 40%. Surgical management of obstruction has been reported to result in spontaneous resolution of disease [8, 9].

In patients for whom conservative management of dysmenorrhea with medical treatment fails, laparoscopic evaluation should be strongly considered for definitive diagnosis and surgical treatment, as this is the gold standard. Goals of surgery should include diagnosis, staging, and excision or destruction of visible disease. It is very important to know that typical surgical findings in adolescents with endometriosis vary from that found in adults, with the classic powder burn and black lesions not often seen in the adolescent population. Adolescents more commonly have red, clear, or white lesions. Peritoneal defects or windows are also commonly found and are diagnostic of endometriosis. These findings, especially the clear vesicular lesions, can be harder to see and may require increased magnification of the laparoscope. Alternatively, filling the pelvis with irrigation fluid then submerging the laparoscope to view the lesions through the fluid medium can be very helpful. Attempt should be made to excise or destroy all visible lesions during surgery, and only fertility-sparing procedures should be offered.

Medical therapy with an oral contraceptive pill should be a first-line treatment for suspected endometriosis however before surgery. The goals of treatment should be suppression of pain, disease progression, and preservation of fertility [3]. Patients can be started on with treatment consisting of continuous oral contraceptives and NSAIDs. Good communication, emotional support, and education are additionally keys to treatment. There is also felt to be a role for complementary and alternative therapies in management of symptoms. If the patient is over the age of 18 years, a trial of GnRH agonist therapy can also be considered prior to surgery. GnRH agonist therapy should be done with add-back therapy to decrease side effects such as vasomotor symptoms, vaginal dryness, mood swings, and most importantly reductions in bone mineral density. Add-back therapy typically consists of 5 mg daily of norethindrone (Aygestin®) or 0.625 mg/2.5 mg of conjugated estrogen. These patients should also be counseled on importance of vitamin D and calcium supplementation for bone health. Progestin-only therapy (Depo-Provera, Aygestin) has also been used in management of endometriosis. In data in the adult population, it is suggested that progestin-only therapy is not particularly effective long term, but there is little data regarding this treatment method in adolescents [10]. Additionally, there is concern regarding bone mineral density loss with long-term use in this population that is still accruing maximum levels of bone mass. The levonorgestrel IUD has been used successfully in the adult population for symptom-related treatment of endometriosis, and a retrospective study by Yoost et al. in 2013 found a reduction in pain in young women with the LNG-IUD placed either at the time of diagnostic laparoscopy [11]. The lack of need for recurrent administration, often improved bleeding patterns, and proven safety in adolescents makes this a promising method for treatment.

There is no long-term published data on outcomes of surgical therapy in adolescents. It was initially suggested in earlier studies that adolescents primarily had stage 1–2 disease, but more recent studies have found as high as 50% of girls undergoing laparoscopy, having stage 3–4 disease [12]. While some of this change in rate of severity has been attributed to improved diagnostic techniques, it underscores the importance of early diagnosis and prevention of disease progression and infertility. Surgical therapy appears to be effective in improving symptoms of endometriosis. There are a few studies looking at symptom relief, progression of disease, and recurrence rates in the current literature, but the data is limited by small sample size, retrospective nature, and lack of controls. However, with surgery alone, up to 80% of patients appear to have symptom relief or improvement [8].

Regarding rate of recurrence, the data is again limited. One study by Yeung et al. found no evidence of recurrence or progression of disease in 8 of 17 girls who had a second-look laparoscopy despite only a third of the patients taking postoperative hormonal maintenance therapy thus asking the question of whether hormonal therapy postoperatively is critical to treatment [13]. Tandoi et al. found a much higher rate of recurrence with 56% recurrence over a 5-year follow-up period in 57 women under the age of 21 years [14]. However, this study did not require visual or histology to make the diagnosis of recurrence but rather relied on symptoms and ultrasound findings. The majority of studies involved use of postoperative hormonal

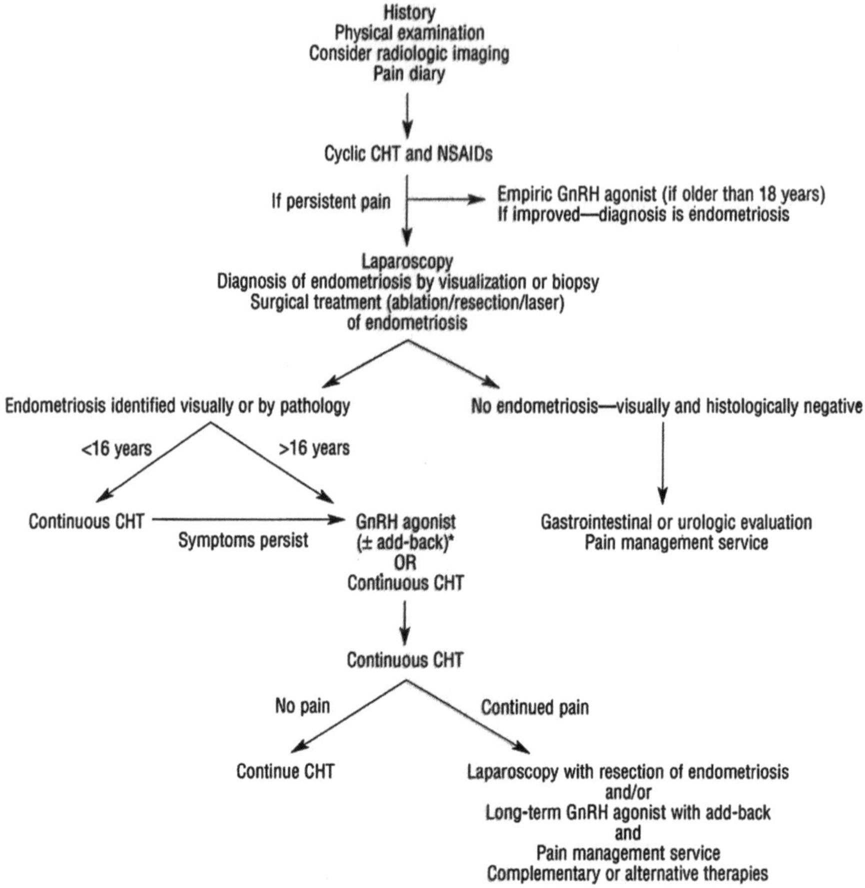

Fig. 7.1 Algorhythm for diagnosis and treatment of endometriosis. Abbreviations: *NSAIDs* non-steroidal anti-inflammatory drugs, *CHT* combination hormone therapy (oral contraceptive pills, estrogen/progestin patch, estrogen/progestin vaginal ring, norethindrone acetate, medroxyprogesterone acetate), *GnRH* gonadotropin-releasing hormone. *Add-back indicates use of estrogen and progestin or norethindrone acetate alone. ACOG Committee Opinion: No 310. Endometriosis in adolescents. Obstet Gynecol 2005;105:921 modified from Bandera CA, Brown LR, Laufer MR. Adolescents and endometriosis. Clin Consult Obstet Gyncol 1995;7:206; with permission

maintenance, and this remains commonplace. More research is needed to better assess long-term outcomes of surgery and medical management (Fig. 7.1).

In summary, endometriosis is a common cause of dysmenorrhea in adolescents and should be on the differential for any patient with chronic pelvic pain. Suspicion should be further heightened in those with pain unresponsive to conservative management with NSAIDs and oral contraceptive pills, which is the first-line therapy for this disease. Surgical diagnosis and treatment should be strongly considered in this population. More data is needed to better elucidate the cause of endometriosis and determine the best options for long-term, postsurgical symptom control and treatment.

Clinical Pearls and Pitfalls

- Acute pelvic pain has a different differential diagnosis than chronic pelvic pain and should elicit a workup to rule out potentially life-threatening or life-altering etiologies.
- Physicians should strongly consider diagnostic laparoscopy to rule out endometriosis in young women with dysmenorrhea refractory to COCPs.
- Endometriosis in adolescents does not have the typical powder burn characteristics seen in adults but are more commonly clear vesicular and red-flame-like lesions.
- Goals of surgery for endometriosis in adolescents should be diagnosis and destruction/removal of visible lesions with care to avoid any procedures that might harm future fertility.
- A multidisciplinary approach to treatment of adolescents with endometriosis may be needed with involvement of psychiatry, pain specialists, and complementary medicine to be considered.
- More research is needed to elucidate standard of care for postsurgical treatment of endometriosis, but most commonly patients are put on hormonal suppression of some type.

References

1. Emans SJ, Laufer MR. Emans, Laufer, Goldstein's pediatric & adolescent gynecology. Chapter 13, Gynecologic pain: dysmenorrhea, acute and chronic pelvic pain, endometriosis, and premenstrual syndrome. 6th ed. Philadelphia, PA: Lippincott Williams & Wilkins; 2012. p. 238–69.
2. Laufer MR. Current approaches to optimizing the treatment of endometriosis in adolescents. Gynecol Obstet. Invest. 2008;66:19–27.
3. ACOG Committee Opinion: No 310. Endometriosis in adolescents. Obstet Gynecol. 2005;105:921.
4. Schroeder B, Sanfillipo JS, Hertweck SP. Musculoskeletal pain in a pediatric and adolescent practice. J Pediatr Adolesc Gynecol. 2000;13:90.
5. Laufer MR. Identification of clear vesicular lesions of atypical endometriosis: a new technique. Fertil Steril. 1997;68:739–40.
6. Goldstein DP, De Cholnoky C, Emansi SJ. Adolescent endometriosis. J Adolesc Health Care. 1980;1:3741.
7. Janssen EB, Rijkers AC, Hoppenbrouwers K, Meuleman C, D'Hooghe TM. Prevalence of endometriosis diagnosed by laparoscopy in adolescent with dysmenorrhea or chronic pelvic pain: a systematic review. Hum Reprod. Update. 2013;19:570–82.
8. Brosens I, Gordts S, Benagiano G. Endometriosis in adolescents is a hidden, progressive and severe disease that deserves attention, not just compassion. Hum Reprod. 2013;28:2026–31.

9. Sanfillipo JS, Wakim NG, Schikler KN, Yussman MA. Endometriosis in association with uterine anomaly. Am J Obstet Gynecol. 1986;154:39–43.
10. Ballweg ML. Big picture of endometriosis helps provide guidance on approach to teens: comparative historical data show endo starting younger, is more severe. J Pediatr Adolesc Gynecol. 2003;16(Suppl 3):S21–6.
11. Yoost J, LaJoie SA, Hertweck P, Loveless M. Use of the levonorgestrel intrauterine system in adolescents with endometriosis. J Pediatr Adolesc Gynecol. 2013;26:120–4.
12. Davies GD, Thillet E, Lindeman J. Clinical characteristics of adolescent endometriosis. J Adolesc Health. 1993;14:362–8.
13. Yeung P Jr, Sinervo K, Winer W, Albee RB Jr. Complete laparoscopic excision of endometriosis in teenagers: is postoperative hormonal suppression necessary? Fertil Steril. 2011;95:1909–12.
14. Tandoi I, Somigliana E, Riparini J, Ronzoni S, Vigano' P, Candiani M. High rate of endometriosis recurrence in young women. J Pediatr Adolesc Gynecol. 2011;24:376–9.

Suggested Educational Reading

ACOG Committee Opinion: No 310. Endometriosis in adolescents. Obstet Gynecol 2005;105:921.

ACOG Committee Opinion: No 114. Management of Endometriosis July 2010. Reaffirmed 2016.

Emans SJ, Laufer MR. Emans, Laufer, Goldstein's pediatric & adolescent gynecology. Chapter 13, Gynecologic pain: dysmenorrhea, acute and chronic pelvic pain, endometriosis, and premenstrual syndrome. 6th ed. Philadelphia, PA: Lippincott Williams & Wilkins; 2012. p. 238–69.

Laufer MR, Goitein L, Bush M, Cramer DW, Emans SJ. Prevalence of endometriosis in adolescent girls with chronic pelvic pain not responding to conventional therapy. J Pediatr Adolesc Gynecol. 1997;110:199–202.

Chapter 8
Case of a Girl with Heavy, Prolonged Periods and Anemia

Risa L. Fridy and Susan M. Coupey

Shelby is an 11-year-3-month-old previously healthy African-American girl who was referred to an adolescent medicine specialist by her primary pediatrician for prolonged, heavy menstrual bleeding. She is accompanied by her mother. Shelby and her mother report that Shelby has had vaginal bleeding daily for the past 25 days. On some days, the bleeding is very heavy, and she passes large clots, often soiling her underwear, and on other days the bleeding is lighter. Today she is only spotting lightly. Shelby's first menstrual period was 9 months prior to this visit. She has had a total of six episodes of vaginal bleeding at irregular intervals ranging from 20 to 54 days between episodes and lasting for as long as 7 to the current 25 days. She has never experienced any abdominal or back pain with the bleeding, nor has she complained of nausea, vomiting, diarrhea, headaches, dizziness, syncope, weakness, or chest pain. She does complain of fatigue and has started taking naps after school. Shelby and her mother deny any other evidences of abnormal bleeding such as nosebleeds, gum bleeding while brushing her teeth, or unusual bruises, and there is no family history of bleeding disorders or autoimmune disease. When interviewed alone without her mother present, Shelby denies ever having sex; she says she "likes boys" but doesn't plan to have sex until she is married. She has never had a romantic relationship, engaged in kissing, or sexual touching. No one has ever touched her inappropriately or made her feel uncomfortable or unsafe.

On physical exam, Shelby is a slim girl in no distress, but she is noted to have mild pallor. Her weight is 90 lb (63rd percentile for age), her height is 60 in.

R.L. Fridy, M.D. (✉)
Mount Sinai Hospital, Icahn School of Medicine, New York, NY, USA
e-mail: rfridy@ayam-nyc.com

S.M. Coupey, M.D.
Professor of Pediatrics, Chief, Division of Adolescent Medicine,
Children's Hospital at Montefiore, The Pediatric Hospital for Albert Einstein
College of Medicine, Bronx, NY, USA
e-mail: scoupey@montefiore.org

H.J. Talib (ed.), *Adolescent Gynecology*,
https://doi.org/10.1007/978-3-319-66978-6_8

(83rd percentile for age), and her body mass index is 18 kg/m^2 (49th percentile for age). Her blood pressure is 97/60 mmHg, and her heart rate is 80 beats/min. Her head, eyes, ears, nose, throat, heart, lung, abdominal, and extremity exams are all within normal limits. She has no thyromegaly or lymphadenopathy on examination of her neck. Her breasts are Tanner stage 4 with no masses, tenderness, or nipple discharge. Her pubic hair is Tanner stage 4. On external genital exam, her vulva has well-estrogenized mucosa with no lesions; she has a normal clitoris and urethral meatus; scant blood is visible at the vaginal introitus. Her skin exam shows mild pustular acne on her forehead with no rash, petechiae, bruises, or hirsutism.

Laboratory testing reveals moderate microcytic anemia with a hemoglobin of 9.6 g/dL, a hematocrit of 31%, and a mean corpuscular volume of 76 fL. White blood cell count of 5.9 k/μL is normal as is the platelet count of 296 k/μL. Hormonal studies are all within normal limits including thyroid-stimulating hormone (TSH) of 2.12 μU/mL, free thyroxine (free T4) of 1.10 ng/dL, follicle-stimulating hormone (FSH) of 4.2 mIU/mL, luteinizing hormone (LH) of 6.48 mIU/mL, prolactin of 14 ng/mL, total testosterone of 28 ng/dL, free testosterone of 2.2 pg/mL, and dehydroepiandrosterone sulfate (DHEAS) of 210 μg/dL. A coagulopathy panel shows a normal prothrombin time (PT), international normalized ratio (INR), and partial thromboplastin time (PTT), and a von Willebrand disease panel is negative. Urine tests for pregnancy as well as nucleic acid amplification testing for gonorrhea and chlamydia are all negative.

Discussion

Menarche and the menstrual cycle are quintessential components of normal adolescent female development. Shelby's pubertal development is on the early side with menarche at age 10 years and 6 months; however, this timing is within the range of normal for girls in the twenty-first century. A national study of a representative sample of adolescents across the United States found the median age at menarche to be 12.43 years and that 10% of girls had attained menarche by 11.11 years [1]. There are notable variations in age at menarche among racial/ethnic groups. Black adolescents have the earliest median age at menarche of 12.06 years, and 10% of black adolescents have attained menarche by 10.52 years. The median age at menarche for Hispanic adolescents is 12.26 years, and for non-Hispanic white adolescents, it is 12.55 years [1].

In addition, Shelby has a young gynecologic age of 9 months (*gynecologic age* is defined as chronological age minus age at menarche) and is very early in her menstrual life, having had only 6 menstrual periods. Her cycles have been prolonged and have occurred at irregular intervals, outside the range of normal even at this early stage of pubertal development. Her excessive bleeding has led to moderate anemia with symptoms of fatigue that must be addressed before the anemia becomes severe with hemodynamic instability requiring hospitalization. Menstrual bleeding should be considered abnormal if it lasts beyond 7 days; the interval between

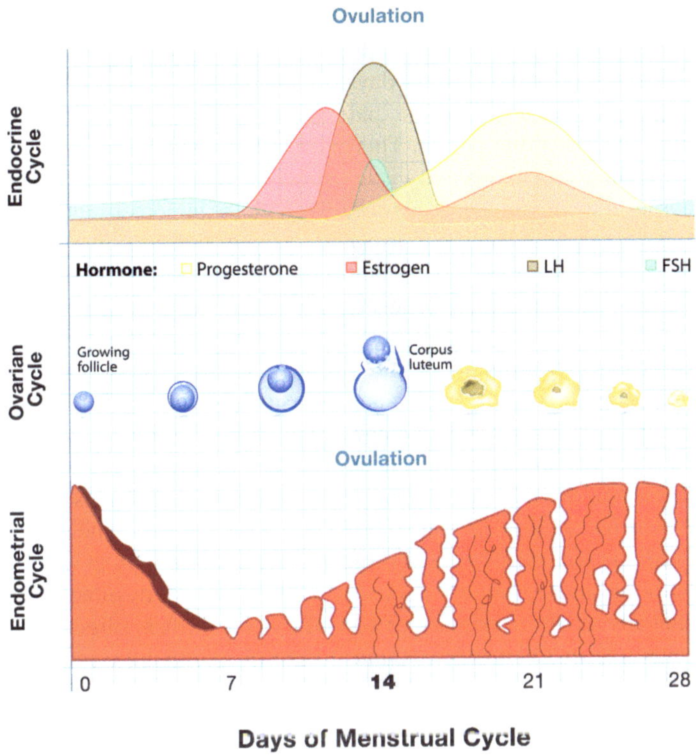

Fig. 8.1 Graphical representation of the menstrual cycle, including gonadotropin levels, steroid hormone levels, the ovarian cycle, and the endometrial cycle

periods is less than 21 or greater than 45 days and requires pad or tampon changes every 2–3 h (typical menstrual flow necessitates using three to six sanitary pads or tampons per day) [2, 3].

Shelby's menstrual symptoms and physical exam are consistent with abnormal uterine bleeding (AUB) due to ovulatory dysfunction, defined as irregular, painless bleeding of endometrial origin that is prolonged, unpatterned, and excessive [4]. The normal menstrual cycle is controlled by a complex interplay of hormonal signals between the hypothalamus, pituitary, and ovaries (the HPO axis), which is susceptible to stimuli from other hormones, behavioral and environmental factors, and other pathophysiological derangements such as polycystic ovary syndrome (PCOS). AUB can occur when the hormonal signaling of the HPO axis is disrupted leading to ovulatory dysfunction or when there is an anatomic, coagulopathic, infectious, or traumatic cause of uterine bleeding.

The normal menstrual cycle (Fig. 8.1 [5]) begins with the follicular phase, during which estrogen secreted by the maturing ovarian follicle stimulates proliferation of the endometrial lining of the uterus. This is followed by a mid-cycle surge of luteinizing hormone (LH), secreted by the pituitary in response to rising estrogen levels, which triggers ovulation. If fertilization does not occur, the follicle is transformed into a corpus luteum which secretes progesterone. This brings about the luteal phase, in which progesterone serves to differentiate and stabilize the endometrium. The corpus luteum involutes after 14 days, and levels of estrogen and progesterone decline resulting in shedding of the endometrial lining of the uterus in what is referred to as the menstrual period. This cyclical hormonal pattern and controlled menstrual bleeding depend on mid-cycle ovulation. Without ovulation and formation of a corpus luteum with progesterone secretion, the endometrium may proliferate in an unstable fashion leading to irregular, uncontrolled shedding and AUB.

In adolescent girls shortly after menarche, the HPO axis is physiologically immature, whereby rising estrogen levels do not positively feedback to trigger an LH surge; therefore, ovulation does not occur. Ovulatory dysfunction due to HPO axis immaturity is very common in girls for the first 2 years after menarche and is often associated with irregular cycles and occasionally with AUB [3, 4, 6]. Given that Shelby has a young gynecologic age of 9 months, it is likely that her AUB is related to physiologic immaturity of the HPO axis.

The differential diagnosis of AUB is broad, and while HPO axis immaturity is the likely cause for Shelby, other diagnoses must be considered. The most common endocrinopathy in women is polycystic ovary syndrome (PCOS), in which elevated levels of ovarian androgens are associated with ovulatory dysfunction and may present clinically as either primary or secondary amenorrhea, oligomenorrhea, or AUB. Women with PCOS may have clinical signs of androgen excess, such as acne and hirsutism, as well as obesity and insulin resistance [7]. Despite the name of the syndrome, adolescents with PCOS may or may not have polycystic ovaries, and this is not used as a criterion for diagnosis in this age group. Rarely, hyperandrogenemia may be related to late-onset adrenal hyperplasia or an androgen-secreting ovarian or adrenal tumor. While Shelby has mild facial acne, her normal body habitus, lack of hirsutism, and normal testosterone and DHEAS levels rule out PCOS or other hyperandrogenic etiologies of AUB. Other endocrinopathies which may cause AUB include thyroid dysfunction, diabetes mellitus, hyperprolactinemia, or elevated cortisol in Cushing's syndrome. Shelby has no past medical history, exam findings, or laboratory evidence to suggest any of these endocrinopathies as cause for her excessive bleeding. Additionally, the HPO axis may be suppressed due to medical illness, emotional stress, weight loss from illness or eating disorders, or overexercising resulting in ovulatory dysfunction. HPO axis suppression typically leads to oligomenorrhea or amenorrhea, but AUB can also occur. While rare in adolescents, primary ovarian insufficiency (e.g., as a result of ovarian toxicity from chemotherapeutic agents) may result in ovulatory dysfunction leading to oligomenorrhea, amenorrhea, or AUB. Given that Shelby is a healthy adolescent of normal weight and mental health, it is unlikely that she has HPO axis suppression or ovarian insufficiency.

Aside from physiologic or endocrine causes of ovulatory dysfunction, AUB may occur in patients with a congenital or acquired bleeding disorder [8, 9]. Von Willebrand disease is a common cause of AUB and should be considered when heavy, prolonged bleeding is present from menarche, especially when it is accompanied by symptoms such as gum bleeding, epistaxis, or abnormal bruising. Other bleeding disorders include coagulation factor deficiencies, fibrinogen disorders, and platelet deficiencies or dysfunction, such as idiopathic thrombocytopenic purpura, aplastic anemia, leukemia, or Glanzmann thrombasthenia. Chronic kidney disease can lead to platelet dysfunction and decreased fibrinogen levels, and liver failure leads to platelet and vitamin K-dependent factor dysfunction, and both conditions can be associated with AUB. Shelby's von Willebrand disease panel is negative, and she has a normal platelet count with no other signs or symptoms of abnormal bleeding; therefore, coagulation or platelet disorders are unlikely causes of her AUB.

Additional pathologic etiologies should be considered, especially in sexually active adolescents and when AUB is associated with lower abdominal pain. Sexually transmitted infections (STIs), especially acute or chronic endometritis with or without salpingitis, caused by pathogens including *N. gonorrhoeae* and *C. trachomatis*, are potential etiologies of AUB, and testing for these STIs should always be done. A miscarriage or ectopic pregnancy could also cause pain and heavy uterine bleeding, so a pregnancy test should always be performed in patients presenting with AUB. Shelby has never had sex, and her negative pregnancy, gonorrhea, and chlamydia tests point against these diagnoses.

Finally, anatomical or structural causes of AUB, while rare in adolescents, must be considered. An external genital exam should be performed on all patients presenting with excessive vaginal bleeding to ensure that the bleeding is coming from the vagina and there are no lesions on the vulva. A full speculum and bimanual pelvic exam should be performed on all sexually active adolescents with AUB. High vaginal lacerations, usually resulting from sexual intercourse, present with profuse sudden bleeding from the vagina and often require examination under anesthesia for diagnosis and suturing. The history of sudden painless bleeding immediately after intercourse is crucial for diagnosis of this lesion, but adolescents are often so frightened and embarrassed by the bleeding that they initially deny sexual activity; a sensitive and private interview with reassurance of confidentiality is essential. Uterine fibroids or polyps are potential causes of AUB, and while they are uncommon in adolescents, a pelvic ultrasound may be useful when evaluating for the etiology of excessive bleeding in unclear cases. In addition, hemangiomas, arteriovenous malformations, and tumors of the genital tract including rhabdomyosarcomas are rare causes of AUB in adolescents.

Shelby has a gynecologic age of less than 2 years, and she had a comprehensive laboratory evaluation, which revealed no pathologic etiology so she was diagnosed with AUB due to physiologic immaturity of the HPO axis. The primary goals of treatment of AUB are to stabilize the endometrium in order to prevent further uncontrolled bleeding, as well as to correct anemia and hemodynamic instability. A combined (estrogen/progestin) oral contraceptive (COC) pill is the treatment of choice to stabilize the endometrium and prevent further bleeding for many different etiologies of AUB in adolescent girls including HPO axis immaturity. Some adolescents have contraindications to estrogen [10], in which case oral progestins alone or an antifibrinolytic medication is a safe alternative.

Combined oral contraceptive (COC) pills are typically dispensed in a pack containing 21 active hormonal pills and 7 placebo pills (Fig. 8.2). During the placebo week of each 4-week cycle, the adolescent should experience a well-controlled,

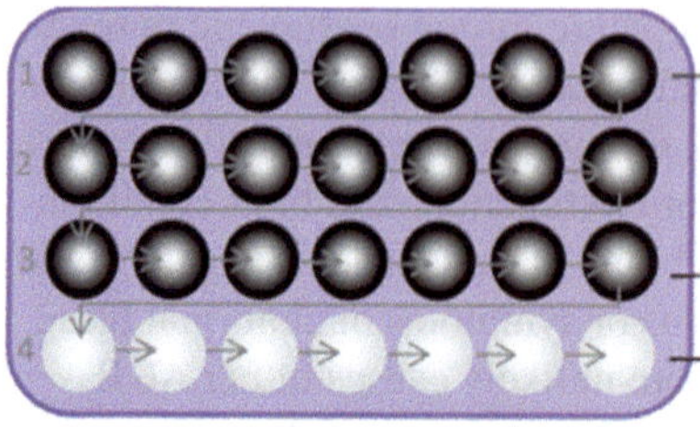

Fig. 8.2 Sample pack of combined oral contraceptive (COC) pills with instructions for how to administer for a 28-day cycle

typically light withdrawal bleed. We recommend that adolescent girls with anemia (Hb < 11 g/dL) take continuous active hormonal pills and discard placebo pills in order to prevent a withdrawal bleed until the anemia resolves. In addition, girls with anemia should take therapeutic doses of oral iron (e.g., ferrous gluconate 325 mg twice per day) accompanied by a stool softener to prevent iron-induced constipation. Once anemia is resolved, the adolescent may begin taking the placebo pills during the fourth week of every cycle allowing for monthly withdrawal bleeds. Therapeutic doses of iron should be discontinued once iron stores are replenished, generally 2–3 months after hemoglobin levels have returned to normal.

If an adolescent with AUB and moderate anemia (Hb 9–11 g/dL) is actively bleeding upon presentation, a COC taper, ranging from four to two pills per day, is an effective means of stopping the current bleed. Once bleeding has ceased, the COC pills should be continued at once daily dosing. Shelby has moderate anemia (Hb 9.6 g/dL) with fatigue, and she currently has light bleeding. An appropriate plan would be to administer a COC pill two times per day for 2 or 3 days to stop her current bleed, followed by once daily dosing, discarding the placebo pills to prevent further bleeding. She should also begin a therapeutic dose of oral iron with a stool softener.

Cases of severe anemia (Hb < 9 g/dL) due to AUB, especially when associated with hemodynamic instability or symptoms such as dizziness, lightheadedness, weakness, or syncope, might require inpatient management for intravenous hydration and, in some cases, blood transfusion. A COC taper is usually an effective means of stopping active bleeding in these patients. However, in cases of profuse bleeding, intravenous conjugated estrogens may be indicated to rapidly manage bleeding by constricting the spiral arteries in the endometrium, stimulating vasospasm of the uterine arteries, and promoting coagulation [4, 11]. Once bleeding has resolved and hemodynamic stability has been achieved, these patients may be managed as an outpatient with continuous COC pills, discarding placebos, and therapeutic doses of oral iron as described above.

All patients with AUB and anemia should be monitored closely in the outpatient setting. In Shelby's case of AUB caused by HPO axis immaturity, we would expect that her menstrual cycles would become ovulatory with regular monthly cycling by a gynecologic age of 2 years. Once her anemia is corrected, she has had several months of regular cycles on COC pills, and she is closer to a gynecologic age of

Table 8.1 Suggested free smartphone-based applications designed for tracking menstrual bleeding, as well as associated premenstrual and peri-menstrual symptoms

Application	Compatible smartphone operating system
Clue	*Free onAndroidandiOS*
Cycles	*Free oniOS*
Eve by Glow	*Free onAndroidandiOS*
iPeriod Tracker Free	*Free oniOS*
Life	*Free oniOS*
MonthPal	*Free onAndroidandiOS*
My Days	*Free onAndroidandiOS*
My Pill	*Free onAndroidandiOS*
Period Diary	*Free oniOS*
Period Log	*Free oniOS*
Period Tracker	*Free onAndroidandiOS*
Spot On	*Free onAndroidandiOS*

2 years, it is reasonable to discontinue the COC pills. AUB should not recur as long as she has no other pathologic causes of abnormal bleeding. Therefore, it will be useful for Shelby, once she discontinues the COC pills, to keep track of her menses very closely on a menstrual calendar. This may be recorded by hand or electronically on web-based or smartphone-based applications designed for tracking menstrual bleeding (Table 8.1). If her cycles do not normalize, further evaluation for alternate causes of AUB should be investigated with additional lab tests and imaging.

Clinical Pearls and Pitfalls

1. Physiologic HPO axis immaturity with ovulatory dysfunction is a common cause of irregular menses and AUB in adolescent girls with a gynecologic age less than 2 years. After 2 years, if menses remain irregular, alternative etiologies should be pursued.
2. Aside from HPO axis immaturity, alternative etiologies of irregular menses and AUB include ovulatory dysfunction due to PCOS, the most common endocrinopathy in women, as well as bleeding disorders, infections, pregnancy, or anatomic abnormalities.
3. In sexually active adolescent girls with AUB, pregnancy and infection must be considered, especially when AUB is accompanied by lower abdominal pain and a pregnancy test and tests for STIs should be done.
4. Combined oral contraceptive pills are first line for managing AUB with resultant anemia. In addition, therapeutic doses of oral iron with a stool softener should be provided to correct anemia.

References

1. Chumlea WC, Schubert CM, Roche AF, et al. Age at menarche and racial comparisons in US girls. Pediatrics. 2003;111:110–3.
2. American Academy of Pediatrics, American College of Obstetricians and Gynecologists. Menstruation in girls and adolescents: using the menstrual cycle as a vital sign. ACOG Committee Opinion No. 651. Obstet Gynecol. 2015b;126:e143–6.
3. World Health Organization multicenter study on menstrual and ovulatory patterns in adolescent girls. II. Longitudinal study of menstrual patterns in the early postmenarcheal period, duration of bleeding episodes and menstrual cycles. World Health Organization Task Force on Adolescent Reproductive Health. J Adolesc Health Care. 1986;7:236–44.
4. Talib HJ, Coupey SM. Excessive uterine bleeding. Adolesc Med. 2012b;23(1):53–72.
5. Hoffman BLSJ, Schaffer JI, Halvorson LM, Bradshaw KD, Cunningham F, Calver LE. Chapter 15: Reproductive endocrinology. In: Hoffman BL, Schorge JO, Schaffer JI, Halvorson LM, Bradshaw KD, Cunningham F, Calver LE, editors. Williams gynecology. 2nd ed. New York: McGraw-Hill; 2012.
6. Apter D, Viinikka L, Vihkho R. Hormonal patterns of adolescent menstrual cycles. J Clin Endocrinol Metab. 1978;47:944–54.
7. Azziz R, Woods KS, Reyna R, et al. The prevalence and features of the polycystic ovary syndrome in an unselected population. J Clin Endocrinol Metab. 2004;89:2745–9.
8. Bevan JA, Maloney KW, Hillery CA, et al. Bleeding disorders: a common cause of menorrhagia in adolescents. J Pediatr. 2001;138:856–61.
9. Kadir RA, Economides DL, Sabin CA, Owens D, Lee CA. Frequency of inherited bleeding disorders in women with menorrhagia. Lancet. 1998;351(9101):485–9.
10. Centers for Disease Control and Prevention. U.S. medical eligibility criteria for contraceptive use. MMWR. 2010;59(RR-4):1–86.
11. Bradley LD, Gueye NA. The medical management of abnormal uterine bleeding in reproductive-aged women. Am J Obstet Gynecol. 2016b;214(1):31–44.

Suggested Reading

American Academy of Pediatrics, American College of Obstetricians and Gynecologists. Menstruation in girls and adolescents: using the menstrual cycle as a vital sign. ACOG Committee Opinion No. 651. Obstet Gynecol. 2015;126:e143–6.

Bradley LD, Gueye NA. The medical management of abnormal uterine bleeding in reproductive-aged women. Am J Obstet Gynecol. 2016;214(1):31–44.

Talib HJ, Coupey SM. Excessive uterine bleeding. Adolesc Med. 2012;23(1):53–72.

Chapter 9
Case of a Girl with Irritability and Mood Swings with Her Periods

Alexandra C. Nevin Lam and Simone Vigod

Case

Anna is a 16-year-old female referred to you with a 1-year history of extreme irritability and mood swings around menses. She had menarche at age 13. She currently has regular monthly menses of normal flow with mild dysmenorrhea on day 1–2 of her period which is controlled with ibuprofen. Other catamenial symptoms include abdominal bloating, breast tenderness, and fatigue. She has mild asthma requiring Ventolin as needed. She has no known medication allergies and has never had surgery. Anna's maternal grandmother suffered from depression.

She denies smoking, alcohol, or recreational drug use. She lives at home with her parents and younger brother; she feels safe there. She is not bullied at school. She is a competitive figure skater, practicing on average 12 h per week. On private questioning, she discloses she has never been sexually active.

Physical examination is unremarkable. Anna becomes upset when she speaks about the impact of her irritability on her relationships. She feels hopeless.

Over the past year, Anna has missed 36 days from school, almost always in the week leading up to her menses, and there are concerns about her passing her exams. She has also missed 20 training sessions for figure skating, and she is worried she will not be ready for her upcoming competition.

Her mother has accompanied her to the visit. She is really concerned and also frustrated with her daughter's mood swings and truancy from school and skating for

A.C. Nevin Lam, M.D. (✉)
Department of Obstetrics and Gynecology, North York General, Toronto, ON, Canada
e-mail: alexandra.nevin@utoronto.ca

S. Vigod, M.D., M.Sc., F.R.C.P.C.
Psychiatry, Reproductive Life Stages Program, Women's Mental Health Program, Women's College Hospital, Toronto, ON, Canada
e-mail: simone.vigod@wchospital.ca

H.J. Talib (ed.), *Adolescent Gynecology*,
https://doi.org/10.1007/978-3-319-66978-6_9

Table 9.1 ACOG diagnostic criteria for PMS

Affective	*Somatic*
Depression	Breast tenderness
Angry outbursts	Abdominal bloating
Irritability	Headache
Anxiety	Swelling of extremities
Confusion	
Social withdrawal	
Timing: at least one of the above symptoms experienced:	
• Prior to menses in each of three prior menstrual cycles	
• Relieved by day 4 of the following cycle	
• No recurrence until at least day 13 (periovulation)	
Symptoms identified prospectively for two cycles	
Identifiable dysfunction in social or economic performance	

Adapted from Premenstrual Syndrome. *ACOG Practice Bulletin* 2000; 15: 1–19
ACOG American College of Obstetricians and Gynecologists [36]

"regular period stuff." As expected, she has lots of questions: "is my daughter depressed?" and "is treatment safe?"

Discussion

Up to 80% of reproductive-aged women with ovulatory cycles report at least one recurring premenstrual physical, affective, cognitive, or behavioral symptom [1]. When these symptoms begin to impact on quality of life and result in functional impairment, then they fall into a class of disorders known as premenstrual disorders (PMDs). PMDs result in a spectrum of impairment, from premenstrual syndrome (PMS) at one end to premenstrual dysphoric disorder (PMDD) at the more extreme end (Tables 9.1 and 9.2). The cardinal feature for both PMS and PMDD is that symptoms occur during the luteal phase of the menstrual cycle, extending potentially from the periovulatory period until the early follicular phase of the next cycle. PMS is defined as a syndrome by the American College of Obstetricians and Gynecologists (ACOG), but it is the extent of symptoms and the marked functional impairment associated with PMDD that differentiates it as a depressive disorder as outlined in the Diagnostic and Statistical Manual of Mental Disorders, Fifth Edition (DSM-5).

Retrospective data document a 20–30% prevalence for PMS, and a 5–8% prevalence for PMDD [2–5], although prospectively collected symptom reporting suggests a much lower prevalence of PMDD [6]. Less robust adolescent studies have documented similar, if not higher, prevalence rates of PMD with one study reporting over 60% of adolescents confirming symptoms consistent with the diagnosis of PMS [7]. The most commonly reported premenstrual symptoms for adolescents are psychological in nature with more than 85% reporting stress and anxiety [7]. Physical symptoms, including fatigue, abdominal bloating, breast tenderness, and

Table 9.2 Diagnostic and statistical manual for mental disorder (fifth edition) criteria for premenstrual dysphoric disorder [17]

The symptoms in criteria A–C must have been met for most menstrual cycles occurring in the preceding year.
A. In the majority of menstrual cycles, at least five symptoms must be present in the final week before the onset of menses, start or improve within a few days after the onset of menses, and become minimal or absent in the week post-menses
B. One or more of the following symptoms must be present:
(a) Marked affective lability (e.g., mood swings)
(b) Marked irritability of anger or increased interpersonal conflicts
(c) Marked depressed mood, feelings of hopelessness, or self-deprecating thoughts
(d) Marked anxiety, tension, and/or feelings of being keyed up or on edge
C. One or more of the following symptoms must additionally be present, to reach a total of five symptoms when combined with symptoms from "B" above:
(a) Decreased interest in usual activities
(b) Difficulty concentrating (subjective)
(c) Marked lack of energy, lethargy, or easy fatigability
(d) Marked change in appetite, overeating, or specific food cravings
(e) Insomnia or hypersomnia
(f) Feeling overwhelmed or out of control
(g) Physical symptoms such as breast tenderness or swelling, joint or muscle pain, a "bloating" sensation, or weight gain
D. Symptoms associated with clinically significant distress or interference with work, school, usual social activities, or interpersonal relationships.
E. Disturbance not merely an exacerbation of the symptoms of another disorder, such as major depressive disorder, panic disorder, or another disorder (although it may co-occur with these disorders)
F. Criterion A should be confirmed by prospective daily ratings in at least two symptomatic cycles (Note: Can make diagnosis provisionally until this is confirmed)
G. Symptoms are not attributable to the physiological effects of a substance or medication or to another medical condition.

dysmenorrhea, are also frequently described by adolescents, with two-thirds reporting abdominal bloating and pain in one study [7]. These symptoms result in a substantial negative functional impact on quality of life in teens, with 88% reporting their symptoms to be of at least moderate severity in one study [8] and another cross-sectional study identifying one in nine female high school students missing more than 1 day of school per month due to premenstrual symptoms [9].

The strongest risk factors for severe PMD such as PMDD include personal and/or family history of depression, suggesting a biological susceptibility to this illness [6]. The leading theory on the etiology of PMDD is that some women appear to have a biological vulnerability to the hormonal fluctuations associated with the menstrual cycle [10]. Specifically, they appear to have differential brain sensitivity to allopregnanolone, a metabolite of progesterone that acts in the central nervous system on GABA receptors implicated in mood disorders [11]. Neuroimaging studies also show evidence of differential brain serotonergic function in response to hormonal fluctuations [12]. It may be that serotonin reuptake inhibitors rapidly ameliorate symptoms of PMDD in some women because they allow for an acute repletion of serotonin in the brain. Hormone fluctuations may also impact other systems implicated in mood disorder etiology such as the hypothalamic-pituitary axis, brain-derived neurotrophic factor (BDNF), and immune function [10].

Two other strong clinical correlates of PMDD symptoms are early childhood sexual abuse [6] and daily life stress. This has led some to suggest that environmental experiences may influence the way that the brain responds to physiologic stimuli, increasing risk for a PMDD phenotype [13]. Early childhood trauma is associated with persistent neurophysiological changes that affect the ability to regulate emotional responses to various internal and external stimuli across the lifespan [14]. It could be that factors such as early childhood trauma sensitize the brain in a manner that makes it more difficult for some women to cope with the biological changes occurring over the menstrual cycle. Females with PMDD appear to more often rely on specific psychological mechanisms for coping with stress such as avoidance or wishful thinking, which are likely to be less effective than problem-focused action strategies such as stress management, lifestyle modification, and behavioral psychological techniques such as relaxation that are known to be effective in managing psychological symptoms associated with the menstrual cycle [15].

The diagnosis of both PMS and PMDD requires prospective evaluation of symptoms for at least two menstrual cycles since there is strong evidence that retrospective reporting of symptoms does not correlate with prospective evaluation in as many as half of women who report PMD symptoms [16]. The premenstrual symptoms screening tool for adolescents (PSST-A), validated for use in adolescents, has been developed to help differentiate adolescents who warrant prospective evaluation, education, and possibly early initiation of treatment in severe cases [3]. PMDs are diagnoses of exclusion. It is important to ensure that the symptoms are not better conceptualized as an exacerbation of another psychiatric disorder such as depression or anxiety that requires a different approach to treatment and that the symptoms are not attributable to the physiological effects of a medication or drug of abuse, nor related to a medical condition requiring treatment such as hypothyroidism or an autoimmune condition [17].

Education plays a central role in the management of PMDs in adolescents. All adolescents, regardless of the severity of their symptoms, should be educated about PMD. This includes education about the menstrual cycle, PMS and PMDD symptoms and their potential impact on functioning, as well as the treatment options. Treatment preferences and potential barriers to treatment should be elucidated. One study showed a sustained reduction in PMS scores 3 months after an educational program involving secondary school students versus uneducated controls [18].

The approach to PMD treatment depends on the severity of symptoms and impact on function, with the least invasive management strategies attempted first [19]. Identified medical and psychiatric comorbidities should be treated and treatment preferences explored. Continued symptom tracking is helpful for assessing treatment response. Symptom trackers available electronically and on mobile devices may provide a more convenient means of symptom tracking for this population over conventional trackers, including the Daily Record of Severity of Problems (DRSP) [20].

While few PMD management strategies have been specifically evaluated in adolescents, with the exception of antidepressant medication use (see below), strategies evaluated in adults are usually applied.

For those with PMS or mild symptoms of PMDD, lifestyle modifications and self-care may be sufficient. Lifestyle modification includes a healthy diet and regular exercise, as well as self-care that includes good sleep hygiene and scheduling stressful activities outside of the premenstrual time period whenever possible. Experts recommend that diet includes adequate intake of fruits, vegetables, whole grains, and water, with reduction (or elimination) of sugar, salty foods, caffeine, red meat, and alcohol. Small, frequent meals high in carbohydrates may help with symptom reduction around the time of menstruation. There is some evidence for non-athlete adolescent girls that regular exercise can improve psychological and physical symptoms of PMS [21], although this has not been investigated among a group with diagnosed PMDD. Other non-pharmacological strategies with some RCT evidence for efficacy in PMS include calcium 600 mg twice daily and chasteberry, or *Vitex agnus-castus* [22]. Some evidence suggests that vitamin B6 (pyridoxine) supplementation (80 mg) reduces PMD symptoms, but this has not been studied in women with diagnosed PMDD. Supplementation with vitamins and other herbal treatments is not necessarily benign; for example, vitamin B6 supplementation has been associated with peripheral neuropathy at higher dosages.

For those with symptoms meeting diagnostic criteria for PMDD, cognitive behavior therapy (CBT) is the most studied psychological treatment. CBT helps to address dysfunctional thinking patterns and enhance coping strategies and is delivered one on one or in groups by a trained therapist. Its effect size on psychological symptoms appears to be only in the small to medium range, but it may appear to have sustained effects over a longer term than medication treatment [23]. There has been increasing interest in behavioral techniques to reduce stress, with some evidence that relaxation therapy and mindfulness-based stress reduction (MBSR) may be helpful for psychological symptoms of PMDs; this requires confirmation in larger RCTs [24, 25].

For women who do not respond to non-pharmacological strategies, or who have more severe symptoms that need to be addressed more quickly, medication treatment may be required. Antidepressant medications such as selective serotonin reuptake inhibitors (SSRIs) and serotonin-norepinephrine reuptake inhibitors (SNRIs) are the mainstay of PMDD treatment in adult women—and in adult women SSRIs are recommended as first-line pharmacological therapy. There is evidence of a moderate to large effect size for daily dosing—with improvements seen within 2–3 menstrual cycles [26, 27]. Some studies also support the effect of luteal phase dosing (where antidepressants are taken in the luteal phase only) or "symptom onset" dosing (where antidepressants are taken with symptom onset and discontinued with menstruation) [28]. Women do not appear to have onset or withdrawal symptoms in intermittent dosing, although PMDD symptoms recur upon discontinuation. The use of antidepressant medication is, however, controversial in adolescents due to a lack of efficacy demonstrated in this population for major depressive disorder and due to an increased risk of side effects that can include increased rates of agitation and suicidal behavior [29]. In a recent large meta-analysis, only the SSRI fluoxetine was more effective than placebo for major depression in adolescents, with evidence of reasonable tolerability. Antidepressants have not been evaluated specifically for the treatment of PMDD in adolescents so they should only be used with extreme caution and likely in situations where symptoms are severe and where other treatments, including hormonal treatments, have been ineffective. If an antidepressant is used, fluoxetine is probably the most defendable choice [30, 31].

The most commonly used alternate pharmacologic treatment for PMD, the combined oral contraceptive pill (COCP), targets the biological vulnerability of affected individuals to periovulatory fluctuations in sex steroids by capitalizing on its ability to maintain a stable hormonal milieu. Two large multicenter, double-blind randomized controlled trials have shown that the 24/4 drospirenone/20 μg ethinyl estradiol (EE) pill combination is significantly effective in treating the mood, physical, and behavioral symptoms of PMDD versus controls [32, 33]. In addition, Pearlstein et al. [33] found a twofold improvement in overall quality of life scores as measured using a validated questionnaire in treated versus placebo controls. Based on the results of these studies, the 24/4 drospirenone/20 μg EE pill is the only US Food and Drug Administration (FDA)-approved COCP for the treatment of PMDD. This specific COCP is theorized to be the most effective due to (1) its novel progestin drospirenone with antimineralocorticoid properties and a longer half-life than conventional androgen-derived progestins and (2) its provision of constant gonadotropin suppression leading to arrest of follicular growth and endogenous estradiol production due to its shortened hormone-free interval (HFI) and its low estrogen content. Extended or continuous use of drospirenone-containing COCPs provides an additional strategy for managing symptoms of premenstrual disorders. The benefit of constant ovulation suppression provided by these regimens was confirmed in one study which showed a significant reduction in such symptoms with extended versus standard cyclic use of the same drospirenone-containing COCP [34]. Although none of the studies discussed above involved adolescents, general expert consensus supports the use of drospirenone-containing COCPs as first-line pharmacologic treatment in the adolescent patient with refractory PMS or PMDD. Of note, in recent years, there has been some concern surrounding the use of drospirenone-containing COCPs and increased venous thromboembolism (VTE) risk. This has been addressed in clinical practice guidelines wherein it has been concluded that their VTE risk is no higher than other COCPs on the market. All COCP use carries an increased risk of 9–10 VTEs/10000 woman years of use versus 4–5 VTEs/10000 woman years of use in women who do not use hormonal contraception [35]. COCPs also have many other benefits including excellent contraceptive efficacy, dysmenorrhea control, and androgenic symptom management that make this a desirable treatment option for PMDs in this population when education, lifestyle and self-care modifications, and non-pharmacologic and psychological treatments are insufficient. Other hormonal treatment options shown to be effective in adults, such as medically (with a gonadotropin-releasing hormone agonist) or surgically induced menopause, would not be considered in adolescents due to their adverse bone and cardiovascular health impact (Fig. 9.1).

Clinical Pearls and Pitfalls

- Premenstrual disorders, including PMS and PMDD, are common, biologically based conditions which cause true physical, behavioral, and psychological impairment to affected individuals.
- Prospective evaluation over 2 months is required for the diagnosis; however, a presumptive diagnosis is possible following administration of the PSST-A.
- Education about the menstrual cycle and perimenstrual symptomatology is key in the adolescent population and may even help improve symptoms.
- Lifestyle optimization including incorporation of adequate aerobic exercise, diet modifications focusing on carbohydrate and calcium intake, and adequate sleep hygiene is a key feature in managing PMDs at baseline.
- Psychotherapy, including CBT, and relaxation techniques should also be considered for those with the diagnosis of a PMD to improve coping strategies. This treatment carries the potential for long-term improvement regarding the psychological impact of this diagnosis.
- First-line pharmacotherapy in adolescents for PMD involves initiation of the 24/4 drospirenone/20 μg EE COCP. Continuous or extended use can be considered.
- A multidisciplinary approach should be employed for refractory cases of PMD when a SSRI is considered due to concerns about using SSRIs in the adolescent population.
- Ongoing tracking of symptoms and regular follow-up allow for appropriate increase in the intensity of interventions prescribed should current management be suboptimal. This symptom-based stepwise management is paramount to minimizing the functional impact of this disorder while also minimizing unnecessary risk and side effects.

Return to Our Case

You have Anna fill out the PSST-A, and based on her responses, including the amount of missed school and other activities, it becomes apparent that she meets criteria for a provisional diagnosis of PMDD (to be confirmed with future prospective charting). You educate Anna and her mother about the symptoms of PMDD, and you explain that many girls experience these symptoms and that the leading theory is that they may be sensitive to the hormonal fluctuations occurring perimenstrually. They are relieved to hear this, and they go away with information about lifestyle changes and self-care. You also give them the name of a psychologist to initiate stress management strategies and CBT if needed. When Anna returns in follow-up about 2 months later, her daily tracking shows that she is clearly experiencing symptoms, and while the lifestyle changes were helpful and she feels that she has made gains in her ability to cope, she continues to have functional impact from her symptoms. The drospirenone/20 μg EE COCP is initiated with instructions to use this in

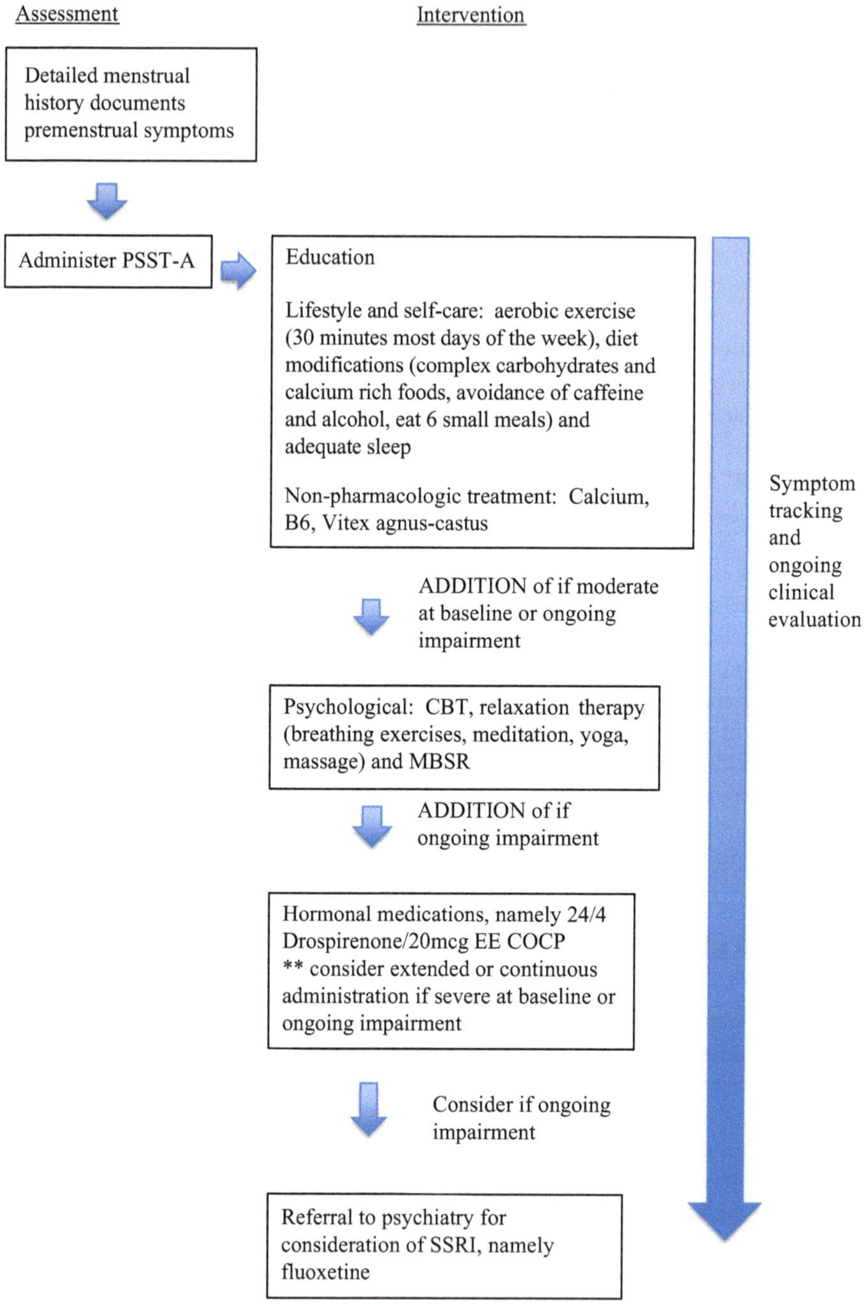

Fig. 9.1 Summarizes the above with a stepwise approach to management based on symptom severity and level of impairment

a continuous fashion, omitting the four placebo pills. Further follow-up in 3 months is made with the understanding that a referral to a psychiatrist will be initiated if ongoing symptom evaluation suggests inadequate treatment.

References

1. Yonkers KA, O'Brien PM, Eriksson E. Premenstrual syndrome. Lancet. 2008; 371(9619):1200–10.
2. Rapkin AJ, Mikacich JA. Premenstrual syndrome and premenstrual dysphoric disorder in adolescents. Curr Opin Obstet Gynecol. 2008;20:455–63.
3. Steiner M, Peer M, Pavlova E, et al. The premenstrual symptoms screening tool revised for adolescents (PSST-A): prevalence of severe PMS and premenstrual dysphoric disorder in adolescents. Arch Womens Ment Health. 2011;14:77–81.
4. Vichnin M, Freeman EW, Lin H, Hillman J, Bui S. Premenstrual syndrome (PMS) in adolescents: severity and impairment. J Pediatr Adolesc Gynecol. 2006;19:397.
5. Allen LM, Nevin Lam AC. Premenstrual syndrome and dysmenorrhea in adolescents. Adolesc Med State Art Rev. 2012;23(1):139–63.
6. Vigod SN, Frey BN, Soares CN, Steiner M. Approach to premenstrual dysphoria for the mental health practitioner. Psychiatr Clin North Am. 2010;33(2):257–72.
7. Derman O, Kanbur NO, Tokur TE, Jutluk T. Premenstrual syndrome and associated symptoms in adolescent girls. Eur J Obstet Gynecol. 2004;116:201–6.
8. Clecker-Smith CS, Doughty AS, Grossman JA. Premenstrual symptoms. Prevalence and severity in an adolescent sample. J Adolesc Health. 1998;22:403–8.
9. Tadakawa M, Takeda T, Monma Y, Koga S, Yaegashi N. The prevalence and risk factors of school absenteeism due to premenstrual disorders in Japanese high school students—a school-based cross-sectional study. BioPsychoSocial Medicine. 2016;10:13–9.
10. Hantsoo L, Epperson CN. Premenstrual dysphoric disorder: epidemiology and Treatment. Curr Psychiatry Rep. 2015;17(11):87.
11. Timby E, Backstrom T, Nyberg S, Stenlund H, Wihlback AC, Bixo M. Women with premenstrual dysphoric disorder have altered sensitivity to allopregnanolone over the menstrual cycle compared to controls—a pilot study. Psychopharmacology (Berl). 2016;233(1):2109–17.
12. Comasco E, Sundstrom-Poromaa I. Neuroimaging the menstrual cyle and premenstrual dysphoric disorder. Curr Psychiatry Rep. 2015;17(10):77.
13. Eisenlohr-Moul TA, Rubinow DR, Schiller CE, Johnson JL, Leserman J, Girdler SS. Histories of abuse predict stronger within-person covariation of ovarian steroids and mood symptoms in women with menstrually related mood disorder. Psychoneuroendocrinology. 2016;67:142–52.
14. Kendler KS, Gardner CO, Prescott CA. Toward a comprehensive developmental mode for major depression in women. Am J Psychiatry. 2002;159(7):1133–45.
15. Peterson N, London ED, Liang L, Ghahremani DG, Gerards R, Goldman L, Rapkin AJ. Emotion regulation in women with premenstrual dysphoric disorder. Arch Womens Ment Health. 2016;19(5):891–8.
16. Halbreich U. The diagnosis of premenstrual syndromes and premenstrual dysphoric disorder—clinical procedures and research perspectives. Gynecol Endocrinol. 2004;19:320–34.
17. American Psychiatric Association. Diagnostic and statistical manual of mental disorders. 5th ed. Washington, DC: Author; 2013.
18. Chau JP, Chang AM. Effects of an educational programme on adolescents with premenstrual syndrome. Health Educ Res. 1999;14:817–30.
19. Nevatte T, O'Brien PM, Backstrom T, et al. ISPMD consensus on the management of premenstrual disorders. Arch Womens Ment Health. 2013;16:279–91.
20. Endicott J, Nee J, Harrison W. Daily Record of Severity of Problems (DRSP): reliability and validity. Arch Womens Ment Health. 2006;9:41.

21. Samadi Z, Taghian F, Valiani M. The effects of 8 weeks of regular aerobic exercise on the symptoms of premenstrual syndrome in non-athlete girls. Iran J Nurs Midwifery Res. 2013;18(1):14–9.
22. Dante G, Facchinetti F. Herbal treatments for alleviating premenstrual symptoms: a systematic review. J Psychosom Obstet Gynaecol. 2011;32(1):42–51.
23. Kleinstauber M, Witthoft M, Hiller W. Cognitive-behavioral and pharmacological interventions for premenstrual syndrome or premenstrual dysphoric disorder: a meta-analysis. J Clin Psychol Med Settings. 2012;19(3):308–19.
24. Jasuja V, Purohit G, Mendpara S, Palan BM. Evaluation of psychological symptoms in premenstrual syndrome using PMR technique. J Clin Diagn Res. 2014;8(4):BC01–3.
25. Bluth K, Gaylord S, Nguyen K, Bunevicius A, Girdler S. Mindfulness-based stress reduction as a promising intervention for amelioration of premenstrual dysphoric disorder symptoms. Mindfulness (NY). 2015;6(6):1292–302.
26. Brown J, O'Brien PM, Marjoribanks J, Wyatt K. Selective serotonin reuptake inhibitors for premenstrual syndrome. Cochrane Database Syst Rev. 2009;(6):CD001396.
27. Shah NR, Jones JB, Aperi J, Shemtov R, Karne A, Borenstein J. Selective serotonin reuptake inhibitors for premenstrual syndrome and premenstrual dysphoric disorder: a meta-analysis. Obstet Gynecol. 2008;111:1175–82.
28. Yonkers KA, Kornstein SG, Gueorguieva R, Merry B, Van Steenburgh K, Alternus M. Symptom-onset dosing of sertraline for the treatment of premenstrual dysphoric disorder. JAMA Psychiat. 2015;72(10):1037–44.
29. Cipriani A, Zhou X, Del Giovane C, et al. Comparative efficacy and tolerability of antidepressants for major depressive disorder in children and adolescents: a network meta-analysis. Lancet. 2016;388(10047):881–90.
30. Silber TJ, Valadez-Meltzer A. Premenstrual dysphoric disorder in adolescents: case reports of treatment with fluoxetine and review of the literature. J Adolesc Health. 2005;37(6):518–25.
31. Nur MM, Romano ME, Siqueira LM. Premenstrual dysphoric disorder in an adolescent female. J Pedatr Adolesc Gynecol. 2007;20(3):201–4.
32. Yonker KA, Brown C, Pearlstein TB, Foegh M, Sampson-Landers C, Rapkin A. Efficacy of a new low-dose oral contraceptive with drospirenone in premenstrual dysphoric disorder. Obstet Gynecol. 2005;106:492–501.
33. Pearlstein TB, Bachmann GA, Zacur HA, Yonkers HA. Treatment of premenstrual dysphoric disorder with a new drospirenone-containing oral contraceptive formulation. Contraception. 2005;72:414–21.
34. Coffee AL, Kuehl TJ, Willis S, Sulak PJ. Oral contraceptives and premenstrual symptoms: comparison of a 21/7 and extended regimen. Am J Obstet Gynecol. 2006;195:1311–9.
35. Reid R, Leyland N, Wolfman W, et al. SOGC clinical practice guidelines: oral contraceptives and the risk of venous thromboembolism: an update: no 252. Int J Gynaecol Obstet. 2010;112:252–6.
36. ACOG American College of Obstetricians and Gynecologist. ACOG practice bulletin: premenstrual syndrome. Obstet Gynecol. 2000;15:1–19.

Suggested Reading

ACOG Practice Bulletin 2000;15:1–19.
Arch Womens Ment Health 2011;14(1):77–81 (PSST-A).
Life (period and symptom tracker available at the App Store by Lovetap LLC) www.aafp.org/afp/2011/1015/afp20111015p918_fig1.pdf (DRSP sheet)
Useful resources for adolescents: https://womensmentalhealth.org/resource/patient-support-services/teen-pms-and-pmdd-guide/ http://youngwomenshealth.org/2013/10/31/pms/

Chapter 10
Case of a Girl with Secondary Amenorrhea and an Eating Disorder

Nancy A. Dodson

Case

Holly is a 13-year-old female who presents with a chief complaint of "I'm not getting my period anymore." She is accompanied by her mother. Holly reports menarche just after her 11th birthday. At first, her periods came every 6–8 weeks. By age 12, she had monthly periods that were 4–5 days long. Some months she would have cramps at the start of menses; these cramps responded well to Motrin and tea. Other months, she would not have any cramps. In the past year, she has started having longer time periods in between menses. She had a menstrual cycle around 8 months ago and then 2 months after that. For the past 6 months, she has not had any period at all.

She reports a normal energy level. She denies any headaches or vision changes. She has no breast discharge or breast tenderness. She denies heat or cold intolerance although her mother notes that she has been wearing more layers even in the very warm weather. She reports constipation. She denies tremors or night sweats. She does not think she is hirsute, and she does not suffer from acne. She is interested in boys but has never had a boyfriend, and she has never had sexual intercourse.

The pediatrician has provided growth charts, which are shown in Fig. 10.1. Her height has tracked along the 90th percentile for her childhood and adolescence and is now between the 75th and 90th percentile. Her weight has tracked along the 75th percentile until around age 12 years; she is now between the 25th and 50th percentile for weight. Her BMI fluctuated between the 50th and 75th percentile but is now at the 16th percentile. In total, she has lost 3 kg from age 12 to age 13. The pediatrician did basic lab work which showed a low white blood cell count of 4.0, a normal Hgb and Hct of 13.6 and 39, and a normal platelet count of 357,000. Her liver

N.A. Dodson, M.D., M.P.H. (✉)
Division of Adolescent Medicine, Department of Pediatrics, Children's Hospital at Montefiore, Bronx, NY, USA
e-mail: ndodson@montefiore.org

H.J. Talib (ed.), *Adolescent Gynecology*,
https://doi.org/10.1007/978-3-319-66978-6_10

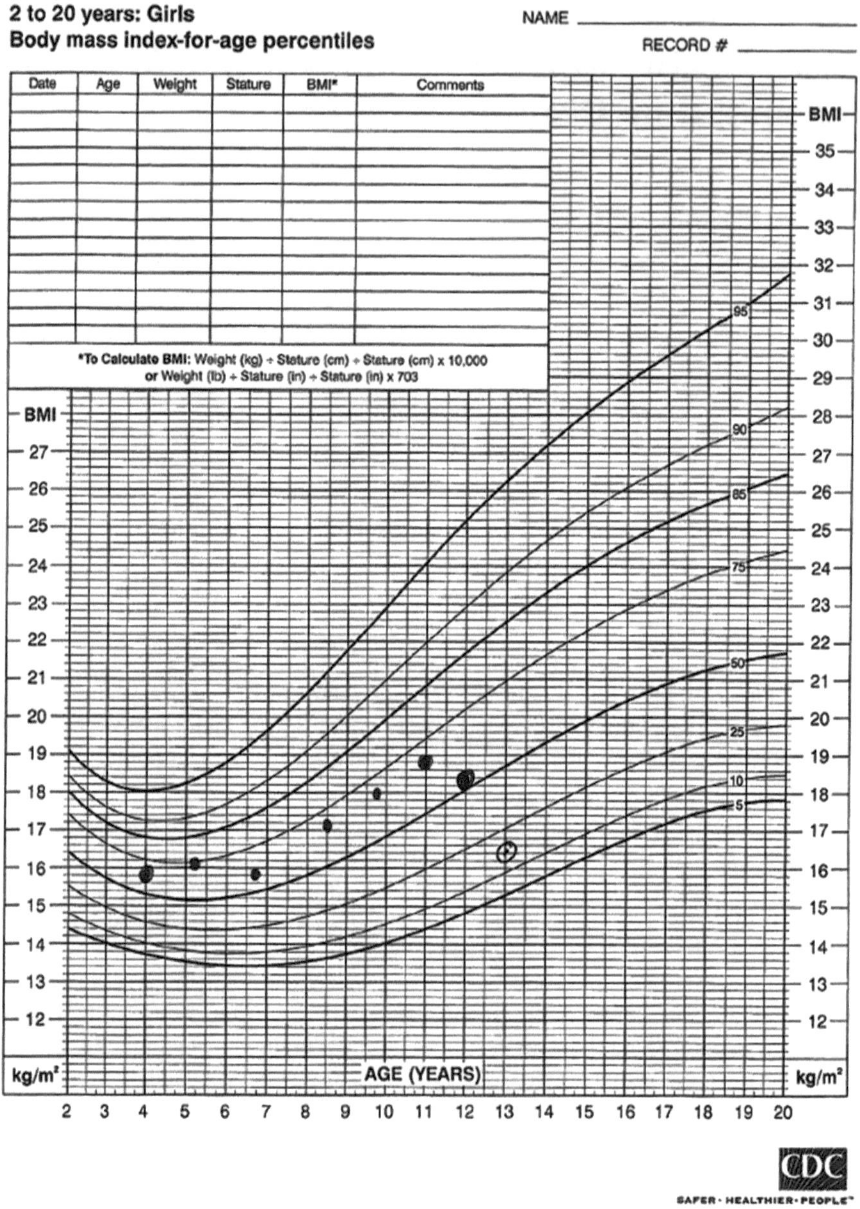

Fig. 10.1 A 3 kg weight loss in the peripubertal period, when patients are naturally supposed to grow in height, weight, and BMI, can cause a steep decline in BMI percentile and profound nutritional deficiency. (**a**) Stature-for-age and weight-for-age percentiles. (**b**) Body mass index-for-age percentiles. Source: Developed by the National Center for Health Statistics in collaboration with the National Center for Chronic Disease Prevention and Health Promotion (2000). http://www.cdc.gov/growthcharts

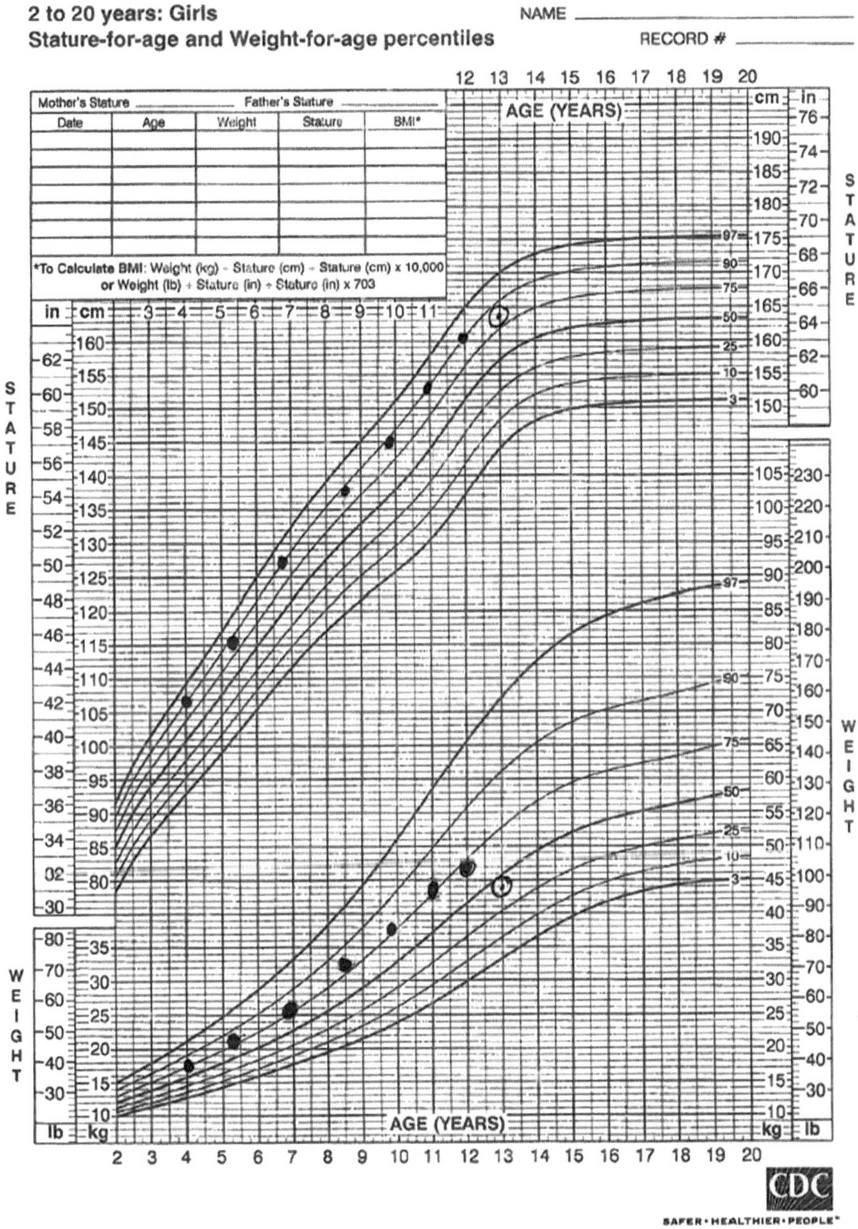

Fig. 10.1 (continued)

function tests show a slight elevation of AST and ALT to 55 and 38. Total and direct bilirubins are normal. Her basic metabolic panel is as follows: sodium of 140, potassium of 4.2, chloride of 102, HCO_3 of 26, BUN of 26, creatinine of 0.6, and glucose of 67. Calcium, magnesium, and phosphorus are all within normal limits. TSH and free T4 are within normal limits, but T3 is low.

When questioned about her decrease in weight, the patient notes that she became concerned that her diet was unhealthy after her health class talked about diabetes and obesity. Around the same time, her father was told by his doctor that he had prediabetes and should lose weight and decrease sugar intake. Her father has lost about 20 lb by decreasing his sugar intake, eating a more plant-based diet, and exercising regularly. Holly started to watch her sugar intake too and joined the gym with her father. She became a vegetarian and is now a vegan, because she is concerned about cruelty to animals. She now exercises at the gym with her father, goes for runs by herself around the school track, and does crunches in her bedroom. She used to think she would be happy at her current weight of 44 kg, but now that she is at this weight, she feels an urge to have a lower weight. She thinks she looks heavy when she looks in the mirror.

Her mother reports that Holly eats a full plate of food at every meal, but the food is very healthful. Holly's diet recall is as follows: for breakfast, she had a bowl of oatmeal made with water and a spoonful of peanut butter. For lunch, she had an entire plate of greens with lentils, slices of avocado, and a bowl of watermelon. For dinner, she had two plain baked potatoes and salad; she did not eat the roast beef that the family had because she does not eat meat. She declined dessert last night as she does on most nights, although she will eat fruit for dessert.

Holly is questioned confidentially about her social history. She reports a good relationship with her mother, father, and two brothers at home. She feels safe and loved. She enjoys school and all of her activities. She is a competitive violinist and is involved in the student community service organization. She has friends and can name a best friend (Her mother later notes that Holly has been spending less time with her friends and avoids a lot of fun outings that she would have enjoyed when she was younger.). Holly denies all substance abuse. Her mood is "fine," and she denies any depression or suicidality. There are no firearms in the home.

Holly's vital signs show bradycardia to 49 bpm supine and a blood pressure of 102/70. Standing vital signs are 88 bpm and 100/72. She has a normal temperature and oxygen saturation. Her weight is 44 kg, height is 163.5 cm, and BMI is 16.5. On physical exam, Holly is very thin and sallow appearing. She has a flat affect and speaks in a high, quiet voice. She has bitemporal wasting and no parotid enlargement. No dental decay is noted. She has shotty lymphadenopathy in her anterior cervical chain, without thyromegaly. She has no acne, hirsutism, or lanugo. Extremities are cool to palpation with good cap refill. Abdomen is scaphoid with hard stool palpated in the lower left quadrant. Spinous processes are prominent with an abrasion noted over the lumbar spine. Breasts are a small tanner 5, and pubic hair is tanner 4. Neurologic exam is within normal limits. Mental status exam is significant for a flattened affect, but Holly is otherwise lucid and communicative. You suspect that Holly has anorexia nervosa.

Questions from Patient and Family

- How can a few pounds of weight loss lead to such malnutrition?
- Can we give her something to make her have a period?
- What can we do to help Holly recover?

Discussion

Holly is a 15-year-old previously healthy young woman who presents with amenorrhea. Her history is significant for an increasingly restrictive diet and compulsive exercise. Holly has only lost 3 kg. However, she is at an age where the slopes of the normal growth curves for height, weight, and BMI all have an increased rate of rise. Therefore, to maintain her normal BMI percentile, she has to gain in height, weight, and BMI. In the peripubertal age range, even a small amount of weight loss or a failure to gain weight can cause a precipitous decline in BMI percentile and lead to profound nutritional deficiency as shown in Fig. 10.1.

Her physical exam shows several signs of nutritional deficiency: bradycardia, an orthostatic pulse, cool distal extremities, cachexia, a sallow appearance, and a flattened affect. The abrasion on her spinous processes results from compulsive stomach crunches in the setting of decreased protective fat over her spine. Her lab work supports a diagnosis of malnutrition: leukopenia with other cell lines being normal, a mild transaminitis, a low T3 with normal thyrotropin, and normal free thyroxine. Holly's diagnosis is anorexia nervosa. The criteria for anorexia nervosa as delineated in the *Diagnostic and Statistical Manual of Mental Disorders 5* (DSM 5) are listed in Table 10.1. It is important to note that although amenorrhea is a common sequela of anorexia, it is no longer required for the diagnosis.

Discussion

Holly has secondary amenorrhea, meaning that she has gone without menses for at least 3 months after the onset of menarche. The differential diagnosis for secondary amenorrhea can be grouped into estrogen-deficient and estrogen-replete conditions.

Table 10.1 Diagnostic criteria for anorexia nervosa (patients must endorse all three)

Restriction of energy intake relative to requirements, leading to a significantly low body weight in the context of age, sex, developmental trajectory, and physical health
Intense fear of gaining weight or of becoming fat, or persistent behavior that interferes with weight gain, even though at a significantly low weight
Disturbance in the way in which one's body weight or shape is experienced, undue influence of body weight or shape on self-evaluation, or persistent lack of recognition of the seriousness of the current low body weight

Adapted from the *Diagnostic and Statistical Manual of Mental Disorders*, 5th edition [1]

Some common estrogen-replete conditions include pregnancy, polycystic ovary syndrome, and physiologic anovulation. These conditions are characterized by endometrial buildup without the regular shedding of the lining that is normally brought on by the proliferative phase of the menstrual cycle.

Estrogen-deficient conditions are characterized by a lack of endometrial buildup. Common estrogen-deficient conditions include hypothalamic amenorrhea from chronic illness, stress, or nutritional deficiency; primary ovarian insufficiency; or hyperprolactinemia. In anorexic patients, the pathophysiology starts with an energy (nutritional) deficit leading to suppression of GnRH secretion, mediated in part by low leptin levels [1]. Suppressed GnRH levels lead to suppressed LH and FSH levels, and thus ovarian estrogen and androgen production returns to prepubertal levels.

Other conditions that cause amenorrhea can usually be swiftly ruled out by history or basic blood work. Anorexic patients are usually bradycardic, and thus their clinical presentation of weight loss with concomitant bradycardia is not consistent with hyperthyroidism. A thyrotropin (TSH) level can rule out both hyper- and hypothyroidism, both of which can cause amenorrhea. A low FSH rules out primary ovarian insufficiency. A normal prolactin and a lack of galactorrhea or visual field deficits rule out hyperprolactinemia. A careful history and physical with judicious blood work can rule out insidious diseases such as celiac disease or lymphoma that can cause cachexia.

Patients with anorexia nervosa often present with a classic constellation of lab abnormalities, and documenting these objective measures of starvation can help crystallize the diagnosis for patients and parents. LH, FSH, and estradiol are suppressed to prepubertal levels. Commonly, a complete blood count shows leukopenia with other cell lines being normal (and in fact, patients have robust hemoglobins because of the cessation of menses). Electrolytes are usually normal while they are in the starved state, but hypophosphatemia can develop rapidly when patients are re-nourished. Thyroid studies show a low T3 with a normal TSH and free T4, as the thyroid gland preferentially creates reverse T3 in lieu of the more metabolically active T3 in the face of nutritional deficiency. Liver function tests can show a mild transaminitis; the etiology is unclear but may include hepatocyte injury due to glutathione depletion or autophagy [2]. Inflammatory markers are very low.

Parents may worry that amenorrhea is causing a dangerous "buildup" of uterine lining. In estrogen-replete conditions such as PCOS, the buildup of endometrial tissue does indeed represent a threat to the long-term health of the uterus and may predispose patients to uterine cancer. However, this does not apply to patients with anorexia. It should be explained to parents and the patient that the lining is not building up at all; rather, there is little-to-no uterine lining because the ovaries are quiescent.

A 10-day course of medroxyprogesterone is often used as a "challenge" to distinguish estrogen-replete vs. estrogen-deficient endometrium, since a patient with an endometrial lining would develop a secretory endometrium under the influence of medroxyprogesterone and then have a withdrawal bleed once the medication was stopped. For a patient with anorexia, a negative response (no withdrawal bleed) certainly supports the diagnosis of estrogen deficiency. However, patients may still have a positive response (a withdrawal bleed) due to earlier endometrial buildup, and so patients with classic signs and symptoms should not be falsely reassured by the presence of a withdrawal bleed. If this test is used, its limitations should be explained to parents ahead of time.

Health Consequences of Amenorrhea from Anorexia Nervosa

The suppression of ovarian activity to prepubertal levels has profound health consequences. The lack of ovarian activity leads to increased bone resorption (from decreased estrogen) and decreased bone deposition (from decreased androgens), at a time of life when patients should be accruing and not losing the bone. Many parents may request hormone replacement. It is important to discuss the profound limits of this treatment modality and to give the clear message that nutritional rehabilitation and weight restoration are the best treatments for bone health. This is because the hormonal derangements of anorexia nervosa go beyond a lack of gonadal steroid production. Anorexia creates an environment that is toxic to the bones. In addition to underproduction of estrogen and androgens, there are lower-than-normal levels of IGF1, insulin, leptin, and oxytocin and overproduction of cortisol, adiponectin, and peptide YY [3]. Each of these hormonal derangements has a deleterious effect on bone accrual. In addition, decreased fat and muscle mass causes decreased skeletal loading of bones, which negatively affects bone turnover.

Combined estrogen-progestin pills have not been shown to decrease fracture risk or improve bone mineral density among anorexic patients [4], possibly because the first-pass liver metabolism of estrogen leads to a further decrease in IGF1. Transdermal estrogen at physiologic levels, with cyclic progesterone to protect the endometrium, has been shown to increase BMD at the hip and spine in adolescents with anorexia [5]. A combination of oral estrogen and progestin with DHEA leads to maintenance of BMD *z*-scores and improvements in bone geometry [6]. However, inducing menses with estrogen and progesterone is often undesired because it obscures the resumption of spontaneous menses which can be an important marker of recovery. No clinical intervention except for nutritional rehabilitation reverses the vast insult to the bone created by derangements in the many hormones listed above.

The initial evaluation of an adolescent patient with anorexia nervosa is a critical time for direct and clear communication with parents. Other organic causes of weight loss can be ruled out with basic blood work and a thorough exam. After swiftly and accurately diagnosing a child with anorexia nervosa, parents should be informed of the profound consequences of untreated anorexia, some of which include low bone density, growth stunting, infertility, and death from cardiac arrest or suicide. Medical providers should also speak to the “big picture” sequelae of

Table 10.2 Principles of family-based treatment

Agnostic view of the eating disorder	Focus is on the treatment of the disorder, and not its etiology
Lack of blame	Parents are empowered to refeed their child, rather than blamed for the disorder
Centrality of parents to treatment	Parents are drivers of treatment, and therapists and physicians act as consultants
The role of siblings	Siblings are brought into treatment in a supportive role
Externalization of the disorder	The disorder and the child are two separate entities, and only the disorder is blamed for the problems that have resulted

Adapted from *Anorexia Nervosa in Adolescents: a Treatment Manual* by James Lock and Daniel LeGrange [2]

anorexia, which include an arrest of typical adolescent development, a retreat from a normal social life, constant psychological distress, and the development of chronic anorexia nervosa which becomes harder to treat and cure as time passes. Parents should understand that patients with chronic, lifelong anorexia do not generally go on to enjoy the "normal" life that most parents envision for their children (school, career, family of one's own, good health, and longevity).

Fortunately, adolescents who are treated early and aggressively often go on to have a full recovery, [7] and so parents and providers should maintain high expectations. After relaying the gravity of the diagnosis, providers should focus parents on a results-oriented, proactive treatment approach centered on rapid, steady weight restoration. Adolescents with eating disorders should be referred to adolescent medicine specialists for management. There is strong evidence to support the treatment modality of family-based treatment (FBT), also known as the Maudsley method, for young adolescents with restrictive eating disorders [7]. FBT empowers parents to refeed children at home, using their own intuition and knowledge of their child's preferences to administer high-fat, nutritionally dense meals which are eaten under parental supervision [8]. Principles of FBT are outlined in Table 10.2. Patients with bradycardia, hypotension, hypothermia, electrolyte derangements, or body weight less than 75% of ideal body weight (or less than 80% for prepubertal patients) may require hospitalization for medical stabilization at the start of treatment. In addition, patients who are not appropriate for FBT or who are not successful at it may need a higher level of care (partial, residential, or inpatient facility). Because early weight gain is the prognosticator of a broader psychological recovery [9], it is imperative that the patient not be allowed to stay low-weighted and restricting, regardless of whether that happens at home or in a facility. It is also critical that parents and patients understand that an initial goal weight, based on the child's premorbid growth chart, will be a fast-moving target. Goal weights will change every few months as the patient gets older, especially if they gain height. Higher percentage body fat is correlated with resumption of menses [10], but it can be hard to predict in any individual patient when menses will resume. Some patients need to reach a higher BMI percentile than they were premorbidly in order to resume menstruation.

Clinical Pearls and Pitfalls

- In young adolescents, small amounts of weight loss or failure to gain weight can cause dramatic drops in BMI percentile and profound nutritional deficiency (Fig. 10.1).
- Amenorrhea in anorexic patients is the result of suppression of gonadotropins with resulting hypoestrogenemia.
- A medroxyprogesterone "challenge" has limited utility in supporting a diagnosis of anorexia; a lack of withdrawal bleed shows a low-estrogen state, but the presence of a withdrawal bleed may indicate that endometrium had built up prior to illness.
- A well-described pattern of lab results, including leukopenia and low T3 can help to support the diagnosis of anorexia.
- Electrolytes are often normal in even profoundly malnourished patients and only become deranged when patients nutritionally rehabilitate. Normal electrolytes are therefore not reassuring when making a diagnosis of anorexia nervosa.
- Anorexia nervosa has profound health consequences that affect many organ systems, cause an arrest of normal adolescent development, and, if left untreated, can become a chronic illness that is increasingly hard to cure.
- Given the many hormonal derangements are harmful to the bone in anorexia nervosa, hormonal replacement has limited utility in restoring bone health. Nutritional rehabilitation is the best strategy to maximize bone health.
- Both primary care providers and adolescent medicine specialists should spend time conveying the gravity of the diagnosis to parents and motivating them to pursue rapid and complete weight restoration.
- Family-based treatment is the most evidence-based treatment modality for anorexic adolescents.

References

1. Golden NH, Carlson JL. The pathophysiology of amenorrhea in the adolescent. Ann N Y Acad Sci. 2008;1135:163–78. https://doi.org/10.1196/annals.1429.014.
2. Winston AP. The clinical biochemistry of anorexia nervosa. Ann Clin Biochem. 2012;49(2):132–43. https://doi.org/10.1258/acb.2011.011185.
3. Misra M, Golden NH, Katzman DK. State of the art systematic review of bone disease in anorexia nervosa. Int J Eat Disord. 2016;49(3):276–92. https://doi.org/10.1002/eat.22451.
4. Golden NH, Lanzkowsky L, Schebendach J, Palestro CJ, Jacobson MS, Shenker IR. The effect of estrogen-progestin treatment on bone mineral density in anorexia nervosa. J Pediatr Adolesc Gynecol. 2002;15(3):135–43. https://doi.org/10.1016/S1083-3188(02)00145-6.
5. Misra M, Katzman D, Miller KK, et al. Physiologic estrogen replacement increases bone density in adolescent girls with anorexia nervosa. J Bone Miner Res. 2011;26(10):2430–8. https://doi.org/10.1002/jbmr.447.
6. DiVasta AD, Feldman HA, Beck TJ, LeBoff MS, Gordon CM. Does hormone replacement normalize bone geometry in adolescents with anorexia nervosa? J Bone Miner Res. 2014;29(1):151–7. https://doi.org/10.1002/jbmr.2005.

7. Lock J, Le Grange D, Agras WS, Moye A, Bryson SW, Jo B. Randomized clinical trial comparing family-based treatment with adolescent-focused individual therapy for adolescents with anorexia nervosa. Arch Gen Psychiatry. 2010;67:1025–32. https://doi.org/10.1001/archgenpsychiatry.2010.128.
8. Lock JD, Legrange D. Anorexia nervosa in adolescents: a treatment manual. 2nd ed. New York: The Guilford Press; 2013.
9. Accurso EC, Ciao AC, Fitzsimmons-Craft EE, Lock JD, Le Grange D. Is weight gain really a catalyst for broader recovery?: The impact of weight gain on psychological symptoms in the treatment of adolescent anorexia nervosa. Behav Res Ther. 2014;56:1–6. https://doi.org/10.1016/j.brat.2014.02.006.
10. Pitts S, Blood E, Divasta A, Gordon CM. Percentage body fat by dual-energy x-ray absorptiometry is associated with menstrual recovery in adolescents with anorexia nervosa. J Adolesc Health. 2014;54(6):739–41. https://doi.org/10.1016/j.jadohealth.2013.12.033.

Suggested Educational Reading and References

Campbell KA, Peebles R. Eating disorders in children and adolescents: state of the art review. Pediatrics. 2014;134(3):582–92.

Katzman DK, Peebles R, Sawyer SM, Lock J, Le Grange D. The role of the pediatrician in family-based treatment for adolescent eating disorders: opportunities and challenges. J Adolesc Health. 2013;53:433–40.

Maudsley Parents website: www.maudsleyparents.org

Chapter 11
Case of a Girl with Primary Amenorrhea, Cyclic Pelvic Pain, and Absent Vagina

Oluyemisi A. Adeyemi-Fowode and Jennifer E. Dietrich

Case

A 16-year-old female presents to clinic with cyclic pelvic pain that has worsened over the past 2 years. There is nothing that makes the pain better or worse, except "just waiting until ibuprofen starts to work." She has begun to miss school at least 1 day every month as well. Past medical history and surgical history are unremarkable. There are no major medical problems in the family. Upon review of her pubertal history, you discover that she began breast development at age 11.5 years and pubarche around age 12 years. Her growth has been normal at the 50% for height, and her BMI is 17 as she is a dancer and practices everyday. She has never had a period. On inquiry about social activities, she reports that she has never been sexually active. Review of systems reveals no evidence of constipation, dysuria, headaches, visual changes, or heat and cold intolerance. On physical exam you note that she has no thyromegaly; she points to pain on her abdomen on both sides. On the right side, she reports pain above the pelvic brim, and on the left, she reports pain low in her pelvis. There is no rebound, guarding or palpable mass on abdominal exam. She also has Tanner 5 breast development and Tanner 5 pubic hair. Skin exam is normal without evidence of severe acne or hirsute features. You note a widely splayed urethra but cannot clearly see a vaginal opening. Probing with a Q-tip below the urethra reveals lack of patency and a vaginal dimple of 1 cm depth. On rectal exam, no bulge effect is appreciated.

O.A. Adeyemi-Fowode, M.D. (✉)
Division of Pediatric and Adolescent Gynecology, Department of Obstetrics and Gynecology, Baylor College of Medicine, Houston, TX, USA
e-mail: adeyemi@bcm.edu

J.E. Dietrich, M.D., M.Sc.
Obstetrics and Gynecology and Pediatrics, Texas Children's Hospital, Baylor College of Medicine, Houston, TX, USA
e-mail: jedietri@bcm.edu

H.J. Talib (ed.), *Adolescent Gynecology*,
https://doi.org/10.1007/978-3-319-66978-6_11

You begin an evaluation by ordering a few tests, including a pregnancy test, which is negative, a pelvic ultrasound, and gonadal hormones. Gonadal hormones are normal. A pelvic ultrasound reveals a normal left ovary, they cannot visualize the right ovary, and they see a possible small uterus in the midline measuring 1.5 cm. You order an abdominal and pelvic MRI to further evaluate her pelvic structures. The MRI shows evidence of two normal ovaries; however, the right ovary is undescended and located above the pelvic brim. There is a small pelvic kidney on the right side with a normal left kidney in the anatomic location and no evidence of a midline uterus or cervix. The MRI does show right and left ovoid-appearing structures near the pelvic sidewalls that enhance with fluid, but this fluid does not appear to follow the path of the ureters or bladder and does not communicate with the intestine. These measure 1 cm × 2.5 cm in size. A karyotype is also ordered and reveals a normal female with results of 46XX.

You bring the patient and her mom back to clinic to discuss these results and explain that she has a condition called uterovaginal agenesis, also known as Mayer-Rokitansky-Kuster-Hauser (MRKH) syndrome, and that it may occur in 1:5000 girls.

Questions

1. Can I ever have a period one day like my friends?
   (a) Unfortunately this is not possible; however you have undergone hormonal changes that are similar to all women. You have undergone stages of puberty with the exception of having a period. That is because you don't have a uterus which is where menstrual blood comes from.
2. If I have no uterus and normal ovaries, why do I have pain?
   (a) Approximately 10–15% of women with this condition will have a remnant uterine horn which is an underdeveloped uterus with a small amount of endometrial lining which may bleed each month in response to your normal ovarian hormones. Because the remnant did not develop normally and does not have a connection to the vagina, it has no way of being released to the outside. This can cause you to have pain.
3. Will I be able to have children in the future?
   (a) Yes, there are many ways in which women with this condition can be a mom. The ovaries developed normally, and therefore with the assistance of a reproductive endocrinologist and infertility specialist, your ovaries can be stimulated with hormones and the eggs retrieved. These eggs can then be mixed with your partner's sperm, and a fertilized egg would result. The fertilized eggs can then be transferred into a surrogate carrier's uterus to carry on your behalf. This is still your baby and contains the genetic material of you and your partner one day.
4. Can I pass this on one day to my children?

(a) In some cases there may be the possibility of passing on the condition, but in the majority of cases, literature shows that this is a multifactorial process that is not a result of a single mutation. Studies thus far have not indicated that the risk to your offspring is any higher.

Puberty occurs as a result of hormonal influences and consists of a series of predictable events that have been studied and described. The earliest noticeable sign of puberty in the majority of females is breast development (thelarche), followed by pubarche (pubic hair), a growth spurt, and lastly the first menstrual period (menarche), which marks the end of puberty. The stages of puberty are orchestrated through the HPO (hypothalamic-pituitary-ovarian) axis. In addition, menstruation requires a patent outflow tract (uterine corpus, cervix, and vagina). Lack of thelarche by age 13 or of menarche by age 15 with or without secondary sexual characteristics warrants investigation [1] as this is considered delayed puberty.

When an adolescent female presents with complaints of primary amenorrhea (lack of menarche), the entire clinical presentation needs to be taken into consideration; as with any clinical complaint, a thorough history and physical examination is crucial as they help guide the clinical decision of expectant management versus immediate investigation. Delayed puberty, specifically, can be the result of a number of etiologies ranging from gonadal dysgenesis and disorders of the hypopituitary system with resulting ovarian dysfunction to outflow tract abnormalities. The most common cause of primary amenorrhea, after gonadal dysgenesis, is Mullerian agenesis [1, 2]. However, all possibilities must be considered during differential diagnosis. The diagnosis of girls and young women with primary amenorrhea requires knowledge of the current functional state of the HPO axis and reproductive tract anatomy of the affected patient.

Embryologically, the paired Mullerian ducts are derived from the mesoderm (intermediate mesenchyme) and develop along the posterior wall of the abdominal cavity. These ducts give rise to the fallopian tube, uterine corpus, cervix, and upper portion on the vagina while the lower vagina is derived from the urogenital sinus [3]. Mullerian agenesis also referred to as Mullerian aplasia or Mayer-Rokitansky-Kuster-Hauser (MRKH) syndrome is estimated to occur in one in 4000–5000 births [1, 3–8]. MRKH results from the embryologic growth failure of the Mullerian ducts with resultant agenesis of the vagina and an absent or rudimentary uterus [1, 9]. Approximately one-third of affected patients have urinary tract abnormalities as well [6]. Although the urinary and genital systems are two very different systems functionally, anatomically, and embryologically, they are closely related. Both are derived from the mesoderm (intermediate mesenchyme), and the Mullerian ducts are positioned in close proximity to the primitive kidneys (mesonephros).

The American Society of Reproductive Medicine (ASRM) classifies MRKH as a class I Mullerian duct anomaly. There are various clinical presentations of this anomaly due to varying degrees of uterine aplasia and simultaneously affected systems; in some cases, there is a rudimentary uterus, which may have functioning or nonfunctioning endometrium [2, 10]. Differentiation between various forms has also been proposed. Type I (typical MRKH) describes the combination of aplasia of the uterus and an absence of the upper two-thirds of the vagina; type II (atypical) includes forms with further malformations affecting the urologic, skeletal, cardiac, or auditory system [4, 5, 11]. No causal association has been established to explain this spectrum of presentation, and there is no known specific genetic cause for Mullerian agenesis [5, 6]; however, multiple genes have been implicated in the normal development of the Mullerian, renal, and bone structures. Genes of interest include HOXA, WNT4, HOX, and SOX9 genes [4, 5].

The typical presentation of MRKH is primary amenorrhea (absent period) in an otherwise normally developed adolescent female around the age of 15–18 years [4, 8]. A smaller number of women may seek medical help because of an inability to have penetrative coitus. A subset will have complaint of chronic or cyclical pelvic pain. This is typically due to a functional uterine remnant. Establishing a pubertal timeline is important, when amenorrhea is found more than 2 SD (about 4 years) after the onset of breast development; without any other symptoms, MRKH should be in the differential diagnosis [5]. History will reveal normal pubertal milestones and the presence of normal secondary sexual characteristics. On physical examination, breast, axillary, and pubic hair development aligns with chronological age. The presence of these secondary sexual characteristics can be reassuring that the HPO axis is intact. There is also a normal appearance to the external genitalia whether there is absent or hypoplastic vagina. In the pediatric and adolescent age group, an internal exam is not always possible; we recommend bilateral labial traction as that will allow visualization of the hymen and inferior vagina. Vaginal length differs in patients with MRKH from a vaginal dimple to shortened vaginal length. If the patient can tolerate a Q-tip exam, the Q-tip can be used to measure the depth of the vaginal dimple. If a rectal examination can be tolerated, the absence of a vaginal bulge will help differentiate MRKH from an imperforate hymen or distal transverse vaginal septum.

Differential Diagnosis

Vaginal agenesis may occur in conjunction with certain disorders of 46XY sexual differentiation such as mixed gonadal dysgenesis (MGD), complete androgen insensitivity syndrome (CAIS), and partial androgen insensitivity syndrome (PAIS) [1, 5]. Differences that can help differentiate MRKH from AIS are summarized in Table 11.1.

Diagnosis

When a Mullerian duct anomaly is suspected, imaging is essential for diagnosis and management and to direct reproductive counseling. As mentioned above, there is a spectrum in presentation due to anatomic variation known to occur with Class I

Table 11.1 Differential diagnosis between MRKH and AIS [1, 4, 6, 12]

MRKH	AIS
Genotype XX	Genotype XY
Normal hormonal profile	Male testosterone levels
Normal height	Increased height compared to female counterparts
Normal secondary sexual characteristics	Abnormal secondary sexual characteristics
– Normal breasts	– Normal breasts
– Normal pubic and axillary hair	– Absent to sparse pubic and axillary hair
Normal ovaries but often in ectopic positions	Intra-abdominal testicles
Normal external genitalia	Normal external genitalia
Variable vaginal length	Variable vaginal length [shortened to normal length]
No increased risk of gonadal malignancy	Gonadectomy recommended due to increased risk of malignancy
Varying degree of uterine hypoplasia	No uterus or cervix
Hereditary unknown	Maternal X-linked recessive, 25% risk of affected child, 25% risk of carrier
	Fair incidence of sporadic mutation
Other anomalies frequent	Other anomalies rare

reproductive tract anomalies. Vaginal agenesis is usually accompanied by cervical and uterine agenesis [10, 12]. However, in 10% of cases, a rudimentary Mullerian structure is identified, which can be functional (endometrial layer present) or non-functional (endometrial layer absent) [10]. A functional uterine remnant can present with chronic cyclic pain due to obstruction of the outflow tract. A pelvic ultrasound (US) is often the initial imaging study of choice, although the transvaginal approach is typically not utilized in this population. A transabdominal or transperineal ultrasound can be obtained instead; however, magnetic resonance imaging (MRI) is the study of choice due to its high accuracy, detailed delineation of anatomy, noninvasive nature, and lack of ionizing radiation exposure to the patient [10]. Evaluation of a uterine remnant may be difficult with US due to the limited acoustic ultrasound window. In contrast, MRI can differentiate between uterine agenesis versus hypoplasia (remnant) [10] quite readily. Among patients with pelvic pain, MRI is the gold standard to evaluate anatomic variants [5, 8]. Pelvic MRI is also useful for the preoperative detection of MRKH-associated malformations in order to help optimize clinical and/or surgical management of patients with MRKH [11]. Once the diagnosis of vaginal agenesis is confirmed, a karyotype may be ordered to rule out 46XY sexual differentiation.

Besides delineating the reproductive anatomy, it is also important to evaluate other systems that might be affected. A renal US and spine radiograph should be ordered because of the possibility of associated anomalies. In addition to approximately one-third of type II MRKH patients having urinary tract abnormalities, an estimated 12% have skeletal anomalies mostly involving the spine [6]. Although the most common associated anomaly in MRKH is unilateral renal agenesis, a pelvic kidney is sometimes seen [8]; other abnormalities include ectopic kidney, horseshoe kidney, and abnormal collecting ducts [6].

Management

Strategies for managing this condition range from nonsurgical to surgical options and really depend upon patient readiness. Once a diagnosis is made, some patients will need time to consider when they would like to further discuss options for neovagina creation and fertility options. This readiness is variable and may be dependent on their ability to discuss their diagnosis with a counselor, psychologist, family members, or similarly affected peers [3, 6, 10, 12].

The majority of patients (90%) will respond to a nonsurgical approach using progressive vaginal dilation with perineal dilators [1, 5, 7, 9, 13]. There is variation in terms of the length of time it takes one to create a neovagina as more consistent use will result in improved vaginal lengthening. There are many strategies experts have recommend for improving vaginal dilation techniques, including the use of lubricants, estrogen creams, relaxation, and a warm bath or shower prior to dilation, all designed to help improve tissue pliability and reduce vaginismus. There is no set length that a patient must reach as a vaginal length may range from 6 to 10 cm but is primarily related to what she is comfortable with. Regardless of consistency with dilation, some patients may require surgical intervention if desired to increase the total vaginal length [1, 5, 7, 9, 13]. A variety of surgical techniques have been described with long-term outcomes varying depending on the technique utilized but can include the use of tissue grafts, as well as laparoscopic and open approaches. One study involving 240 patients with MRKH undergoing vaginoplasty via laparoscopic Vecchietti procedure is the largest series looking at outcomes in patients with regard to sexual function, HPV acquisition, and clearance and postoperative complications [14]. This study demonstrated that over a median timeframe of 16 months, all patients maintained a mean total vaginal length of 9.5 cm. There were no long-term complications other than granulation tissue in 2.9% of patients, and sexual function was maintained in all patients. Another interesting finding was that the mean time to HPV acquisition was similar to that of all women, and approximately 2.9% of women in this study were shown to have acquired HPV once they initiated intercourse within 3–6 months [14]. No single technique is necessarily the best way in which to approach vaginal lengthening as it is most important that the surgeon has expertise in the surgical management and individualizes for each patient [1, 5, 7, 9, 13].

For patients with chronic cyclic pain, remnant functional horns may be suspected. These horns may sometimes be seen on MRI studies; however due to the streak appearance of these horns and lateralized location along the pelvic sidewall, occasionally they are not seen except at the time of laparoscopy. Nonetheless several studies suggest this is more common than previously thought. One study of 61 patients with MRKH and pelvic pain who underwent diagnostic MRI alone, 89%

had bilateral remnants, and 11% had a unilateral remnant present [15]. The major diagnostic feature on imaging reported in this study was that of describing that all remnants were found just caudal to the paired ovary on that side even if the ovary was in an ectopic location [15]. For some patients they are easily suppressed with combined or progesterone-only hormone pills. These pills can be administered continuously without a placebo week for breakthrough, since the placebo break could result in breakthrough bleeding within the closed space of the underdeveloped remnant horn [5]. When patients fail medical management or prefer not to take additional hormones for symptom management, surgical excision of the horn can be offered. One surgical study looked at nine women with MRKH who underwent a diagnostic laparoscopy, and 89% were found to have some type of functional horn remnant [8]. Frequently these can be removed laparoscopically with primary excision. Care must be taken to carefully map out the ureters, and therefore knowledge of the renal anatomy is very important prior to offering excision as the ureters can occasionally track close to the remnant horns [5, 11]. Other findings at the time of laparoscopy can include endometriosis and undescended ovaries. Endometriosis occurs in approximately 40% of patients with any type of Mullerian anomaly; however among patients with uterovaginal agenesis, no exact incidence is yet known, though there are many case reports in the literature exhibiting this [2]. This suggests that perhaps endometriosis has an origin related to Mullerian degeneration rather than the retrograde hypothesis alone [2]. In the case that an undescended ovary is discovered, there is not a need to move the undescended ovaries to a new location as they will function normally. However, it is important to know the location of the ovaries as abdominal pain related to the ovary will present in a non-pelvic location in the future [3, 10, 11].

Discussions regarding fertility typically come later; however, patients should be reassured to know that among patients with this condition, the ovaries have a normal appearance and function normally as well. Nonetheless, approximately 10–25% of patients will have undescended ovaries. This is important for the future in terms of anatomic planning for egg retrieval, and in the setting of ovarian-related pain, pain may not occur deep within the pelvis but rather above the pelvic brim in these cases. Women with MRKH are candidates for in vitro fertilization techniques whereby the oocytes can be retrieved from the ovaries once stimulated with hormones, mixed with a partner's spermatocyte, and then a fertilized embryo is created. The fertilized embryo can then be replaced into a surrogate uterus. A number of successful pregnancies and deliveries have been accomplished in this fashion. Nonetheless, not all women worldwide may have access to surrogacy, and as a result, new research is underway to explore uterine transplant and tissue bioengineering of uterine organs. These are still very much in research phase and the long-term implications still not fully understood. Many women will still have questions with regard to their offspring and risk of other females having similar conditions. Thus far the literature supports that among women with MRKH type 1, this is thought to be multifactorial and does not appear to increase risk for offspring. Among women with MRKH type 2, more somatic mutation may be involved, and therefore the risks to offspring have been reported as increased by 25% [3, 5, 12].

Clinical Pearls

- Lack of thelarche by age 13 or of menarche by age 15 with or without secondary sexual characteristics warrants investigation.
- MRKH results from the embryologic growth failure of the Mullerian ducts with resultant agenesis of the vagina and an absent or rudimentary uterus. Approximately one-third of affected patients have urinary tract abnormalities as well.
- There is no known specific genetic cause for Mullerian agenesis; however, multiple genes have been implicated in the normal development of the Mullerian structures.
- The typical presentation of MRKH is primary amenorrhea (absent period) in an otherwise normally developed adolescent female.
- There is also a normal appearance to the external genitalia whether there is absent or hypoplastic vagina. We recommend bilateral labial traction as that will allow visualization of the hymen and inferior vagina. If the patient can tolerate a Q-tip exam, the Q-tip can be used to measure the depth of the vagina.
- A pelvic ultrasound is the initial imaging study of choice; magnetic resonance imaging (MRI) is the study of choice due to its high accuracy and detailed delineation of anatomy.
- Strategies for managing this condition range from nonsurgical to surgical. The majority of patients (90%) will respond to a nonsurgical approach using progressive vaginal dilation with perineal dilators.
- A variety of surgical techniques have been described with long-term outcomes varying depending on the technique utilized but can include the use of tissue grafts, as well as laparoscopic and open approaches.
- For patients with chronic cyclic pain, remnant functional horns may be suspected. Some patients are easily suppressed with hormonal therapy. When patients fail medical management or prefer not to take additional hormones for symptom management, surgical excision of the horn can be offered.
- Women with MRKH are candidates for in vitro fertilization techniques whereby the oocytes can be retrieved from the ovaries once stimulated with hormones, mixed with a partner's spermatocyte, and then a fertilized embryo is created. The fertilized embryo can then be replaced into a surrogate uterus.

References

1. ACOG Committee Opinion. Number 562. Mullerian agenesis: diagnosis, management, and treatment. Obstet Gynecol. 2013 May;121(5):1134–7.
2. Troncon JK, et al. Endometriosis in a patient with Mayer Rokitansky Kuster Hauser Syndrome. Case Rep Obstet Gynecol. 2014;2014:376231. https://doi.org/10.1155/2014/376231.
3. Breech LL, Laufer MR. Mullerian anomalies. Obstet Gynecol Clin North Am. 2009;36:47–68.
4. Laundry L, Choung S, Kolp L. Mayer-Rokitansky-Kuster-Hauser Syndrome: a review. Int J Womens Health. 2015;7:865–70.

5. Dietrich JE, Millar DM, Quint EH, NASPAG Committee Opinion. Non-Obstructive Mullerian anomalies. J Pediatr Adolesc Gynecol. 2014;27(6):386–95.
6. Speroff L, Fritz MA. Clinical gynecologic endocrinology and infertility. 7th ed. Philadelphia: Lippincott Williams & Wilkins; 2005. p. 419–20.
7. Edmonds DK, Rose GL, Lipton MG, Quek J. Mayer Rokitansky Kuster Hauser syndrome: a review of 245 consecutive cases managed by a multidisciplinary approach with vaginal dilators. Fertil Steril. 2012;97(3):686–90.
8. Will MA, et al. Surgical pearls: laparoscopic removal of uterine horn remants in patients with Mayer Rokitansky Kuster Hauser Syndrome. J Pediatr Adolesc Gynecol. 2013;26(4):224–7.
9. Mcquillan SK, Grover SR. Dilation and surgical management in vaginal agenesis: a systematic review. Int Urogynecol J. 2014;25(3):299–311.
10. Junqueira BL, Allen LM, Spitzer RF, Lucco KL, Babyn PS, Doria AS. Müllerian duct anomalies and mimics in children and adolescents: correlative intraoperative assessment with clinical imaging. Radiographics. 2009;29(4):1085–103.
11. Preibsch H, et al. Clinical value of magnetic resonance imaging in patient with Mayer-Rokitanksy-Kuster-hauser (MRKH) syndrome: diagnosis of associated malformation, uterine rudiments and intrauterine endometrium. Eur Radiol. 2014;24(7):1621–7.
12. Emans SJ, Laufer MR. Pediatric and adolescent gynecology. 5th ed. Philadelphia: Lippincott Williams & Wilkins; 2005. p. 239–40.
13. McQuillan SK, Grover SR. Systematic review of sexual function and satisfaction following the management of vaginal agenesis. Int Urogynecol J. 2014;25(10):1313–20.
14. Rall K, et al. Laparoscopically assisted neovaginoplasty in vaginal agenesis: a long term outcomes study in 240 patients. J Pediatr Adolesc Gynecol. 2014;27(6):379–85.
15. Hall-Craggs MA, et al. Mayer Rokitansky Kuster Hauser Syndrome: diagnosis with MR imaging. Can Assoc Radiol J. 2013;64(3):269–73.

Suggested Reading

ACOG Committee Opinion. Number 562. Mullerian agenesis: diagnosis, management, and treatment. Obstet Gynecol. 2013;121(5):1134–7.

Dietrich JE, Millar DM, Quint EH, NASPAG Committee Opinion. Non-Obstructive Mullerian anomalies. J Pediatr Adolesc Gynecol. 2014;27(6):386–95.

Emans SJ, Laufer MR. Pediatric and adolescent gynecology. 5th ed. Philadelphia: Lippincott Williams & Wilkins; 2005. p. 239–40.

Junqueira BL, Allen LM, Spitzer RF, Lucco KL, Babyn PS, Doria AS. Müllerian duct anomalies and mimics in children and adolescents: correlative intraoperative assessment with clinical imaging. Radiographics. 2009;29(4):1085–103.

Chapter 12
Case of a Girl with Primary Amenorrhea, Delayed Puberty, and High Gonadotropin Levels

Rula V. Kanj and Catherine M. Gordon

Case

A 16-year-old female presents because she has never had a menstrual period. She had normal development throughout childhood; however, she notes that she has been the shortest student in her class at school for the past 3 years. She has no other medical problems except that she recently sustained an ankle fracture after a minor fall.

On physical examination, she has Tanner stage I breasts and no axillary or pubic hair. Her height is 150.9 cm (height *Z*-score = −1.8), and her weight is 49.8 kg (weight *Z*-score = 0.5) [1] (Fig. 12.1). A pregnancy test is negative, and prolactin (PRL) and thyroid-stimulating hormone (TSH) levels are normal.

The follicle-stimulating hormone (FSH) level is greater than 36 U/L; on repeat 4 weeks later, it is 40 U/L. A lumbar spine bone density by dual-energy X-ray absorptiometry (DXA) reveals a bone mineral density (BMD) *Z*-score of −2.2 SD. Her karyotype is 46,XX, and she has negative testing for *FMR1* premutation and adrenal autoantibodies.

The diagnosis of primary ovarian insufficiency (POI) is made, and the patient's mother asks you: What condition does my daughter have? What does this mean for her future health? Will I be a grandmother someday?

R.V. Kanj, M.D. (✉)
Division of Pediatric and Adolescent Gynecology, Department of Obstetrics and Gynecology, University of Cincinnati College of Medicine, Cincinnati Children's Hospital Medical Center, Cincinnati, OH, USA
e-mail: rula.kanj@cchmc.org

C.M. Gordon, M.D., M.Sc.
Division of Adolescent and Transition Medicine, Department of Pediatrics, University of Cincinnati College of Medicine, Cincinnati Children's Hospital Medical Center, Cincinnati, OH, USA
e-mail: catherine.gordon@cchmc.org

H.J. Talib (ed.), *Adolescent Gynecology*,
https://doi.org/10.1007/978-3-319-66978-6_12

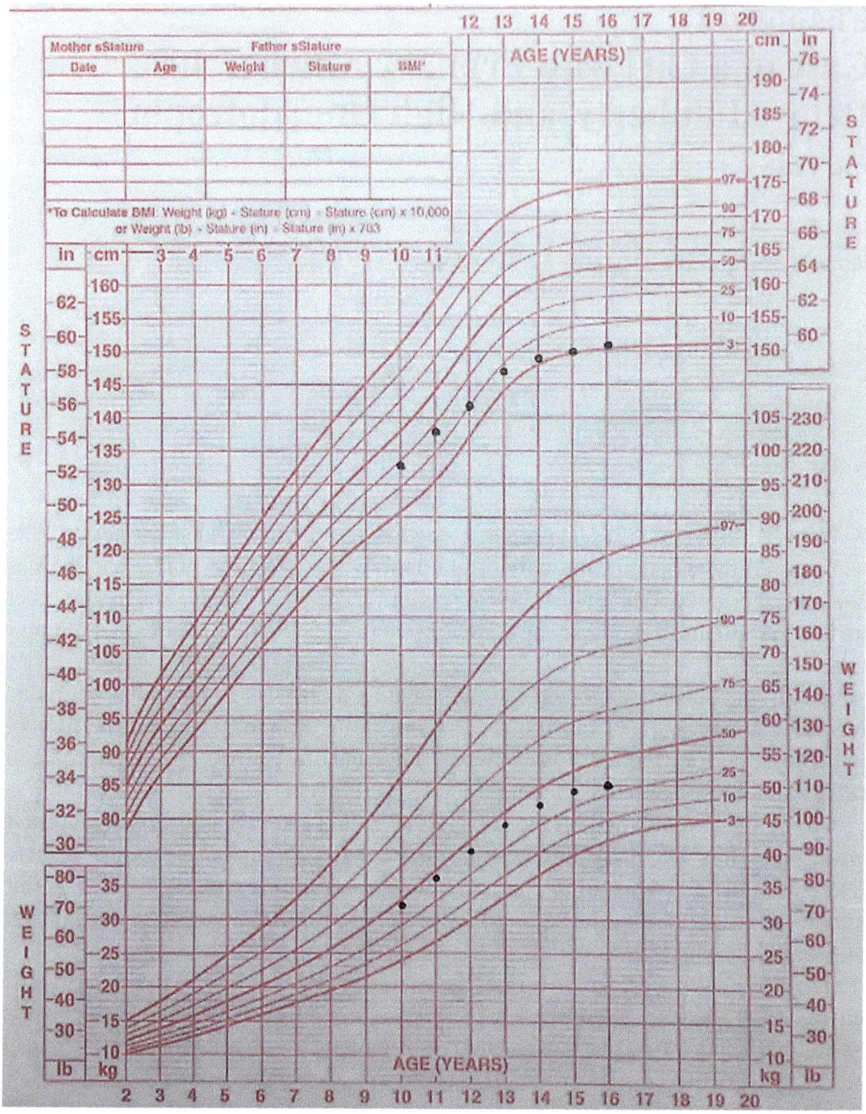

Fig 12.1 Growth chart depicting decrease in growth velocity prior to menarche (*Source*: CDC 2001. Form No. 100125: Growth chart, 2–20 years, girls, stature for age, weight-for-age percentiles. http://www.cdc.gov/growthcharts)

Discussion

POI is "the depletion or dysfunction of ovarian follicles with cessation of menses before age 40" [2]. The condition was formerly known as premature menopause or premature ovarian failure. However, ovarian function is often intermittent and

Table 12.1 Causes of hypogonadism

Hypogonadotropic hypogonadism	Hypergonadotropic hypogonadism
Isolated GnRH deficiency	Idiopathic primary ovarian insufficiency (POI)
– Kallmann syndrome	
– Other	
GnRH insensitivity	Gonadal dysgenesis (e.g., Turner syndrome)
Functional hypothalamic amenorrhea (due to disordered eating, excessive exercise, and/or psychological stress)	Ovarian insufficiency secondary to cytotoxic agents (e.g., chemotherapy)
Brain tumor	Fragile X syndrome
Pituitary adenomas	Autoimmune disorders
	– Isolated POI
	– Component of autoimmune polyglandular syndrome
Hypopituitarism	Alcohol abuse
Cranial irradiation or injury	Gonadal torsion

unpredictable in affected adolescents and women, and ovarian reserve is decreased rather than depleted. Thus, POI is a distinct condition from premature menopause [3].

The differential diagnosis for a female patient with slowing of growth velocity prior to menarche is broad. Several conditions should be considered. Systemic illnesses such as inflammatory bowel disease and hypothyroidism, and central nervous system lesions such as craniopharyngiomas, can lead to dysfunction of the hypothalamic-pituitary axis. Various endocrinopathies, including growth hormone deficiency and adrenal insufficiency, can also lead to slowing of growth velocity or cessation of growth entirely.

In cases where the delay in physical development is found to be due to dysfunction of the hypothalamic-pituitary-gonadal axis, the differential diagnosis includes hypogonadotropic hypogonadism and hypergonadotropic hypogonadism, which are broad categories with various subtypes (Table 12.1). In either category, patients may present with delayed puberty, delayed menarche, and/or amenorrhea.

The distinction between primary and secondary amenorrhea should be made, because this decision affects the level of suspicion for certain conditions. Patients with primary amenorrhea need to have anatomic anomalies (e.g., transverse vaginal septum, imperforate hymen) ruled out early on. Patients with secondary amenorrhea can be assumed to have typical reproductive anatomy with a patent outflow tract, and the focus should be on ruling out endocrinopathies.

POI is a form of hypergonadotropic hypogonadism: that is, the dysfunction is at the level of the ovary rather than within the hypothalamus or pituitary [4]. The diagnosis of POI is made when a female less than 40 years old has amenorrhea or menstrual irregularity for at least 3 months and has FSH levels of greater than 40 U/L on at least two occasions 1 month apart [3].

POI is associated with low levels of serum estradiol [5]. Because ovarian function tends to be intermittent, however, patients may have intermittent hypoestrogenism, with normal levels of serum estradiol at other times. Therefore, a progestin withdrawal challenge is not appropriate and may lead to delay in diagnosis, as patients with POI may have withdrawal bleeding in response to progesterone.

While most patients with POI will present with secondary amenorrhea, younger women may present with primary amenorrhea. These younger patients are more likely to have a chromosomal abnormality: approximately 50% of patients with POI who present with *primary* amenorrhea will have an abnormal karyotype [4].

The diagnostic workup for POI has multiple aspects including genetic testing and antibody testing for ovarian and adrenal autoantibodies [6]. However, even after a thorough evaluation, approximately 90% of cases of spontaneous POI (i.e., those not secondary to cytotoxic therapy such as chemotherapy or radiation) will remain without an identifiable cause [5].

At the time of diagnosis, patients may already have encountered the effects of intermittent hypoestrogenism. These include temporary, reversible effects such as vaginal dryness and hot flashes, which often will completely resolve with hormone replacement therapy. On the other hand, the effects of low serum estradiol on bone density may not be as easily reversed. When patients are diagnosed with POI in adolescence, this is an even more significant issue, as adolescence (up to age 19) is the time of peak accumulation of bone mass for women.

Thus, an important component of the initial evaluation for POI is the measurement of bone density, obtained via DXA. Patients should have a DXA BMD measurement of the lumbar spine as early as possible in their workup (Fig. 12.2). The spine is rich in metabolically active trabecular bone and is typically the first site to exhibit skeletal losses. This measurement will help guide initial medical therapy, including hormone replacement, as well as calcium and vitamin D supplementation. As the variance in an individual's bone density is 70–80% predicted by genetic factors, it can be helpful to obtain a baseline bone density by DXA as an initial assessment of bone health.

A history of bone fractures should raise concern for the presence of a long-term hypoestrogenic state such as can occur with POI. These could include atraumatic fractures or vertebral compression fractures, each of which raises concern for a diagnosis of osteoporosis. However, multiple fractures in any adolescent or young woman, in the presence or absence of trauma, should raise concern [7].

The management of POI is multifaceted and longitudinal. In all cases of POI, the various components of this chronic condition must be considered, including effects on physical, emotional, and mental health in these patients [8]. Important members of the care team for patients with POI may include several of the following specialties: adolescent medicine, endocrinology, gynecology, social work, and psychiatry.

Medical therapy for POI includes hormone replacement therapy, specifically estrogen and progesterone. Without estrogen therapy, patients with POI are at risk for menopausal symptoms (vasomotor flushes, vaginal dryness), decreased bone density, impaired endothelial function, impaired cognition, and decreased sexual satisfaction [7].

Currently, patients with POI are treated with hormone replacement that closely mimics typical physiology within their age group. A recommended form of hormone replacement therapy is transdermal estrogen, which provides the levels of serum

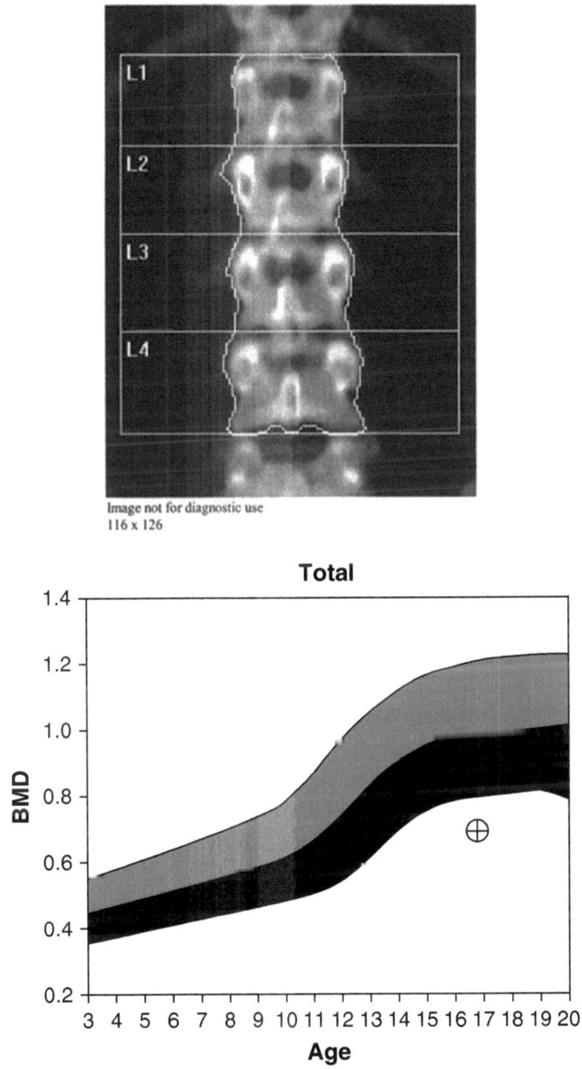

DXA Results Summary:

Region	Area (cm²)	BMC (g)	BMC (g/cm²)	T - score	Z - score
L1	10.72	6.84	0.638		
L2	10.93	7.67	0.702		
L3	12.62	9.02	0.715		
L4	14.96	10.86	0.725		
Total	**49.23**	**34.39**	**0.699**		**–3.3**

Total BMD CV 1.0%

Fig. 12.2 (**a–c**) Lumbar spine bone density by DXA: example of bone mineral density consistent with osteoporosis. *Z*-score vs. white female (*Source*: BMDCS/Hologic White Female)

estradiol that are closest to circulating physiologic levels and are safer than oral therapy as they avoid hepatic bypass metabolism. Therefore, clotting factors are less likely to be altered.

The long-term goals of hormone replacement include achieving adult serum levels of sex steroids for protection of bone density and prevention of endothelial dysfunction, which in turn contributes to risk of cardiovascular disease. Patients who present with delayed puberty and/or primary amenorrhea have additional short-term goals, including achievement of secondary sexual characteristics and induction of growth spurt to achieve their height potential [3].

The emotional and psychological components of POI can have a significant impact on patients [9]. This is especially important to consider when patients are initially informed of their diagnosis. The risk of depression and anxiety increases with menstrual irregularity, and the loss of spontaneous fertility can represent a significant loss and exacerbate mood disorders in young women [10, 11].

Another important aspect of management of POI, especially in the adolescent and young adult population, is the need for and use of contraception. As ovarian function is decreased rather than absent, there is the potential for spontaneous pregnancies in patients with POI. Paradoxically, treatment with hormone replacement therapy may improve fertility for temporary, unpredictable time periods. Thus patients that believe they are not at risk for pregnancy may have unplanned pregnancies [12].

Unfortunately, hormonal contraception such as combined oral contraceptives may not work effectively, as these medications function by suppressing the hypothalamic-pituitary-ovarian axis [13]. Therefore, emphasis should be placed on using barrier contraception (condoms) consistently and consideration of long-acting reversible contraceptive intrauterine devices (IUD), including the levonorgestrel and copper IUD. The levonorgestrel IUD serves the dual purpose of contraception and endometrial protection—the latter function by providing an intrauterine source of progestin.

On the other hand, some patients will express interest in fertility preservation options. It should be noted that most patients, due to markedly elevated follicle-stimulating hormone (FSH) levels, will not be able to undergo oocyte cryopreservation. The process of freezing oocytes requires the ability to stimulate the ovaries to produce follicles, and these menopausal levels of FSH are often impossible to overcome [14]. However, as previously noted, ovarian function in patients with POI is intermittent and unpredictable—thus fertility preservation may be an option for some patients, who should be referred to a reproductive endocrinology and infertility (REI) specialist if they so desire.

Discussion with Patient and Family

What Does My Daughter Have?

She has POI, meaning that her ovaries are not working as well as they should be for her age. Most of the time, we do not know why this happens.

What Does This Mean for Her Future Health?

It means that her levels of ovarian hormones (estrogen and progesterone) will be too low to protect her bones, heart, and brain. So she will need to take hormone replacement therapy until she reaches the age when women typically have menopause.

Will I Be a Grandmother Someday?

Her ovarian reserve (meaning the number of healthy eggs that she can use for future pregnancies) will run out faster than it typically would. So she may not be able to use her own eggs to have a pregnancy. However, she can carry a pregnancy, using donor eggs for in vitro fertilization (IVF).

Clinical Pearls and Pitfalls

- The diagnosis of POI is often delayed in teenagers. These patients may present with primary or secondary amenorrhea.
- Most cases of POI will not have an identified cause even after a complete evaluation.
- The diagnosis of POI often has effects on physical, mental, and emotional health. An interdisciplinary approach to management is recommended.
- POI represents an example of primary hypogonadism with estrogen deficiency. One of the major medical complications can be skeletal losses and lack of bone accrual.
- Hormone replacement therapy is the central component of treatment. However, the optimal dose and delivery system are still under investigation.

References

1. Centers for Disease Control and Prevention NCfHS. CDC Growth Charts: Z-score Data Files. 2009. http://www.cdc.gov/growthcharts/zscore.htm
2. Primary ovarian insufficiency in adolescents and young women. Committee Opinion No. 605. American College of Obstetricians and Gynecologists. Obstet Gynecol. 2014;123:193–7.
3. Nelson LM. Primary ovarian insufficiency. N Engl J Med. 2009;360(6):606–14. https://doi.org/10.1056/NEJMcp0808697
4. Nelson LM, Covington SN, Rebar RW. An update: spontaneous premature ovarian failure is not an early menopause. Fertil Steril. 2005;83(5):1327–32. https://doi.org/10.1016/j.fertnstert.2004.11.059
5. Gordon CM, Kanaoka T, Nelson LM. Update on primary ovarian insufficiency in adolescents. Curr Opin Pediatr. 2015;27(4):511–9. https://doi.org/10.1097/mop.0000000000000236
6. Baker VL. Primary ovarian insufficiency in the adolescent. Curr Opin Obstet Gynecol. 2013;25(5):375–81. https://doi.org/10.1097/GCO.0b013e328364ed2a

7. Anasti JN, Kalantaridou SN, Kimzey LM, et al. Bone loss in young women with karyotypically normal spontaneous premature ovarian failure. Obstet Gynecol. 1998;91(1):12–5.
8. Cooper AR, Baker VL, Sterling EW, Ryan ME, Woodruff TK, Nelson LM. The time is now for a new approach to primary ovarian insufficiency. Fertil Steril. 2011;95(6):1890–7. https://doi.org/10.1016/j.fertnstert.2010.01.016
9. Rafique S, Sterling EW, Nelson LM. A new approach to primary ovarian insufficiency. Obstet Gynecol Clin North Am. 2012;39(4):567–86. https://doi.org/10.1016/j.ogc.2012.09.007
10. Covington SN, Hillard PJ, Sterling EW, Nelson LM. A family systems approach to primary ovarian insufficiency. J Pediatr Adolesc Gynecol. 2011;24(3):137–41. https://doi.org/10.1016/j.jpag.2010.12.004
11. Tsimaris P, Vrachnis N, Iliodromiti Z, Deligeoroglou E. Long-term followup of adolescent and young adult females with hypergonadotropic hypogonadism. Int J Endocrinol. 2012;2012:862892. https://doi.org/10.1155/2012/862892
12. Welt CK. Primary ovarian insufficiency: a more accurate term for premature ovarian failure. Clin Endocrinol (Oxf). 2008;68(4):499–509. https://doi.org/10.1111/j.1365-2265.2007.03073.x
13. Alper MM, Jolly EE, Garner PR. Pregnancies after premature ovarian failure. Obstet Gynecol. 1986;67(3 Suppl):59S–62S.
14. Tartagni M, Cicinelli E, De Pergola G, et al. Effects of pretreatment with estrogens on ovarian stimulation with gonadotropins in women with premature ovarian failure: a randomized, placebo-controlled trial. Fertil Steril. 2007;87(4):858–61.

Suggested Educational Reading, References, and Policies

Covington SN, Hillard PJ, Sterling EW, Nelson LM. A family systems approach to primary ovarian insufficiency. J Pediatr Adolesc Gynecol. 2011;24(3):137–41. https://doi.org/10.1016/j.jpag.2010.12.004
Gordon CM, Kanaoka T, Nelson LM. Update on primary ovarian insufficiency in adolescents. Curr Opin Pediatr. 2015;27(4):511–9. https://doi.org/10.1097/mop.0000000000000236
Menstruation in girls and adolescents: using the menstrual cycle as a vital sign. Committee Opinion No. 651. American College of Obstetricians and Gynecologists. Obstet Gynecol. 2015;126.
Nelson LM. Primary ovarian insufficiency. N Engl J Med. 2009;360(6):606–14. https://doi.org/10.1056/NEJMcp0808697
Primary ovarian insufficiency in adolescents and young women. Committee Opinion No. 605. American College of Obstetricians and Gynecologists. Obstet Gynecol. 2014;123:193–7.

Part III
Sexually Active Adolescents

Chapter 13
Case of a Girl with Vaginal Discharge Who Has Sex with Boys

Alison Eliscu and Gale R.Burstein

Sara is a 16-year-old female who presented to her primary care doctor's office for evaluation of vaginal discharge which started a few days ago. Sara reported that her yellow-green discharge was different than her typical vaginal discharge. She denied vaginal itching, odor, or urinary symptoms such as dysuria, urinary frequency, or urgency. Sara noted that her periods had been irregular recently, which was atypical for her. She usually had a monthly period which lasted for 5 days. Sara's last menstrual period was 3 weeks ago. However, she was now reporting irregular spotting over the last few days, especially after intercourse. On review of systems, Sara denied fever, abdominal pain, nausea, vomiting, or diarrhea.

Sara told her physician that she was not overly concerned about her discharge because she did not think she was particularly at risk for contracting a sexually transmitted infection (STI). Sara's sexual debut was at 14 years old, and she has had 3 lifetime male sexual partners, aged 15, 16, and 20 years old, respectively. She reported that she had been monogamous with her 20-year-old partner for the past 6 months. Although she had used condoms consistently in the past, Sara admitted to inconsistent condom use lately with her boyfriend. Sara believed her boyfriend had also been monogamous during this time, and she did not believe that he was experiencing any discharge, dysuria, or testicular pain. Upon further sexual history, Sara reported that she had never been pregnant and had not been treated for any prior STIs though she was not sure the last time she had been tested for infections. Sara had also never used contraception except for condoms.

A. Eliscu, M.D., F.A.A.P. (✉)
Division Chief of Adolescent Medicine, Department of Pediatrics
Stony Brook Children's Hospital, Stony Brook, NY, USA
e-mail: Allison.eliscu@stonybrookmedicine.edu

G.R. Burstein, M.D., M.P.H.
Erie County Department of Health, Buffalo, NY, USA
e-mail: gale.burstein@erie.gov

H.J. Talib (ed.), *Adolescent Gynecology*,
https://doi.org/10.1007/978-3-319-66978-6_13

Sara's physician recommended a pelvic examination to evaluate for STIs. Speculum examination revealed mucopurulent discharge from the cervix and endocervical bleeding induced by light touch with a cotton swab. Sara's physician collected endocervical samples via cotton swabs for gonorrhea, chlamydia, and trichomonas nucleic acid amplification testing. Sara's physician also performed a bimanual examination which was normal; no cervical motion tenderness, uterine tenderness, or adnexal tenderness appreciated. Sara's physician prepared a wet mount slide by placing a drop of discharge on a slide, combining it with a drop of normal saline and examined the slide under the microscope at low and high power. The wet mount slide contained multiple polymorphonuclear leukocytes, but no clue cells, trichomonads, or hyphae appreciated. The whiff test was negative. Sara's physician decided to treat her empirically for mucopurulent cervicitis with ceftriaxone 250 mg via intramuscular injection and a single oral dose of azithromycin 1 g. Before leaving the office, Sara had several questions for her physician: (1) Would she have any long-term consequences from this infection? (2) Did her boyfriend require treatment for this infection even though he reported no symptoms? (3) How could her boyfriend receive treatment since he did not have a primary care doctor?

Overview

Vaginal discharge is an extremely common complaint among adolescent females and is responsible for many primary care and gynecologic office visits. Assessment of a patient with vaginal discharge should begin with a detailed history, including the discharge color, consistency, volume, and the presence of an odor. Providers should inquire about the presence of vaginal itching or burning and the presence of any associated symptoms such as abdominal pain, nausea or vomiting, diarrhea, fever, or urinary complaints, such as dysuria, frequency, urgency, or hesitancy. Additionally, patients should be asked about recent use of antibiotics or over-the-counter products, such as douches, feminine washes, or topical antifungal medication as different products may induce vaginal irritation. Providers should also obtain a thorough sexual history to determine if an adolescent is at significant risk for contracting an STI. A detailed sexual history includes screening for the number and gender of sexual partners (both lifetime partners and within the past 2 months), types of sexual contact (oral, vaginal, and anal sex), prior STI history, consistency of condom use, and use of other forms of contraception. Having new sexual partners, multiple partners, older sexual partners, and inconsistent condom use all increase an adolescent's risk of acquiring an STI.

Differential Diagnosis

Vaginal discharge may be a marker of an STI; however, physiologic leukorrhea, which is a normal discharge comprised of mucous and desquamated cells, is more commonly responsible for discharge complaints. Physiologic leukorrhea tends to appear clear or slightly yellowish, odorless, and frequently changes in consistency and volume throughout the menstrual cycle [1]. Conversely, vaginal discharge which is malodorous or has an abnormal color is usually pathologic. Discharge can be categorized based on its source as discharge can originate from the vagina or cervix. Vaginal discharge can be further grouped into noninfectious and infectious etiologies. Noninfectious pathologic vaginal discharge may be the result of mechanical irritation from an intrauterine device; a retained foreign body like a tampon, tissue paper, or condom; chemical irritation from the use of lubricants, douches, spermicides, feminine washes, or other scented products; or an allergic reaction to products used in the genital region.

Infectious Etiologies of Vaginal Discharge

Pathologic vaginal discharge in adolescents is commonly attributed to an infectious etiology, especially among sexually active adolescents. Bacterial vaginosis (BV) is the most common infectious etiology of vaginal discharge and is caused by a shift in the normal vaginal flora, whereby anaerobic organisms (most prominently *Gardnerella vaginalis*, *Prevotella* species, *Mycoplasma hominis*, and *Mobiluncus* species) replace normal vaginal lactobacilli. Analysis of vaginal discharge in the general population demonstrated BV infection in almost one quarter of tested adolescents, though many did not report any symptoms [2]. BV is sexually associated, meaning sexual activity is a risk factor for developing BV, but the associated organisms do not appear to be sexually transmitted. Additionally, rates of bacterial vaginosis are significantly lower among females who are not sexually active. The discharge associated with BV is described as a malodorous, thin, white, or gray discharge which adheres to the vaginal walls. Bacterial vaginosis is diagnosed when at least three of the four Amsel criteria are met: (1) presence of a thin, white discharge adherent to vaginal walls; (2) presence of clue cells (epithelial cells studded by bacteria) on wet mount microscopy (Fig. 13.1); (3) vaginal pH > 4.5; and (4) presence of fishy odor before or after 10% potassium hydroxide is added to the

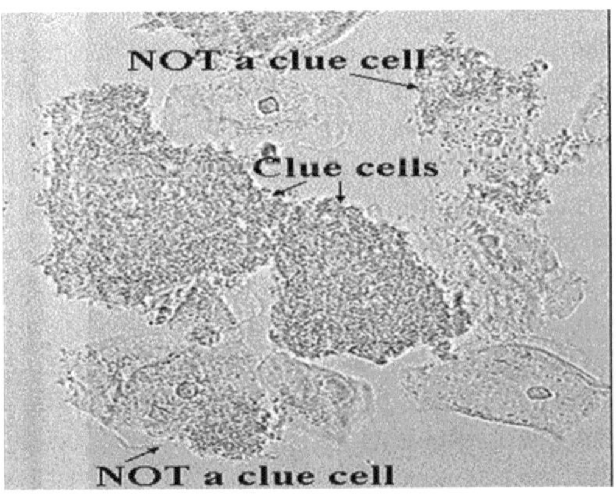

Fig. 13.1 Bacterial vaginosis on wet mount. From [18]. Seattle STD/HIV prevention training center at the University of Washington. Centers for disease control and prevention division of STD prevention. Available at http://www2a.cdc.gov/stdtraining/self-study/. Accessed August 2, 2016

discharge (positive whiff test). BV can also be diagnosed with a Clinical Laboratory Improvement Amendments (CLIA)-waived, OSOM BVBlue Test (Sekisui Diagnostics, Framingham, MA) that detects elevated levels of sialidase activity produced by BV organisms. Results are available within 10 min. The Affirm VPIII Microbial Identification Test (Becton Dickinson, Sparks, MD) is a DNA probe test that can detect *Candida* species, *Gardnerella vaginalis*, and *Trichomonas vaginalis* nucleic acid in vaginal fluid specimens from patients with symptoms of vaginitis. Results are available within 45 min. A BV vaginal culture is not recommended as it lacks specificity since many asymptomatic females are colonized with these organisms. BV can be treated with metronidazole orally or intravaginally, clindamycin intravaginally or alternatively, tinidazole or clindamycin orally [3] (see Table 13.1).

The second most common infectious etiology of vaginal discharge is vulvovaginal candidiasis (VVC), more commonly referred to as a yeast infection. VVC is caused by overgrowth of the fungal organism *Candida albicans* or less commonly *Candida glabrata* or *Candida parapsilosis*, which are all part of the normal vaginal flora. Like BV, VVC is not considered to be sexually transmitted. Risk factors for developing VVC include frequent intercourse, use of oral contraceptives, IUD use, antibiotic use, uncontrolled diabetes, immunosuppression, and pregnancy [4]. Most females are diagnosed with a yeast infection at least once during their reproductive years and frequently have recurrences. VVC presents with thick, cottage cheese-like, white, odorless vaginal discharge which tends to be pruritic. VVC is diagnosed by the presence of hyphae, pseudohyphae, or budding yeast on wet mount (Fig. 13.2), by a positive fungal culture. The Affirm VPIII Microbial Identification Test (Becton Dickinson, Sparks, MD) is a DNA probe test that can detect *Candida* species, as well as BV and *T. vaginalis*. VVC can be treated with intravaginal application of over-the-counter azole antifungal creams (such as clotrimazole 1% cream, 5 g intravaginally for 7 days or miconazole 2% cream, 5 g intravaginally for 7 days), prescription antifungal creams (like terconazole 80 mg vaginal suppository daily for 3 days), or a single oral dose of fluconazole 150 mg [3]. For a complete list of all Centers for Disease Control and Prevention (CDC)-recommended VVC treatment regimens, see www.cdc.gov/std/tg2015/candidiasis.htm.

The third most common infectious cause of vaginal discharge is trichomoniasis, caused by the sexually transmitted parasite, *T. vaginalis*. Clinical hallmarks of this infection include frothy gray or green vaginal discharge, vaginal itching, and a "strawberry cervix" caused by cervical petechiae (Fig. 13.3). Trichomonas infection can be diagnosed with trichomonas NAAT testing which is extremely sensitive (clinical sensitivity of 95–100%) and can detect the parasitic infection three to five times more often compared to wet mount microscopy [5]. The CLIA-waived OSOM Trichomonas Rapid Test (Sekishi Diagnostics, Framingham, MA) provides results in approximately 10 min with sensitivity of 82–95%. The Affirm VPIII (Becton Dickinson, Sparks, MD) is a DNA hybridization probe test that evaluates for *T. vaginalis*, *G. vaginalis*, and *Candida albicans*. The results are available within 45 min; however, sensitivity for trichomonas is only 63%. Trichomonas infection can be diagnosed by visualization of motile trichomonads on wet mount (Fig. 13.4), but alternative tests are preferred since wet mount sensitivity is incredibly low.

Table 13.1 Summary of vaginal discharge

	Physiologic leukorrhea	Bacterial vaginosis	Vulvovaginal candidiasis	Trichomoniasis	Cervicitis
Risk factors	None	Douche, new partner, multiple sexual partners, inconsistent condom use	Diabetes, antibiotic use, pregnancy, HIV disease, corticosteroid use	Multiple sexual partners, inconsistent condom use, low socioeconomicstatus	Adolescent age, new or multiple sexual partners, inconsistent condom use
Symptoms	None	Most asymptomatic, pruritus may be present	Pruritus, dysuria, dyspareunia	Pruritus, burning, dyspareunia, dysuria	Frequently asymptomatic, pruritus, dyspareunia, irregular vaginal bleeding
Discharge	Clear or white, no odor	Thin, white, or gray, malodorous, adherent to vaginal walls	Thick, white, cottage cheese-like, odorless	Gray/green, frothy, malodorous	Purulent or mucopurulent
Vulvar	Normal	Normal	Erythema, excoriations, fissures	Irritation	Normal
Cervix	Normal	Normal	Normal	Strawberry cervix	Friable
Discharge pH	<4.5	>4.5	<4.5	5–6	<4.5
Wet mount					
• WBCs	• Occasional	• Occasional	• Increased	• Increased	• Increased
• Epithelial cells	• Normal	• Clue cells	• Normal	• Normal	• Normal
• Organism	• Lactobacilli	• Bacteria adherent to cells	• Budding yeast or hyphae	• Motile trichomonads	• Normal
Whiff test	Negative	Positive	Negative	Positive	Negative
Other recommended tests		OSOM BVBlue Test, Affirm VP III, culture	Affirm VP III, culture	OSOM Trichomonas test, NAAT, Affirm VP III, culture	NAAT
Preferred treatment	None	Metronidazole oral or topical, clindamycin topical	OTC or Rx azole creams topically, fluconazole oral single dose	Single-dose oral metronidazole or tinidazole	Doxycycline × 7 days or azithromycin single dose; add ceftriaxone for GC coverage if high risk (including females <25 years)
Partner treatment	None	None	None	Recommended	Recommended

WBCs white blood cells, *NAAT* nucleic acid amplification test, *OTC* over the counter, *Rx* prescription, *GC* gonorrhea

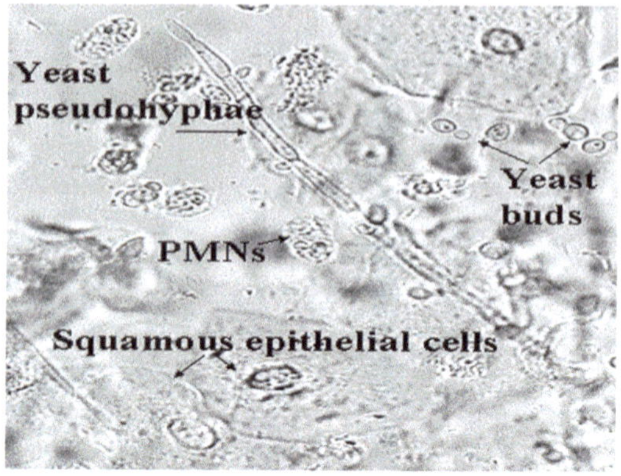

Fig. 13.2 Polymorphonuclear leukocyte and yeast pseudohyphae. From [18]. Seattle STD/HIV prevention training center at the University of Washington. Centers for disease control and prevention division of STD prevention. Available at http://www2a.cdc.gov/stdtraining/self-study/. Accessed August 2, 2016

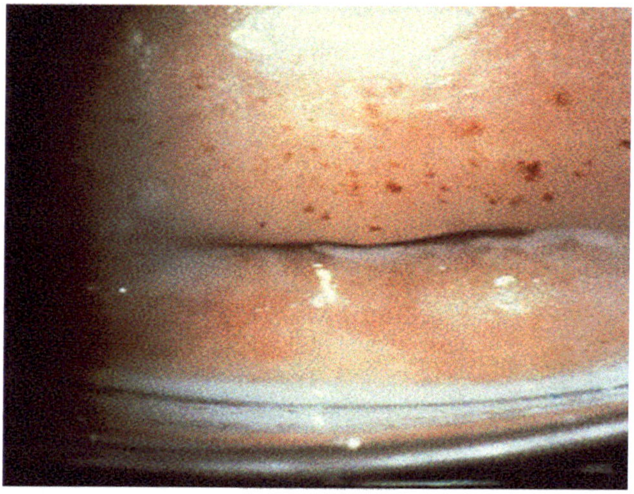

Fig. 13.3 Strawberry cervix due to trichomonas vaginalis. From [18]. Seattle STD/HIV prevention training center at the University of Washington. Centers for disease control and prevention division of STD prevention. Available at http://www2a.cdc.gov/stdtraining/self-study/. Accessed August 2, 2016

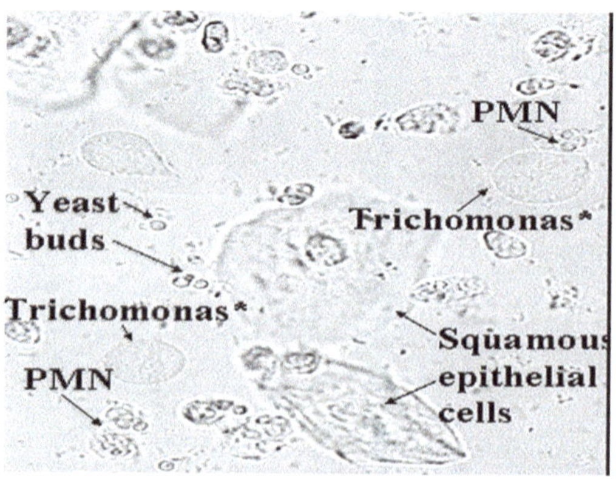

Fig. 13.4 Trichomonads and yeast buds on wet mount. From [18]. Seattle STD/HIV prevention training center at the University of Washington. Centers for disease control and prevention division of STD prevention. Available at http://www2a.cdc.gov/stdtraining/self-study/. Accessed August 2, 2016

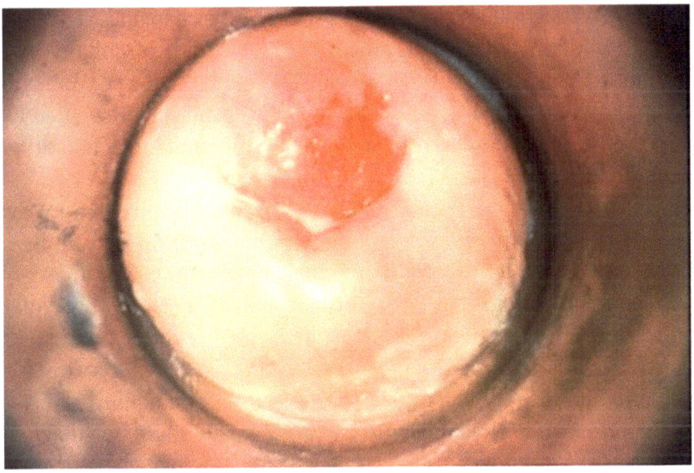

Fig. 13.5 Mucopurulent cervicitis. From [18]. Centers for Disease Control and Prevention. STD clinical slides. Atlanta, GA: U.S. Department of Health and Human Services, May 2011. Available at http://www.cdc.gov/std/training/clinicalslides/slides-dl.htm. Accessed August 2, 2016

Trichomoniasis is treated with a single oral dose of metronidazole or tinidazole and requires treatment of exposed sexual partners.

In the case described at the start of this chapter, Sara did not have malodorous discharge or clue cells on wet mount, making BV an unlikely diagnosis. She also did not have thick, cottage cheese-like discharge or green frothy malodorous discharge making VVC and trichomoniasis, respectively, unlikely as well. Sara's provider did however notice mucopurulent discharge exuding from the cervical os (Fig. 13.5) and endocervical bleeding induced by gentle touch with a swab, known as friability. With these two clinical signs, Sara meets criteria for mucopurulent cervicitis, defined as an inflammation of the cervix with mucopurulent cervical discharge. Patients with gonorrhea or chlamydial cervicitis are frequently asymptomatic though they may experience discharge, dysuria, urinary frequency, dyspareunia (pain with intercourse), or irregular vaginal bleeding most commonly following intercourse. The underlying etiology of mucopurulent cervicitis is frequently unidentified. However, when an underlying cause is determined, *Chlamydia trachomatis* and *Neisseria gonorrhoeae* are the most common infections responsible for cervicitis. Less frequently, herpes simplex virus 2 and *Trichomonas vaginalis* infections can also cause similar clinical signs. Additionally, these same symptoms can be produced by irritation from retained foreign bodies or products like douche or feminine washes.

Chlamydia trachomatis is the most common reportable communicable disease in the United States and is most prevalent among adolescents and young adults. In 2014, 66% of reported cases occurred in 15–24 year olds with over three times more infections reported among female adolescents and young adults compared to males [6]. Traditionally, risk factors for acquiring a chlamydia infection have included younger age, having a new sexual partner, earlier sexual debut, having a prior STI, or having a lower education level [7]. Additionally, non-Hispanic African American females and Latina females have significantly higher rates of chlamydia infection compared to non-Hispanic Caucasian young females [7]. Newer studies have also revealed that early smoking initiation [8], use of substances other than alcohol or marijuana weekly, and human papillomavirus infection detected at preceding appointment are also risk factors for chlamydia infection [9].

Females infected with *C. trachomatis* may present with discharge, dysuria, or irregular menstrual bleeding 7–21 days after exposure, though almost 80% of chlamydia infections are asymptomatic. Females presenting with these symptoms should be tested for *C. trachomatis* with a urine, vaginal, or cervical specimen nucleic acid amplification test (NAAT). NAAT testing, which amplifies particular nucleic acid sequences for the specific organism, is the most sensitive testing available to diagnose chlamydia. NAATs can detect shed organisms on noninvasively collected specimens like urine and self-collected vaginal swabs. Self-collected vaginal swabs are good alternatives to endocervical samples since they have been shown to be at least as accurate [10] and more acceptable to patients [11] compared to provider-obtained endocervical specimens. Despite its high specificity levels, culture testing for chlamydia is no longer used very frequently because it is expensive, requires viable organisms, and has precise transport time and media requirements so is less sensitive and has long turnaround time.

NAATs are not FDA approved for use on extragenital specimen (like oral and rectal swabs) testing despite studies demonstrating improved accuracy for NAATs compared to culture for these sites. Labs may establish CLIA-regulated specifications for use on extragenital specimens to be able to perform the test. Given that the majority of *C. trachomatis* cases are asymptomatic, it is imperative that high-risk adolescent and young adult females are screened regularly for chlamydia infections. The CDC [3], US Preventative Services Task Force [12], American Academy of Pediatrics [13], American College of Obstetricians and Gynecologists, and Society for Adolescent Health and Medicine [13] unanimously agree that all sexually active females under 25 years of age should be screened for chlamydia infections annually. In fact, some experts recommend testing high-risk females (those with multiple partners, prior STIs, or sex workers) every 6 months for chlamydia. With the use of noninvasive testing on urine or self-collected vaginal swabs, routine screening can be easily incorporated into routine annual physical exams without requiring a pelvic exam.

Females diagnosed with a *Chlamydia trachomatis* infection should be treated as soon as possible with a single dose of azithromycin 1 g orally or doxycycline 100 mg orally twice daily for 7 days. Partners of treated individuals exposed within the prior 60 days should also receive appropriate treatment, even if their chlamydia test is negative. Infected individuals should abstain from having intercourse, even with a condom, until 7 days following their treatment and all partners' treatments. A test of cure, which was traditionally collected 3–4 weeks following treatment to detect treatment failure, is not recommended for adequately treated individuals since recommended antibiotic regimens are very effective in treating chlamydia infections. In fact, performing a NAAT test within 3 weeks of treatment may produce a false-positive result since the test can detect persistent nonviable organisms which have not been cleared yet. Alternatively, patients treated for chlamydia should receive a test of reinfection 2–3 months after treatment to detect reinfection of individuals whose partners were not appropriately treated or were reexposed to chlamydia by new partners.

Rapid and appropriate treatment of chlamydia infections is of utmost importance to prevent ascension of persistent infections into the pelvic region leading to pelvic inflammatory disease (see Chap. 3, Case of a Girl with Delayed Puberty and Inflammatory Bowel Disease). Additionally, prompt treatment decreases the risk of transmission to sexual partners. Preventing transmission requires treatment of both index patient and all sexual partner(s) from the prior 60 days or most recent partner if longer than 60 days. Ideally, partners exposed to an STI are notified by the index patient, provider, or health department and referred for complete clinical evaluation with STI testing and empiric treatment for the exposed infection. However, local and state health departments usually do not have resources to undertake partner notification for chlamydia infection. Untreated partners contribute to high rates of chlamydia reinfection, especially among adolescents and young adults. One strategy which can facilitate partner treatment is expedited partner therapy (EPT), whereby providers treat the partner(s) of an STI-infected individual without examining the partner. EPT usually involves providing the index patient with medication or a prescription to deliver to their exposed partner(s). The medication is usually accompanied by an information packet describing the prescribed medication, the underlying infection to which they have been exposed, and recommending a complete STI evaluation by a provider. EPT is not an ideal method of partner treatment since partners may assume that they have been treated for all exposed infections and may not get tested for other concomitant asymptomatic infections. EPT is only recommended for use among heterosexual individuals since data are limited on the efficacy of EPT use in same gender relationships, and men who have sex with men (MSM) who are exposed to an STI have a higher risk of having an undiagnosed coinfection like HIV, which may go undiagnosed if EPT is used. As of July 2017, EPT is legally permissible in 41 states in the United States, potentially allowable in 7 states and prohibited in only 2 states (see www.cdc.gov/std/ept/legal/default.htm) [14].

Adolescents and young adults should receive counseling regularly to reduce their risk of contracting an STI like chlamydia. Providers should obtain a detailed, confidential, sexual history on individuals presenting for an annual well visit as well as those presenting for a pregnancy test and gynecological complaint (like vaginal discharge or irregular menses) or to start birth control. Additionally, young women should also receive risk reduction counseling encouraging consistent condom use, limiting the number of sexual partners, and encouraging regular STI screens to detect asymptomatic infections and prevent further transmission. Client-centered counseling and motivational interviewing can be used effectively by clinicians and trained staff to move adolescent and young adult patients toward achievable risk reduction goals. CDC provides additional information on these and other effective behavioral interventions at http://effectiveinterventions.org. Free condoms should also be easily accessible for adolescents.

Gonorrhea is the second most common reportable STI diagnosed in the United States. Like chlamydia, gonorrhea is most prevalent among young women 15–24 years of age, though young males 20–24 years of age also have fairly high rates of infection. Gonorrhea rates are also disproportionally higher in specific racial/ethnic groups: with almost 13 times higher rates in African American adolescent females compared to white females and 1.5 times higher rates in Hispanic adolescent females compared to white peers [6]. Also similar to chlamydia infections, young women infected with gonorrhea are frequently asymptomatic. When symptomatic, presenting symptoms vary based on the infection site. Females infected in the genital region may develop cervicitis with profuse mucopurulent cervical discharge and irregular vaginal bleeding. Females may also develop pharyngitis or proctitis (rectal inflammation associated with pain, rectal discharge, and tenesmus) when gonorrhea is contracted via receptive oral or anal sex, respectively.

Gonorrhea infections may be diagnosed by cell culture or NAAT testing. NAAT tests are more sensitive than culture for detection of gonorrhea but are only FDA approved for endocervical, urine, and vaginal (patient- or provider-collected) specimens. Since the majority of gonorrheal infections, especially in the adolescent and young adult populations, are asymptomatic, sexually active young females under 25 years of age should be screened annually for a gonorrhea infection [3, 12, 13]. This screening test can easily be performed on noninvasively collected specimens like urine or self-collected vaginal swabs and incorporated into a routine annual physical exam without requiring a pelvic exam. Additionally, females with symptoms of or at risk for acquiring gonococcal proctitis or pharyngitis should receive appropriate extragenital testing. NAATs are not currently FDA approved for use on extragenital specimens, though studies have demonstrated increased sensitivity for NAATs compared to culture for these sites. Some clinical labs, including the large, national, clinical labs, such as QUEST and Lab Corps, have met CLIA-specified requirements to run NAAT testing on these extragenital specimens in their lab. If NAAT testing is not available for testing extragenital sites, gonorrhea culture should be used instead. Gonorrhea culture requires specific medium (such as Thayer-Martin medium), and results are optimized when specimens are directly plated and incubated. One benefit of obtaining a gonorrhea culture is the ability to obtain antibiotic sensitivities when there is the potential for antibiotic resistance. This is especially beneficial when patients are unable to receive first-line treatments (due to cephalosporin allergy or unavailability of injectable medications) or have persistent infection despite appropriate treatment raising the suspicion of cephalosporin resistance.

Recommended antibiotic treatment regimens for the treatment of a gonococcal infection have changed over the past 10 years in response to increased gonococcal antibiotic resistance. In 1986, the Gonococcal Isolate Surveillance Project (GISP) was created as a national surveillance system to monitor antibiotic resistance among gonorrhea strains in the United States. Resistance was initially noted to quinolones with quinolone-resistant strains increasing from <1% in 1999 to 15% in 2007 [15]. In response to this change in resistance patterns, CDC subsequently recommended against the use of quinolone antibiotics to treat gonorrhea infections. In 2010, decreased cephalosporin susceptibility was noted among gonorrhea strains so the CDC recommended increased cephalosporin dosage and dual treatment with azithromycin or doxycycline in addition to a cephalosporin. Most recently, in 2015, resistance levels to cefixime increased, compelling CDC to recommend only one preferred treatment regimen for uncomplicated gonococcal infections: ceftriaxone 250 mg via intramuscular injection and a single oral dose of azithromycin 1 g [15]. Sexual partners potentially exposed to gonorrhea during the 60 days prior to treatment should be tested and receive appropriate empiric antibiotic therapy. Since injectable ceftriaxone is the only recommended treatment for gonorrhea, recommended usage of EPT for partner treatment of gonococcal-exposed individuals has changed. Ideally, partners exposed to gonorrhea should be referred for complete STI evaluation and empiric treatment with injectable ceftriaxone and oral azithromycin. If this referral is not feasible, in states where EPT is legally permissible for gonorrhea, heterosexual partners who are unlikely to receive prompt treatment can be treated via patient-delivered expedited partner therapy with a single oral dose of cefixime 400 mg and a single oral dose of azithromycin 1 g. These prescriptions should be accompanied by an information packet including information about the medications and the exposed infection and recommending complete STI evaluation [16].

STI Prevention

STIs occur in adolescent and young adults at disproportionally high rates compared to the adult populations (Fig. 13.6). Decreasing infection rates in this population hinges on risk reduction and education. Providers should regularly screen patients

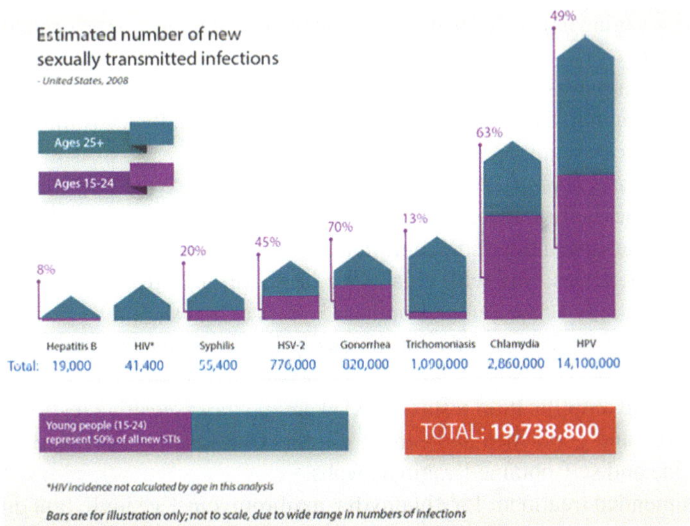

Fig. 13.6 Estimated number of new sexually transmitted infections in the United States, 2008. From [19]. Centers for Disease Control and Prevention. Available at https://www.cdc.gov/std/stats/sti-estimates-fact-sheet-feb-2013.pdf. Accessed August 2, 2016. Source: U.S. Centers for Disease Control and Prevention

with a detailed sexual history to determine their risk of contracting an infection. Individuals engaging in high-risk behaviors (such as those with multiple sexual partners, older partners or engaging in substance use or sex work) should receive brief risk reduction counseling or motivational interviewing recommending behavioral changes to decrease their risk of contracting infections. Research has shown that client-centered or motivational interviewing techniques for risk reduction counseling can increase condom use and subsequently decrease STIs in a study population [17]. Patients should be encouraged to limit their number of sexual partners and ask sexual partners to get STI tested before engaging in sexual activity. Additionally, providers should recommend consistent condom use, instruct males and females on correct condom usage techniques, and make condoms easily accessible. At-risk individuals should also be screened regularly for STIs via NAAT testing when available. For example, all sexually females under 25 years of age should be screened for chlamydia and gonorrhea annually and potentially more often if engaging in high-risk behaviors. Partners exposed to an infection should receive a complete STI evaluation and appropriate treatment, and expedited partner therapy may be an option to facilitate partner treatment.

Clinical Pearls and Pitfalls

- A common cause of vaginal discharge in adolescents is physiologic leukorrhea, presenting as clear-yellowish, odorless discharge which fluctuates in consistency and volume throughout the menstrual cycle.
- Vaginal discharge can originate from the vagina (i.e., physiologic leukorrhea, bacterial vaginosis) or from the cervix (chlamydia or gonorrhea mucopurulent cervicitis).
- Bacterial vaginosis and vulvovaginal candidiasis are the two most common causes of vaginal discharge. These entities are not sexually transmitted, but rates may be increased among sexually active individuals.
- *Chlamydia trachomatis* and *Neisseria gonorrhoeae* are the two most common reportable sexually transmitted infections. Rates of these infections are highest among adolescent and young adult females.
- Majority of adolescents with chlamydia or gonorrhea infection are asymptomatic. All sexually active females under 25 years of age should be screened annually for these infections; this can be easily incorporated into a routine annual physical.
- Nucleic acid amplification tests (NAATs) are the most sensitive tests to diagnose chlamydia and gonorrhea and can be run on noninvasively collected specimens like urine and self-obtained vaginal swabs.
- Recommended treatment for chlamydia, azithromycin 1 g single oral dose; gonorrhea, ceftriaxone 250 mg IM injection + azithromycin 1 g single oral dose.
- Expedited partner therapy (EPT) involves treating the partner(s) of an STI-infected individual without examining the partner. As of July 2017, EPT is

legally permissible in 41 states for the treatment of heterosexual individuals infected with gonorrhea or chlamydia.

- Individuals diagnosed with gonorrhea or chlamydia should receive a test of reinfection 3 months after treatment to detect individuals who were inadequately treated or reexposed to infected partner.
- It is no longer recommended to routinely perform a test of cure 3–4 weeks after treatment of gonorrhea or chlamydia to detect antibiotic treatment failures since antibiotic resistance rates to recommended regimens are fairly low.

References

1. Spence D, Melville C. Vaginal discharge. Br Med J. 2007;335(7630):1147–51.
2. Allsworth JE, Peipert JF. Prevalence of bacterial vaginosis: 2001-2004 National Health and Nutrition Examination Survey data. Obstet Gynecol. 2007;109(1):114–20.
3. Workowski KA, Bolan GA, Centers for Disease Control and Prevention. Sexually transmitted diseases treatment guidelines, 2015. MMWR Recomm Rep. 2015;64(RR-03):1–137.
4. Goncalves B, Ferreira C, Alves CT, Henriques M, Azeredo J, Silva S. Vulvovaginal candidiasis: epidemiology, microbiology and risk factors. Crit Rev Microbiol. 2015;42(6):905–27.
5. Roth AM, Williams JA, Ly R, Curd K, Brooks D, Arno J, et al. Changing sexually transmitted infection screening protocol will result in improved case finding for trichomonas vaginalis among high-risk female populations. Sex Transm Dis. 2011;38(5):398–400.
6. Centers for Disease Control and Prevention. Sexually transmitted disease surveillance, 2014. Atlanta: US Dept Health Hum Services; 2016.
7. Datta SD, Sternberg M, Johnson RE, Berman S, Papp JR, McQuillan G, et al. Gonorrhea and chlamydia in the United States among persons 14 to 39 years of age, 1999-2002. Ann Intern Med. 2007;147(2):89–96.
8. Hansen BT, Kjaer SK, Munk C, Tryggvadottir L, Sparen P, Hagerup-Jenssen M, et al. Early smoking initiation, sexual behavior and reproductive health—a large population-based study of Nordic women. Prev Med. 2010;51(1):68–72.
9. Hwang LY, Ma Y, Moscicki AB. Biological and behavioral risks for incident Chlamydia trachomatis infection in a prospective cohort. Obstet Gynecol. 2014;124(5):954–60.
10. Fang J, Husman C, DeSilva L, Chang R, Peralta L. Evaluation of self-collected vaginal swab, first void urine, and endocervical specimens for the detection of Chlamydia trachomatis and Neisseria gonorrhoeae in adolescent females. J Pediatr Adolesc Gynecol. 2008;21(6):355–60.
11. Chernesky MA, Hook EW 3rd, Martin DH, Lane J, Johnson R, Jordan JA, et al. Women find it easy and prefer to collect their own vaginal swabs to diagnose Chlamydia trachomatis or Neisseria gonorrhoeae infections. Sex Transm Dis. 2005;32(12):729–33.
12. Lefevre ML. U.S. Preventive Services Task Force. Screening for chlamydia and gonorrhea: U.S. Preventive Services Task Force recommendation statement. Ann Intern Med. 2014;161(12):902–10.
13. Committee on Adolescence, Society for Adolescent Health and Medicine. Screening for nonviral sexually transmitted infections in adolescents and young adults. Pediatrics. 2014;134(1):e302–11.
14. Centers for Disease Control and Prevention. Legal status of expedited partner therapy (EPT). http://www.cdc.gov/std/ept/legal. Accessed 28 July 2016.
15. Centers for Disease Control and Prevention. 2014 sexually transmitted diseases surveillance gonorrhea. http://www.cdc.gov/std/stats14/gonorrhea.htm. Accessed 28 July 2016.
16. Centers for Disease Control and Prevention. Guidance on the use of expedited partner therapy in the treatment of gonorrhea. http://www.cdc.gov/std/ept/gc-guidance.htm. Accessed 28 July 2016.

17. Kamb ML, Fishbein M, Douglas JM Jr, Rhodes F, Rogers J, Bolan G, et al. Efficacy of risk-reduction counseling to prevent human immunodeficiency virus and sexually transmitted diseases: a randomized controlled trial. Project RESPECT Study Group. JAMA. 1998;280(13):1161–7.
18. Seattle STD/HIV prevention training center at the University of Washington. Centers for disease control and prevention division of STD prevention. http://www2a.cdc.gov/stdtraining/self-study/. Accessed 2 Aug 2016.
19. Centers for Disease Control and Prevention. https://www.cdc.gov/std/stats/sti-estimates-fact-sheet-feb-2013.pdf. Accessed 2 Aug 2016.

Recommended Reading

Centers for Disease Control and Prevention. Sexually transmitted diseases treatment guidelines, 2015. MMWR Recomm Rep. 2015;64(RR-3):1–137.
Centers for Disease Control and Prevention. Legal status of expedited partner therapy (EPT). http://www.cdc.gov/std/ept/legal. Accessed 27 September 2017.
Committee on Adolescence, Society for Adolescent Health and Medicine. Screening for nonviral sexually transmitted infections in adolescents and young adults. Pediatrics. 2014;134(1):e302–11.

Chapter 14
Case of a Girl with Vaginal Discharge Who Has Sex with Girls

Chanelle Coble and Donna Futterman

Case

Karla is a healthy 16-year-old adolescent girl who presents for her annual physical exam with complaints of vaginal discharge. She reports 6 months of daily, malodorous, thick, yellow, vaginal discharge that has worsened in recent weeks. She notices a slight reduction in the amount and consistency of the discharge during her menses but continues to have persistent discharge that stains her undergarment. She denies the use of feminine hygiene products or douching, but she does regularly take bubble baths. She also denies any associated vulvar lesions or pruritus, dysuria, hematuria, increased urinary frequency, abdominal or pelvic pain, or intermenstrual spotting or bleeding.

Her menstrual history includes menarche at age 12 years with monthly interval cycles with up to 1 week of bleeding with mild cramping on the first 2 days of her menses, for which she takes ibuprofen as needed. Her last menstrual period was 2 weeks ago with normal flow. On confidential sexual history, she reports that she is not currently sexually active with male partners but endorsed one episode of vaginal intercourse with a male partner over 1 year ago. When asked about current sexual partners, she reluctantly discloses that she has one current female sexual partner, with whom she engages in receptive and active oral sex, genital fingering, and genital touching, without the use of barrier protection methods. She does not want her mother to know about her current partner, and she states she is "unsure" about her

C. Coble, M.D. (✉)
Department of Pediatrics, NYU School of Medicine/Bellevue Hospital, New York, NY, USA
e-mail: coblec01@nyumc.org

D. Futterman, M.D.
Adolescent AIDS Program, Einstein College of Medicine, Children's Hospital at Montefiore, Bronx, NY, USA
e-mail: DFutterman@adolescentaids.org

H.J. Talib (ed.), *Adolescent Gynecology*,
https://doi.org/10.1007/978-3-319-66978-6_14

sexual orientation and is attracted to both girls and boys. She is concerned about the discharge but is convinced it is a yeast infection because she believes that there is no way that the discharge is related to a sexually transmitted infection because she "doesn't have sex with boys anymore." She has never been pregnant and has never been tested for sexually transmitted infections.

Past medical history is unremarkable. She is not currently taking any medications and denies prior hospitalizations, ER visits, or surgeries. She lives at home with her parents and two younger sisters and reports feeling safe at home. She is an honor student and recently completed the 11th grade at a public high school. She is a member of the dance and softball teams and participates in a youth group at her church. She denies any history of suicidal thoughts but reports some depression and anxiety about her family finding out that she is exploring her sexuality and attraction to both genders. She has only disclosed this attraction to her current sexual partner but does not feel her parents will accept this.

On physical examination, she is a well-appearing healthy girl who is in no acute distress with a weight of 52 kg, height of 160 cm, and BMI of 20.3. She is afebrile with a blood pressure and heart rate of 116/72 mmHg and 72 bpm, respectively. Her HEENT and CV exams are within normal limits. On breast exam she is found to have Tanner 5 breasts without any masses or nipple discharge. Her abdomen is soft, nontender, without any suprapubic tenderness or fullness. Pelvic examination revealed normal external female genitalia with Tanner 4 pubic hair and no visible genital lesions or erythema. Speculum exam revealed thick gray malodorous discharge in the vaginal vault, nonfriable and normal appearing closed cervix. There was no cervical motion or adnexal tenderness on bimanual exam. The vaginal discharge was evaluated under direct microscopy and sent for NAAT testing for gonorrhea, chlamydia, and trichomoniasis. Her urine was sent for dipstick microscopy and HCG. After obtaining consent, her blood was screened for HIV. Karla wonders, what is the likely cause of her vaginal discharge? Is she at risk for sexually transmitted infection given that she only has a female sexual partner? Is there any routine gynecologic care that girls with female sexual partners should have at their annual health visits?

Discussion

Adolescent young women who have sex with women (WSW) and women who have sex with women and men (WSWM) are a subpopulation of women with unique sexual and health concerns [1]. Many of these young women are often not identified as such by health-care providers because of the providers' assumption of heterosexuality when taking sexual histories and the lack of sexual behavior disclosure [2]. Although these women were commonly believed to be at low risk for STIs, studies have demonstrated that WSW have disease rates similar to their heterosexual counterparts [3]. According to the National Survey of Family Growth, about 12.5% of American women aged 15–44 years have engaged in sexual activities with

Table 14.1 Obtaining a culturally sensitive sexual history

Dimension assessed	Sample questions
Sexuality	• Are you dating anybody?
	• Are you involved in any romantic relationship?
	• Tell me about your partner
Sexual behavior	• Have you ever had sex? What have you done sexually with a partner?
	• Have you ever had oral sex? Has a partner ever "gone down" on you or have you ever "gone down" on a partner?
	• Have you ever had vaginal sex? Have you ever engaged in penile-vaginal sex or insertive sex with hands or sex toys?
	• Have you ever had anal sex? Did you put your penis in your partner's anus or did your partner put his penis in your anus?
	• *If there was any insertive or receptive sex:* Do you use condoms? What percentage of the time? What about last time?
	• *If there was any oral-genital contact:* Do you use dental dam or another barrier? What percentage of the time? What about last time?
Sexual attraction	• Tell me about your partner?
	• Are you sexually attracted to men, women, both, or unsure?
Sexual orientation	• Do you consider yourself to be: heterosexual or straight, gay or lesbian, bisexual, questioning, queer, trans, something else?

Adapted from Levine DA, Adolescence CO. Office-based care for lesbian, gay, bisexual, transgender, and questioning youth. Pediatrics 2013;132:e297–313 and SMART 2009 guidelines (pp. 25–26)

other women at some point during their lifetime, while only 4.1% of those surveyed (ages 18–44) self-identify as being homosexual, gay, lesbian, or bisexual [4]. The discordance between sexual behavior and sexual identity can make it challenging to correctly identify this population. Also, the emergence and visibility of transgender and gender nonconforming youth within the past decade has further complicated the picture for youth and providers seeking to properly provide care. For example, a young female who is having sex with a female partner may not disclose that her partner is a transgender female (born male) which can impact the needed health screening and anticipatory guidance.

That is why is it important for clinicians who care for sexual minority adolescent young women to obtain an accurate and culturally sensitive sexual history that explores all three dimensions of sexual identity: sexual attraction, sexual behavior, and sexual orientation. Table 14.1 includes a summary of questions that can be used by providers to obtain a culturally sensitive sexual history. Using gender neutral terms and open-ended questions can help to facilitate a conversation with the adolescent patient that allows for honesty and trust. For all adolescents, confidentiality should be ensured and must be emphasized at all levels of the clinic staff [5]. Written confidentiality statements should be made available to patients, but it is also important for medical providers to verbalize confidentiality to their adolescent patients.

If a young woman has expressed history of sexual activity, it is important to explore the various types of sexual behaviors she engages, as well as, the gender of those partners. Assessment of sexual behavior should be done first by starting with an open-ended question like, "have you ever had sex?" or "what have you done sexually with a partner?" [5]. Once a young woman discloses that she has a female sexual partner, it is important to explore her specific sexual practices with that partner. While research is limited about the prevalence of specific sexual practices that adolescent WSW engage in with their female sexual partners, accurate histories should be sought in each clinical encounter. Qualitative research in adult WSW has shown that these women frequently report oral sex, digital penetration "fingering," and vaginal grinding or bumping as common sexual practices and less frequently the use of sexual toys [6]. It is important to note that not all WSW engage in oral sexual intercourse with their female partners, and providers should not assume that this is a sexual behavior for their WSW patients. Table 14.1 also includes detailed sexual behavior questions that include the types of sexual intercourse (oral, vaginal, anal, etc.) that young women may engage in. If practicing oral sex, patients should be encouraged to use a barrier such as a dental dam or plastic wrap. When using sex toys, such as dildos and vibrators, patients should be instructed to clean and disinfect them after use and cover them with a condom during sex when possible.

Although WSW may have lower risk of HIV/AIDS than women who have sex with men (WSM), it is important for these women to practice safe sex. There is limited data on the risk for STI transmission between female sexual partners. The risk of STI is thought to vary by the specific STI and sexual practice (e.g., oral-genital sex; vaginal or anal sex using hands, fingers, or penetrative sex items; oral-anal sex) [3]. Practices involving digital-vaginal or digital-anal contact, particularly with shared penetrative sex items, present a possible means for transmission of infected cervicovaginal secretions [7]. This is complicated by the fact that majority of WSW also report sexual history with male partners, therefore, increasing the risks acquiring STIs from their male partners and transmitting them to their female partners [8]. Report of same-sex behavior in women should not deter providers from considering and performing screening for STIs [8].

Several studies have shown that adult populations of WSW have significant rates of STIs such as chlamydia and trichomoniasis. The CDC recommends screening *T. vaginalis* in women seeking care for vaginal discharge and also recommends screening once for HIV in all persons older than 13 years of age and annually or sooner for those at high risk for infection that includes women who have new or multiple partners, have a history of STDs, exchange sex for payment, or use injection drugs [7]. In large study of over 9000 sexually active women, ages 15–24, presenting for care at a family planning clinic, *C. trachomatis* positivity among the WSW and WSMW participants was 7.1% compared with 5.3% among the purely WSM [9]. Risks for *C. trachomatis* positivity were comparable across groups and included younger age (<20 years), nonwhite race/ethnicity, new sex partner, symptomatic sex partner, and current clinical symptoms [9]. The reports of same-sex only behavior in women should not deter providers from screening these women for STIs including chlamydia [7]. The CDC and the USPSTF recommend routine annual screening for *C. trachomatis* in all sexually active female aged ≤25 years (Grade B recommendation) [7].

Table 14.2 Summary of STI and other infections affecting WSW can site USPSTF and CDC

Infection/condition	Recommend screening test(s)	Screening frequency
Trichomoniasis	NAAT (APTIMA *T. vaginalis* Assay)	Annually and if symptomatic
	Clinical diagnosis (wet mount)	
C. trachomatis	NAAT	Annual screening for all sexually active women age ≤25 (Grade B recommendation)
	Chlamydia culture	
Human papillomavirus (HPV)	HPV DNA detection via PCR	Screening as per CDC guidelines
HSV-2	Clinical diagnosis	No routine screening recommended (Grade D recommendation)
	Cell culture	
	PCR	
	HSV-2 serology(IgG)	
Human immunodeficiency Virus (HIV)	Antigen/antibody combination immunoassay that detects HIV-1 and HIV-2 antibodies	Universal screening at baseline and annually if ongoing risk
Bacterial vaginosis	Clinical diagnosis (wet mount)	No routine screening in nonpregnant women or adolescents recommended
	Amsel's criteria or Gram stain	
	DNA probe assay for detecting *G. vaginalis*	
Candida vulvovaginitis	Clinical diagnosis (wet mount)	No routine screening recommended
	Gram stain	

Other common causes of vaginal discharge in WSW are bacterial vaginosis (BV) and candidiasis [10, 11]. The etiology of BV remains uncertain, but is characterized by disruption of the normal vaginal microbiome which includes a depletion of lactobacilli and overgrowth of anaerobic and highly fastidious bacteria that include *Gardnerella*, *Prevotella* species, *Mycoplasma hominis*, *Bacteroides* spp., *Peptostreptococcus* spp., *Fusobacterium* spp., *Mobiluncus* spp., and *Atopobium vaginae* [12]. A large representative sample of US adolescent and adult women ages 14–49 found that almost one third of women (29%) were positive for BV and that higher prevalence rates were associated with increasing age, Black and Hispanic race, low socioeconomic status, and recent history of douching [12]. A convenience sample of African-American WSW women seeking care at a STD clinic in Mississippi found that of the almost 200 women recruited, almost half (47.4%) were diagnosed with BV [10]. They also found that BV infection was almost twice as likely in women with bisexual identity, douching in the past 30 days, and report of more than one lifetime male partner [10]. There is no routine screening recommended for BV in asymptomatic WSW (see Table 14.2 for summary of diagnostic testing for BV), but we recommend that any WSW who presents with complaints of vaginal discharge should be screened for BV.

Vulvovaginal candidiasis (VVC) is a common vaginal syndrome among WSW and is often associated with larger number of female partners, but there has been debate about whether VVC can be sexually transmitted [11]. Risk of VVC is increased in women who identify as being bisexual, women who have large number of female sexual partners and history of sexual intercourse with a male partner in the past 12 months, as well as women who have recently used antibiotics leading to a disruption in the normal vaginal microbiome and overgrowth of candida [11]. The contribution of sexual transmission of genital *Candida* spp. among female sexual partner remains unclear with little evidence to support the link between sexual activity among women and symptomatic or asymptomatic VVC [11]. A British study of over 700 WSW found that there were increasing odds of candidiasis with greater numbers of female sexual partners suggesting the possibility that *Candida* species could be sexually transmitted between women [11]. However, a recent mixed methods study by Munzy et al. demonstrated that there is lack of evidence for sexual transmission of genital *Candida* species among WSW [13].

There are also other sexual and health disparities exist among WSW that include having higher rates of unplanned pregnancies, depression, and intimate partner violence (IPV) than non-WSW women. A national representative samples of high school girls in the USA have shown that lesbian and bisexual girls are less likely to use condoms or other pregnancy prevention methods during recent sexual intercourse [14]. These high school girls also have unplanned pregnancy rates comparable and in some cases higher rates than their heterosexual peers. Adolescent WSW are vulnerable to unplanned pregnancy when engaging in sex with male partner, and the American Academy of Pediatrics (AAP) recommends that medical providers for adolescents provide access to comprehensive sexual health information and for sexually active adolescents, including gay and lesbian adolescents [15]. The American College of Obstetricians and Gynecologists (ACOG) and the AAP recommend offering long-acting reversible contraception (LARC) methods as a first-line contraception option for sexually active adolescent girls [15, 16]. It is recommended that medical providers that provide care for adolescent WSW offer the same contraception counseling that he/she would for adolescents reporting opposite sex behaviors. Counseling should start with the highly effective LARC methods first. Do not assume that adolescent girls reporting same-sex behaviors are not interested in contraception counseling. On the other hand, resistance to discussion of birth control might be a signal to the provider to find out why the young woman is not interested and may lead to disclosure about same-sex only experience. This is a clear example of the "art" of medicine, as young women who identify as a lesbian but also have sex with men may believe the myth that their lesbian identity is sufficient for birth control.

There is a strong link between adolescent sexual orientation and suicidal thoughts and behaviors [17]. The strong effect of sexual orientation on suicidal thoughts is mediated by critical youth suicide risk factors, including depression, hopelessness, alcohol abuse, recent suicide attempts by a peer or a family member, and experiences of victimization [17]. Research among sexual minority youth shows that these teens have anywhere from two to three times greater risk of depression and suicidality than their heterosexual peers [18]. The updated ACOG statement on depression screening in 2015 highlighted how depression also impacts women who aren't pregnant and the unique advantage gynecologist have in identifying and diagnosing depression in their patients [19]. Their recommendation is routine mental health screening in all routine gynecologic visits [19].

Intimate partner violence (IPV) is a significant preventable public health problem that affects millions of women regardless of age, economic status, race, religion, ethnicity, sexual orientation, or educational background [20]. IPV describes a pattern of coercive behavior that establishes power and control and may include physical violence, sexual violence and assaults, emotional violence, progressive isolation, deprivation, intimidation, and reproductive coercion [21]. Research has demonstrated that sexual minority adolescents have greater of odds of IPV and physical dating violence victimization than their heterosexual peers [22, 23]. Among sexual minority youth, those who have had sexual contact with both sexes (behaviorally bisexual) have greater odds of IPV than youths with same-sex-only sexual contact [23]. The US Department of Health and Human Services has recommended that IPV screening and counseling should be a core part of women's preventive health visits [20]. ACOG recommends that physicians screen all women and adolescents for IPV at periodic intervals, offer ongoing support, and review available preventative and referral options [20].

Conclusions

Results from direct microscopy of the vaginal discharge from our case were consistent with a diagnosis of bacterial vaginosis. Karla was treated with a 7-day course of metronidazole and her symptoms resolved. Her STI screening for gonorrhea and chlamydia and HIV were all negative. Her depression and screening for IPV were also negative. Although not indicated for our current case, the CDC recommends routine cervical cancer screening to all women over the age of 21 years, regardless of sexual preference or sexual practices in accordance with the current guidelines [7]. She was counseled on her contraceptive options and declined initiating a hormonal contraceptive at this visit. She was encouraged to use barrier protection when engaging in sexual intercourse with her partner and given information about community-based LGBTQ peer support groups for high school girls in her city.

Adolescent WSW are a unique group of young women with diverse sexual health needs and who are often presumed to be at low or no risk for STIs because of medical provider bias and presumptions of heterosexuality. Sexual histories for adolescent girls should include all three dimensions of sexual identity, and reporting same-sex behavior should not deter providers from considering and performing screening for STIs, offering contraception counseling including provision of LARC methods, and screening for depression and IPV. Problematic vaginal discharge may be a common gynecologic complaint among these girls, and anticipatory guidance and counseling on the use of barrier methods, hand and sexual instrument hygiene, and the risk of acquisition of sexually transmitted infections should be included in the counseling for these girls. Even with the unique challenges faced by sexual minority youth, the majority grow up healthy and lead happy, productive lives.

Clinical Pearls and Pitfalls

- Adolescent WSW are a unique group of young women with diverse sexual experiences and sexual identities.
- These girls may be at increased risk of unplanned pregnancies and STIs.
- Sexual histories for these girls should include the use of gender neutral terms, open-ended questions, and the three dimensions of sexual identity in a manner that facilitates honesty and trust while ensuring confidentiality. Never assume heterosexuality!
- A detailed sexual history should also include questions on the specific types of sexual behaviors, as well as, the gender of sexual partners.
- Problematic vaginal discharge may be a common gynecologic complaint among these girls, and they should be evaluated for BV and candida vulvovaginitis as appropriate.
- All adolescent WSW should be offered annual chlamydia screening and HIV testing as per CDC guidelines.
- Adolescent WSW should routinely be offered contraception counseling, including provision of LARC methods.
- Universal screening for depression and IPV should be included in routine gynecologic care visits.
- Adolescent WSW should be encouraged to use barrier contraceptive methods.
- Referral to local community-based LGBTQ peer support groups for these girls could also be helpful in ensuring their health and wellbeing.

References

1. Institute of Medicine Committee on Lesbian GBaTHIaRGaO. The National Academies Collection: reports funded by National Institutes of Health. The Health of Lesbian, Gay, Bisexual, and Transgender People: building a foundation for better understanding. Washington, DC: National Academies Press (US) National Academy of Sciences; 2011.
2. Diamant AL, Schuster MA, McGuigan K, Lever J. Lesbians' sexual history with men: implications for taking a sexual history. Arch Intern Med. 1999;159:2730–6.
3. Fethers K, Marks C, Mindel A, Estcourt CS. Sexually transmitted infections and risk behaviours in women who have sex with women. Sex Transm Infect. 2000;76:345–9.
4. Chandra A, Mosher WD, Copen C, Sionean C. Sexual behavior, sexual attraction, and sexual identity in the United States: data from the 2006-2008 National Survey of Family Growth. Natl Health Stat Rep. 2011:1–36.
5. Levine DA, Adolescence CO. Office-based care for lesbian, gay, bisexual, transgender, and questioning youth. Pediatrics. 2013;132:e297–313.
6. Muzny CA, Harbison HS, Pembleton ES, Austin EL. Sexual behaviors, perception of sexually transmitted infection risk, and practice of safe sex among southern African American women who have sex with women. Sex Transm Dis. 2013;40:395–400.
7. Workowski KA, Bolan GA. Sexually transmitted diseases treatment guidelines, 2015. MMWR Recomm Rep. 2015;64:1–137.

8. Gorgos LM, Marrazzo JM. Sexually transmitted infections among women who have sex with women. Clin Infect Dis. 2011;53(Suppl 3):S84–91.
9. Singh D, Fine DN, Marrazzo JM. Chlamydia trachomatis infection among women reporting sexual activity with women screened in Family Planning Clinics in the Pacific Northwest, 1997 to 2005. Am J Public Health. 2011;101:1284–90.
10. Muzny CA, Sunesara IR, Austin EL, Mena LA, Schwebke JR. Bacterial vaginosis among African American women who have sex with women. Sex Transm Dis. 2013;40:751–5.
11. Bailey JV, Benato R, Owen C, Kavanagh J. Vulvovaginal candidiasis in women who have sex with women. Sex Transm Dis. 2008;35(6):533.
12. Allsworth JE, Peipert JF. Prevalence of bacterial vaginosis: 2001-2004 National Health and Nutrition Examination Survey data. Obstet Gynecol. 2007;109:114–20.
13. Muzny CA, Rivers CA, Parker CJ, Mena LA, Austin EL, Schwebke JR. Lack of evidence for sexual transmission of genital Candida species among women who have sex with women: a mixed methods study. Sex Transm Infect. 2014;90:165–70.
14. Riskind RG, Tornello SL, Younger BC, Patterson CJ. Sexual identity, partner gender, and sexual health among adolescent girls in the United States. Am J Public Health. 2014;104:1957–63.
15. Ott MA, Sucato GS, COMMITTEE ON ADOLESCENCE. Contraception for adolescents. Pediatrics. 2014;134:e1244–56.
16. Committee on Adolescent Health Care Long-Acting Reversible Contraception Working Group, The American College of Obstetricians and Gynecologists. Committee opinion no. 539: adolescents and long-acting reversible contraception: implants and intrauterine devices. Obstet Gynecol. 2012;120:983–8.
17. Russell ST, Joyner K. Adolescent sexual orientation and suicide risk: evidence from a national study. Am J Public Health. 2001;91:1276–81.
18. Marshal MP, Dietz LJ, Friedman MS, et al. Suicidality and depression disparities between sexual minority and heterosexual youth: a meta-analytic review. J Adolesc Health. 2011;49:115–23.
19. ACOG Statement on Depression Screening. 2015. http://www.acog.org/About-ACOG/News-Room/Statements/2015/ACOG-Statement-on-Depression-Screening. Accessed 22 Dec 2015.
20. ACOG Committee Opinion No. 518: intimate partner violence. Obstet Gynecol. 2012;119:412–7.
21. Chamberlain L, Levenson R. Reproductive health and partner violence guidelines: an integrated response to intimate partner violence and reproductive coercion. San Francisco: Family Violence Prevention Fund; 2010.
22. Martin-Storey A. Prevalence of dating violence among sexual minority youth: variation across gender, sexual minority identity and gender of sexual partners. J Youth Adolesc. 2015;44:211–24.
23. Luo F, Stone DM, Tharp AT. Physical dating violence victimization among sexual minority youth. Am J Public Health. 2014;104:e66–73.

Suggested Reading

CDC Sexually Transmitted Disease Treatment Guidelines 2015—Special Populations: WSW

Workowski KA, Bolan GA. Sexually transmitted diseases treatment guidelines, 2015. MMWR Recomm Rep. 2015;64:1–137. http://www.cdc.gov/std/tg2015/specialpops.htm

ACOG Committee Opinion 525: Health Care for Lesbians and Bisexual Women

ACOG Committee on Health Care for Underserved Women. ACOG Committee Opinion No. 525: health care for lesbians and bisexual women. Obstet Gynecol. 2012;119(5):1077. http://www.acog.org/Resources-And-Publications/Committee-Opinions/Committee-on-Health-Care-for-Underserved-Women/Health-Care-for-Lesbians-and-Bisexual-Women

Chapter 15
Case of a Girl with Lower Abdominal Pain

Megan Jacobs and Paritosh Kaul

Case

Juliet is a 16-year-old female who presents to the office complaining of lower abdominal pain for 5 days. Her pain increased progressively and was mildly relieved by ibuprofen. Juliet denies fevers, nausea, vomiting, diarrhea, constipation, back pain, dysuria, or hematuria. In addition, she denies vaginal discharge and does have some discomfort during sexual activity. She has been with her current partner for the past 6 months. She has had oral and vaginal sex, and they use condoms. Juliet is also using a 52 mg levonorgestrel intrauterine device (IUD) for birth control for the past 1 year with very light irregular menses about every 2–3 months since its placement. Her last menstrual period was 2 weeks ago and has a typical light period without cramping. She had chlamydia 1 year ago with a previous partner for which she was treated. Juliet has had three lifetime male sexual partners since coitarche at the age of 15. She denies history of sexual abuse or assault.

Physical exam: Temperature 38.2 °C, pulse 82 bpm, blood pressure 106/74 mmHg, weight 142 lb, and BMI 23.6 kg/m^2.

Significant physical findings: Right lower quadrant (RLQ) abdominal tenderness and no rigidity or guarding or rebound tenderness. Normal bowel sounds. No masses palpable. No costovertebral angle tenderness. Head and neck, cardiac, lung, and musculoskeletal examinations are normal.

Pelvic exam: Normal appearing vulva and no lesions nor visible discharge. Speculum exam reveals normal vaginal mucosa and moderate amount of thin white fluid adherent to the mucosa of the vagina and vulva. Cervix: ectropion present

M. Jacobs, M.D., F.A.A.P. (✉) • P. Kaul, M.D.
Section of Adolescent Medicine, Department of Pediatrics, University of Colorado – School of Medicine, Children's Hospital Colorado, Aurora, CO, USA
e-mail: megan.jacobs@childrenscolorado.org; paritosh.kaul@childrenscolorado.org

H.J. Talib (ed.), *Adolescent Gynecology*,
https://doi.org/10.1007/978-3-319-66978-6_15

Table 15.1 Differential diagnosis of lower abdominal pain in an adolescent female [1]

Gynecologic
Pregnancy—intrauterine or ectopic
Ovarian torsion
Ovarian cyst—simple, complex, or ruptured
Cervicitis
Pelvic inflammatory disease ± abscess
Fitz-Hugh-Curtis syndrome
Dysmenorrhea
Endometriosis
Fibroadenoma/leiomyoma
Vaginal foreign body
Vaginal trauma
Sexual assault/abuse
Gastrointestinal
Small bowel obstruction
Postoperative adhesions
Inflammatory bowel disease
Irritable bowel syndrome
Constipation
Urinary
Cystitis
Pyelonephritis
Nephrolithiasis
Oncologic
Tumor

friable and thicker yellowish discharge seems to be coming from the os. Blue IUD strings are visible ~2 cm in length. On bimanual exam, Juliet has cervical motion tenderness and right adnexal tenderness.

Clinical Decision-Making Considerations

1. What Is Your Differential Diagnosis and Why?

   The differential diagnosis for Juliet's presentation is pelvic inflammatory disease (PID), ovarian cyst, cystitis, or pregnancy. Other etiologies that are less common for this patient are listed in Table 15.1. These should be considered in the differential diagnosis for general presentations of lower abdominal pain in an adolescent female (Fig. 15.1).

   (a) PID is the best fitting diagnosis because the patient is sexually active and complaining of dyspareunia (pain with sex) and lower abdominal pain without overt symptoms of alternative diagnostic process that can be evaluated in

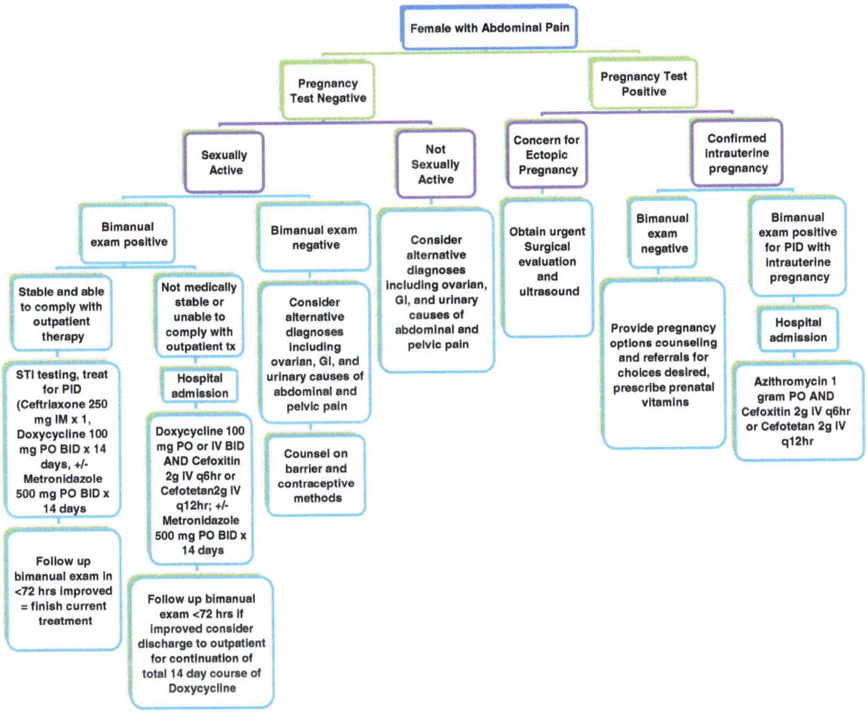

Fig. 15.1 Algorithm for diagnosis and management of pelvic inflammatory disease

the office. She has cervical motion tenderness and right adnexal tenderness as well as evidence of cervical inflammation on speculum exam with purulent discharge.

(b) Ovarian simple and hemorrhagic cysts with or without rupture can cause a ranging severity of focal lower abdominal pain and should be evaluated by ultrasound. If ruptured, the cystic fluid can settle to the retro-uterine pouch and become irritating to the surrounding tissue until it is reabsorbed. Rupture of a cyst is often exquisitely painful and can be followed by vaginal bleeding. On bimanual exam, ovarian pain or pain at the posterior fornix can be difficult to differentiate from PID. The patient in this case also has evidence of purulent discharge and a friable-appearing cervix. Neither of which would be present if pelvic pain was secondary to an ovarian cyst.

(c) Cystitis should be considered based on the location of the patient's pain. This is often difficult for patients to differentiate from uterine compression discomfort on exam. Key features of typical urinary tract infection include dysuria, urgency, frequency, and hematuria. The pain is often described as colicky in nature and limited to the suprapubic region. Juliet's history and exam were not consistent with this diagnosis.

(d) Pregnancy, including the potential of an ectopic pregnancy, should always be ruled out in all cases. Since Juliet has an IUD, her risk of pregnancy is

Table 15.2 Diagnostic tests in the work-up for pelvic inflammatory disease [1]

Pregnancy test
Gonorrhea and chlamydia NAAT test
Wet mount microscopic exam of vaginal fluid
Additional but not required for PID: CBC with differential, CRP, ESR, pelvic ultrasound
Additional testing for STIs: HIV, syphilis, and trichomonal testing

extremely low. Additionally, she is not experiencing abnormal bleeding, vital sign abnormalities, nor is her pain severe. She has a nonsurgical abdomen, making an ectopic pregnancy, as well as other emergent processes such as ovarian torsion, appendicitis, or ileus, less likely.

2. What Is the Most Likely Diagnosis in Juliet's Case and Why?

   Pelvic inflammatory disease is the patient's diagnosis. Juliet's lower abdominal pain in the setting of sexual activity and lack of other symptoms suggesting an alternative process brings PID to the top of the diagnostic list. Diagnostic criteria for PID are met by findings of the bimanual exam, which is indicated in all sexually active patients presenting for abdominal pain. Diagnostic criteria for PID are described in "Discussion" section of this chapter. An incidentally concomitant process has not been ruled out, such as ovarian cyst, constipation, or cystitis. Clinical judgment should be utilized at the time of the visit to determine if further work-up is required.
3. What Diagnostic Tests Are Indicated? (Table 15.2)

   In all patients presenting with abdominal pain, a pregnancy test should always be performed. Juliet has an IUD; therefore, it is highly unlikely that she is pregnant and is confirmed by the negative pregnancy test. During the pelvic exam, a vaginal swab of the discharge is obtained to test for gonorrhea and chlamydia via nucleic acid amplification test (NAAT). This test result will not be available during the patient encounter and should not change management. Juliet should be treated on the day of presentation as should all patients when the diagnosis is PID. Sexually transmitted infection (STI) testing should always be obtained prior to any treatment.

   Additionally during the exam, a second swab of vaginal fluid is obtained to perform a wet mount. Microscopic exam demonstrates >30 white blood cells per high-power field (hpf), 5 red blood cells/hpf, >20% clue cells, no trichomonad visualized, and a pH of 6.0 with a positive "whiff test" on KOH application. Juliet has just been diagnosed with a second condition based on these findings: bacterial vaginosis (BV) by Amsel criteria. The Amsel criteria are a set of four conditions that must be present: a homogenous, nonviscous milky-white discharge adherent vaginal walls, vaginal pH >4.5, >20% per hpf of "clue cells" (epithelial cells speckled with bacteria), and positive amine or "whiff" test when 10% KOH solution is applied to vaginal fluid. Greater or equal to three out of the four of these criteria indicates a diagnosis of bacterial vaginosis (a vaginal bacterial overgrowth syndrome). BV on its own does not cause inflammation in the vagina,

Table 15.3 Diagnostic criteria for pelvic inflammatory disease [1, 4]

Minimal criteria for diagnosis	*Additional diagnostic criteria*	*Definitive diagnostic criteria*
If 1+ of the following are found	Fever >101 °F or 38.3 °C	Endometrial biopsy with evidence of endometritis
Cervical motion tenderness	Abundant white blood cells on wet mount of vaginal fluid	Transvaginal ultrasound/MRI showing thickened fluid-filled fallopian tubes ± free pelvic fluid or tubo-ovarian complex
Adnexal tenderness	Elevated ESR or CRP	Gold standard: Laparoscopy demonstrating fallopian tube erythema or mucopurulent exudates
Uterine tenderness	Mucopurulent discharge or cervical friability	
	Positive cervical *Neisseria gonorrhea* or *Chlamydia trachomatis* documentation	

which makes the amount of white blood cells seems concerning and even more consistent with PID. The presence of an IUD can increase the number of WBC seen on vaginal fluid smear due to the induction of a mild local foreign body reaction [2]. However, seeing large amounts of WBC is concerning for sexually transmitted infection [3].

See Table 15.3: PID diagnostic criteria

4. What Treatment, if Any, Is Indicated at Today's Visit?

Treatment guidelines for PID cover presumed gonorrhea and chlamydia with consideration for anaerobic bacteria as well. In the clinic, the patient should receive 250 mg ceftriaxone intramuscularly and be given a prescription for doxycycline 100 mg twice a day for a 2-week (14 day) course. In this case, Juliet also has BV, which, in isolation, is treated with 500 mg of metronidazole orally for 7 days twice a day. However, in the setting of PID, the Center for Disease Control (CDC) recommends extending the treatment for a total of 14 days. Studies have found aerobic bacteria associated with BV in the fallopian tubes on laparoscopy of asymptomatic women treated with standard second-generation cephalosporin and doxycycline antibiotics [5]. There is, therefore, a suggested recommendation to broaden PID treatment to triple antibiotic therapy by adding metronidazole for a 14-day course to cover for anaerobic bacteria [1].

See Table 15.4 for antibiotic treatment recommendations in PID.

5. Intrauterine Devices in Adolescents with PID

PID is often diagnosed in locations and by providers who may not be as familiar with intrauterine devices (IUDs). Important knowledge for this case is that IUDs are not only safe and effective in adolescents but that if present during PID diagnosis should be left in place. The American College of Obstetricians and Gynecologists (ACOG) and the American Academy of Pediatrics (AAP) both have approved of these contraceptives in the teen and young adult populations as well as older women [6, 7]. If PID is diagnosed in an individual with an IUD

Table 15.4 Antibiotic treatment for PID [1, 4]

Outpatient therapy regimens				
Ceftriaxone 250 mg IM × 1	+	Doxycycline 100 mg PO q12 h × 14 days	±	Metronidazole 500 mg PO q12 h × 14 days
Cefoxitin 2 g IM × 1 AND probenecid 1 g PO	+	Doxycycline 100 mg PO q12 h × 14 days	±	Metronidazole 500 mg PO q12 h × 14 days
Other third-generation cephalosporin (ceftizoxime or cefotaxime)	+	Doxycycline 100 mg PO q12 h × 14 days	±	Metronidazole 500 mg PO q12 h × 14 days
Inpatient therapy regimens				
Cefotetan 2 g IV q12 h[a]	±	Doxycycline 100 mg PO or IV[b] q12 h		
Cefoxitin 2 g IV q6 h[a]	±	Doxycycline 100 mg PO or IV[b] q12 h		
Clindamycin 900 mg IV q8 h[a]	±	Gentamicin 2 mg/kg loading dose IV/IM	Gentamicin maintenance dose 1.5 mg/kg q8 h or 3–5 mg/kg/day single dose	

[a]Duration of therapy for 24–48 h after clinical improvement; oral doxycycline should be continued for a total treatment course of 14 days
[b]IV doxycycline infusions are known to be painful, when able administer PO

in place, the device does not have to be removed prior, during, or after antibiotic treatment. There is even evidence to suggest that women with IUDs have decrease risk of acquiring PID by thinning the endometrium and thickening cervical mucus [8]. It is important to keep the patient's highly effective method of pregnancy prevention and treat her infection separately.

6. What Are the Next Steps in Management?

   Juliet should return within 72 h for repeat vital signs and abdominal and bimanual exams. If symptoms and exam are improved at that time, then Juliet should continue her doxycycline and metronidazole treatment and have repeat STI testing in 3 months if either gonorrhea or chlamydia was positive at the time of PID diagnosis. Additionally, sexual partners within the past 60 days of Juliet's symptom onset should be evaluated, tested, and empirically treated for gonorrhea and chlamydia infections (ceftriaxone 250 mg IM + azithromycin 1 g PO for urethritis/cervicitis) [1]. If the last time Juliet had sex was >60 days ago, then her most recent sexual partner should still be treated. Juliet and any partners should be advised to abstain from sexual intercourse during symptoms and treatment and for 7 days after current partner is treated, whichever is longer.

7. When Would Juliet Require Hospitalization?

   See Ta le 15.5 for hospitalization criteria for PID.

Table 15.5 Hospitalization criteria for pelvic inflammatory disease [1]

Pregnancy
Surgical emergency
Tubo-ovarian abscess
Severe illness (i.e., sepsis)
Dehydration requiring parenteral fluids
Inability to take oral medications
Failure of outpatient treatment

The criteria for hospitalization for PID include pregnancy (at any stage), surgical emergencies (i.e., appendicitis or ovarian torsion) that cannot be ruled out at the time of diagnosis, tubo-ovarian abscess, severe illness with concern for sepsis, or failure of outpatient therapy. Additionally, if there is no improvement on oral antibiotics, patients should be evaluated for other etiologies and are recommended to switch to parenteral antibiotic therapy in the hospital. Prior to 1998, being an adolescent was a criterion for inpatient management of PID [9]. There is no evidence to suggest specialized treatment methods. Therefore, the criteria for hospitalization should be the same regardless of age [1].

Patient and Family Questions

All adolescents should have a confidential discussion and exam with the provider. During the visit, the provider should explore what could be discussed with the parents. It is best to discuss this prior to having the guardians return to discuss the assessment and plan. If the patient requires hospitalization, these issues need to be further clarified and handled. While engaging in private discussions, as a mandated reporter, the provider must identify limits of confidentiality.

How Did I Get This?

Providers should tailor their conversation depending on the developmental stage of the patient. They should be direct and polite, stating the evidence and facts. Information regarding the etiology and pathogenesis of PID should be discussed with the help of pictures or models. At the end of the visit, it is helpful to ask the patient to explain their understanding of the disease process.

There are many organisms that can cause this infection, and some of these are associated with sexual activity. The ones tested for and treated regularly are sexually transmitted, i.e., gonorrhea and chlamydia. Even if sexual partners use condoms, there is a risk of transfer. Not using regular condoms increases this risk. This is why it's important that the patient notifies their sexual partner(s) to be treated and tested as well. These infections very frequently show no symptoms, and it is possible that a sexual partner does not know he/she is infected. If the STI testing is still pending, be clear that other infections or conditions may be causing the presenting pain. Despite lack of causal pathogen at diagnostic visit, it is extremely important for the patient and partner to be treated.

Will This Affect My Ability to Have Future Children?

Sequelae of PID should be shared with the patient with careful wording for long-term fertility. Many adolescents leave their appointments thinking that they will be infertile and are at risk of declining further use of contraception. Emphasize that the reason to treat the day of diagnosis is to attempt to reduce any damage to the reproductive organs as quickly as possible. There is evidence of mucosal scarring and adhesions in the fallopian tubes on biopsy of individuals with a history of pelvic inflammatory disease. If enough scarring, blockages, or narrowing of the fallopian tubes occurs, it can lead to what is described in the evidence as tubal factor infertility. This condition is thought to be caused by multiple etiologies, only one of which is infectious (PID), and within that group sexually transmitted diseases are implicated. One or both fallopian tubes can be affected leading to difficulty of moving eggs to the uterus. Not only can this lead to difficulty becoming pregnant, but it also is associated with higher incidence of ectopic pregnancy. Ectopic pregnancy is ten times higher in individuals with a history of PID. Studies show that both severity and number of PID episodes have been associated with infertility [10]. The studies and details are less important to the patient than clear points: Concern for possibility of fertility issues is why treatment is so immediate and broad, and we do not know for sure if a patient's current diagnosis will have any long-term sequelae on her fertility.

What Can I Do to Prevent This in the Future?

The patient should be given positive reinforcement for asking this thoughtful question. She demonstrates concern and baseline understanding of her diagnosis by inquiring. It is a valuable topic for the provider to cover. If the patient does not ask this question, then the provider can suggest this question to invite a conversation regarding their education and understanding. Discussion should include the use of barrier methods, regular STI screening tests, and encouragement of open communication between the patient and their partner(s) regarding their sexual history and risks. Condom use 100% of the time is recommended to help prevent transmitting or receiving infections. Regular STI screening is recommended by the CDC for all sexually active individuals every 6–12 months depending on number and new sexual partners. With increasing number of partners and with new sexual partners, screening is recommended more frequently.

Juliet's Follow-Up Visit

Juliet returns 48 h after her initial visit for scheduled follow-up. The vaginal NAAT gonorrhea and chlamydia tests are negative. She has been adherent with taking her medications two times a day and reports that her lower abdominal pain has improved significantly though is not completely resolved. On examination, the abdomen is normal with no tenderness. Repeat bimanual exam is negative for CMT and adnexal tenderness.

As Juliet's symptoms have improved and she is adherent to her treatment, the diagnosis of PID is supported. There is no need for additional antibiotics or hospitalization, and she should be instructed to continue her doxycycline and metronidazole medications to complete the entire 14-day course.

Clinical Question

If Juliet's gonorrhea and chlamydia testing are negative, was she diagnosed and treated correctly?

Yes, Juliet was diagnosed and treated correctly. There are multiple organisms that have been implicated in cases of PID (see Table 15.6 and "Discussion" section for further details). Gonorrhea and chlamydia are the most commonly tested organisms but are not necessarily the most common. This patient met the PID diagnostic criteria, and empiric treatment is recommended even when the patient has tested negative. The goal of treatment is to preserve fertility by decreasing upper reproductive organ inflammation and scarring. Hence, providers should maintain a low threshold for diagnosis specifically in adolescents.

Table 15.6 Microbial pathogens implicated in pelvic inflammatory disease [1, 4]

Sexually transmitted diseases	• *Chlamydia trachomatis*
	• *Neisseria gonorrhea*
	• HSV and *Trichomonas vaginalis* (rare)
Genital mycoplasmas	• *Mycoplasma genitalium, Mycoplasma hominis*
	• *Ureaplasma urealyticum*
Anaerobic organisms	• *Bacteroides* spp.
	• *Peptostreptococcus* spp.
	• *Prevotella* spp.
Aerobic gram-positive and gram-negative organisms	• *Escherichia coli*
	• *Gardnerella vaginalis*
	• *Haemophilus influenzae*
	• *Streptococcus* spp.

Discussion

Definition of PID

Pelvic inflammatory disease is a syndrome of inflammation of the uterus, fallopian tubes, ovaries, and peritoneum that is triggered by an ascending infection from the lower reproductive tract of females. PID is a clinical diagnosis.

Incidence

In the United States, every year, almost 1 million people are diagnosed with PID. Twenty percent of these diagnoses are estimated to occur in adolescents and young adults. The National Survey of Family Growth estimates that approximately 8% of women have or will acquire PID at some point in their lives [11].

Etiology

PID is caused by organisms ascending into the pelvis from the lower genital tract. The absolute etiology is unknown in most cases; however, sexually transmitted pathogens such as *Chlamydia trachomatis* and *Neisseria gonorrhoeae* have been detectable in 30–50% of cases [11]. Despite reports from both the CDC and European CDC implicating *Chlamydia trachomatis* as the main etiological agent identified in causing PID, the low detection rates of pathogens in PID cases indicate other non-sexually transmitted etiologies [12]. See Table 15.6.

It is estimated that there are 820,000 new cases of gonococcal infections in the United States [13]. It is the second most common communicable disease in the United States [1]. *N. gonorrhoeae* is a gram-negative intracellular diplococcus and is spread by sexual activity or vertically from mother to child by mucous membrane contact. The risk of transmission from female to male partner is 20% per exposure and increases to >50% with more than four occurrences. A female's risk of contracting gonorrhea from her male partner is ≥50% at each encounter. The highest incidence of gonorrhea is among 14–19-year-old adolescent females. Antimicrobial-resistant *N. gonorrhoeae* has become more prevalent since 2007 when resistance to fluoroquinolones was reported. From 2006 to 2011, treatment failures with cefixime and other oral cephalosporins were reported worldwide. Dual therapy for uncomplicated gonococcal infections is now recommended as a cephalosporin (ceftriaxone 250 mg IM once) plus azithromycin 1 g PO once [14]. Annual screening should be performed utilizing samples from all areas involved in sexual activity regardless of the presence or absence of symptoms. More frequent testing is encouraged in high-risk populations [1].

Chlamydia is the most common STIs detected in the United States with the highest prevalence in youth aged ≤24 years [1]. Specifically between 1999 and 2008,

6.8% of US sexually active females between the ages of 14 and 19 years tested positively for chlamydia. Routine annual screening of <25-year-old women for chlamydial infections has given a way to reduce rates of PID [15]. Details regarding chlamydia are discussed in Chap. 10 in this book.

As previously stated, PID is polymicrobial, and pathogens other than *C. trachomatis* and *N. gonorrhoeae* are likely to be implicated in >50% of PID cases. Further discussion of newly emerging literature on mycoplasma as an implicated organism will take place later in this section. A complete list of pathogens involved in PID will not be reviewed. There is growing evidence that *Mycoplasma genitalium* may have a role in PID cases. Due to current lack of FDA-approved diagnostic test for *M. genitalium* population, rates of infection are estimated and variable. The organism was first identified in the 1980s as a cause of male urethritis. It has been found in the urethra, vagina, cervix, and endometrium of mostly asymptomatic women. In available PID studies, approximately 10% of cases have detected mycoplasma [16, 17]. It lacks a cell wall and is slow growing, taking up to 6 months to culture in the laboratory. The CDC suggests considering mycoplasma infection when patients do not respond to standard PID treatments within 7–10 days. Recommended treatment for *M. genitalium* in patients with PID is moxifloxacin 400 mg/day for 14 days [18]. There have also been randomized controlled trials indicating that 1 g of azithromycin is significantly more effective than doxycycline; however, resistance is emerging. Therefore, a longer course of azithromycin has been proposed: 500 mg on day 1 and followed by 250 mg daily for 4 days [19, 20].

Associations

Bacterial vaginosis has been implicated as a potential cause of PID as it has been found in fallopian tubes and abscess diagnosis and treatment of PID. However, BV does not induce an inflammatory response in the vagina. White blood cells are not found on wet mount when BV is diagnosed alone; thus, it is unlikely to cause inflammation in other areas of the body. The group of bacterial species termed as BV has been found to secrete sialidases. These sialidase enzymes have the ability to break down cervical mucus. The proposed theory is the incidental thinning of cervical mucous that occurs in the presence of bacterial vaginosis, allowing an incidental pathogen to gain access to the upper genital tract. Patients are counseled on avoiding behaviors associated with higher incidence of BV, i.e., douching and smoking [1]. Consistent and correct use of condoms reduces rates of STIs and thus PID [21].

Specific Issues Regarding PID in Adolescents

The highest rates of gonorrhea and the second highest rates of chlamydia are found in adolescent girls between 15 and 19 years of age [22]. The normal social and sexual development of this age group includes impulsive decision-making and higher numbers of romantic partners in shorter periods of time. This combination of behaviors increases a youth's risk of being exposed to a sexually transmitted disease. The diagnosis of PID lacks specificity and sensitivity. PID is likely highly underdiagnosed due to many asymptomatic and/or mild cases. In addition, adolescents do not commonly seek out regular healthcare. They are often seen in emergency departments and urgent care facilities, potentially after prolonged duration of symptoms. Due to the permanent fertility implications of PID, the standard of care is to default to low threshold for diagnosis and treatment. Compliance to medication prescription is difficult for most people, but youths statistically struggle with this. Assessing the issues that might keep young people from taking twice daily medication is extremely important. Examples of these barriers include financial costs, lack of transportation to go to the pharmacy, privacy at home (lack of a place to keep the medication), organizational or memory concerns, or simply lack of understanding of importance of medication and reason for treatment.

Clinical Pearls

- Testing for pregnancy and most recent unprotected sexual activity should be the primary assessment for a female with abdominal or pelvic pain.
- PID is a clinical diagnosis. Providers should have a low threshold for diagnosis and treatment.
- Ensure confidential adolescent services.
- Confirm that the youth has access to the healthcare services while keeping in mind nontraditional medical settings.

References

1. MMWR Recomm Rep. 2015;64(3):1–82.
2. Shulman LP, Nelson AL, Darney PD. Recent developments in hormone delivery systems. Am J Obset Gynecol. 2004;190(4 Suppl):S39–48.
3. Moore SG, et al. Clinical utility of measuring white blood cells on vaginal wet mount and endocervical gram stain for the prediction of chlamydial and gonococcal infections. Sex Transm Dis. 2000;27(9):530–8.
4. British Columbia Treatment Guidelines: Sexually Transmitted Infections in Adolescents and Adults (2014) Section 4.
5. Sweet RL. Treatment of acute pelvic inflammatory disease. Infect Dis Obstet Gynecol. 2011;2011:561909. https://doi.org/10.1155/2011/561909.
6. The American College of Obstetricians and Gynecologists, Committee Opinion Number 539, October 2012, reaffirmed 2014.
7. Committee on Adolescence. Contraception for adolescents. Pediatrics. 2014. https://doi.org/10.1542/peds.2014-2299.
8. Toivonen J, Luukkainen T, Allonen H. Protective effect of intrauterine release of levonorgestrel on pelvic infection: three years' comparative experience of levonorgestrel- and copper-releasing intrauterine devices. Obstet Gynecol. 1991;77:261–4.

9. Kaul P, Stevens-Simon C, Saproo A, Coupey SM. Trends in illness severity and length of stay in inner-city adolescents hospitalized for pelvic inflammatory disease. J Pediatr Adolesc Gynecol. 2008;21:289–93.
10. Weström L, et al. Pelvic inflammatory disease and fertility. A cohort study of 1,844 women with laparoscopically verified disease and 657 control women with normal laparoscopic results. Sex Transm Dis. 1992;19(4):185–92.
11. United States Census Bureau. Current Population Survey (CPS). Fertility; 2012.
12. Short V, et al. Clinical presentation of *Mycoplasma genitalium* infection versus *Neisseria gonorrhoeae* infection among women with pelvic inflammatory disease. Clin Infect Dis. 2009;48(1):41–7. https://doi.org/10.1086/594123.
13. Abu Raya B, et al. Beyond "safe sex"—can we fight adolescent pelvic inflammatory disease? Eur J Pediatr. 2013;172(5):581–90.
14. Satterwhite CL, Torrone E, Meites E, et al. Sexually transmitted infections among US women and men: prevalence and incidence estimates, 2008. Sex Transm Dis. 2013;40:187–93.
15. Burnett AM, Anderson CP, Zwank MD. Laboratory-confirmed gonorrhea and/or chlamydia rates in clinically diagnosed pelvic inflammatory disease and cervicitis. Am J Emerg Med. 2012;30:1114–7.
16. Scholes D, Stergachis A, Heidrich FE, et al. Prevention of pelvic inflammatory disease by screening for cervical chlamydial infection. N Engl J Med. 1996;334:1362–6.
17. Cohen CR, Manhart LE, Bukusi EA, et al. Association between *Mycoplasma genitalium* and acute endometritis. Lancet. 2002;359:765–6.
18. Cohen CR, Mugo NR, Astete SG, et al. Detection of *Mycoplasma genitalium* in women with laparoscopically diagnosed acute salpingitis. Sex Transm Infect. 2005;81:463–6.
19. Ross JD, Cronje HS, Paszkowski T, et al. Moxifloxacin versus ofloxacin plus metronidazole in uncomplicated pelvic inflammatory disease: results of a multicentre, double blind, randomised trial. Sex Transm Infect. 2006;82:446–51.
20. Mena LA, Mroczkowski TF, Nsuami M, et al. A randomized comparison of azithromycin and doxycycline for the treatment of Mycoplasma genitalium-positive urethritis in men. Clin Infect Dis. 2009;48:1649–54.
21. Schwebke JR, Rompalo A, Taylor S, et al. Re-evaluating the treatment of nongonococcal urethritis: emphasizing emerging pathogens—a randomized clinical trial. Clin Infect Dis. 2011;52:163–70.
22. Warner L, et al. Condom use and risk of gonorrhea and Chlamydia: a systematic review of design and measurement factors assessed in epidemiologic studies. Sex Transm Dis. 2006;33(1):36–51.

ACOG committee opinion statements:

1. Number 539, October 2012 *Adolescents and Long-Acting Reversible Contraception: Implant Adolescents and Long-Acting Reversible Contraception: Implants and Intrauterine Devices*
2. Number 672, September 2016 *Clinical Challenges Of Long-Acting Reversible Contraceptive Methods*
3. Number 626, March 2015 *The Transition from Pediatric to Adult Health Care: Preventative Care for Young Women Aged 18–26 Years*

Chapter 16
Case of a Girl with Vulvar Ulcers

Marina Catallozzi, Susan L. Rosenthal, and Lawrence R. Stanberry

Case

A 17-year-old young woman for whom you recently started oral contraception walks in today for a female complaint. Your medical assistant said that the patient refused to discuss it with her and finally reported that she has some irritation and maybe a pimple in her private area. Upon reviewing the chart and before seeing the patient, you note that she became sexually active approximately 6 months ago with a male partner that she considers her boyfriend. About 2 months ago, she came in for oral contraception and STI testing because they wanted to stop using condoms. Her partner had two prior partners and had been "tested for everything" and was negative. He was about to leave for college, but she planned to see him during his breaks. While her mother was aware of her recent sexual debut and knew the patient's partner well, she was not aware that her daughter stopped using condoms. The patient is accompanied by her mother at the visit today, who is in the waiting area. Your chart review also revealed that her mother has been ill in the last year with a new diagnosis of lupus.

M. Catallozzi, M.D., M.S.C.E. (✉)
Division of Child and Adolescent Health, Department of Pediatrics, Heilbrunn Department of Population and Family Health, Columbia University Medical Center, Morgan Stanley Children's Hospital at New York Presbyterian, New York, NY, USA
e-mail: mc2840@cumc.columbia.edu

S.L. Rosenthal, Ph.D., A.B.P.P.
Division of Child and Adolescent Health, Department of Pediatrics, Columbia University Medical Center, Morgan Stanley Children's Hospital at New York Presbyterian, New York, NY, USA
e-mail: slr2154@cumc.columbia.edu

L.R. Stanberry, M.D., Ph.D.
Department of Pediatrics, Columbia University Medical Center, Morgan Stanley Children's Hospital at New York Presbyterian, New York, NY, USA
e-mail: lrs2155@columbia.edu

H.J. Talib (ed.), *Adolescent Gynecology*,
https://doi.org/10.1007/978-3-319-66978-6_16

In speaking with the patient alone, she reports that she has not been feeling very well over the last week. She visited her boyfriend at college this past weekend (about 6 days ago), and since then she has been very tired and felt warm but never took her temperature. They had unprotected sex even though he was just getting over a cold. She was fine the first few days after she got home but then about 2 days ago noticed that her vaginal area was very itchy, like the time she had a yeast infection. It seemed to get worse, and at first she thought it was because she scratched the area so much, but this morning in the shower, she felt something that felt like pimples in her vaginal area. She reports that she waxed her pubic area prior to visiting her boyfriend. She has had a low-grade headache that responds to over-the-counter medicine, no cold symptoms, no cough, no abdominal pain, no vomiting or diarrhea, some pain with urinating, and no joint pain. She has never had lesions in her genital area before and has never had any cold sores or mouth ulcers.

On physical examination, the patient is afebrile with stable vital signs. She is generally well appearing. She has no oral lesions and her oropharynx is nonerythematous. Her lung and heart exams are normal. Her abdomen is soft and nontender with no hepatosplenomegaly. She has no cervical or axillary lymphadenopathy but does have some mobile palpable nodes in the bilateral inguinal region. Her skin other than in her genital region has no rashes. Her genitourinary exam is significant for vulvar erythema. There is no vaginal discharge, but there are multiple lesions on the labia majora and minora bilaterally. Some of the lesions are vesicular on an erythematous base, and some are ulcers that are shallow and are grouped with other ulcers. There are no necrotic areas. Cervical examination is not performed. There are no perianal tags, fissures, or lesions. You collect specimens during the examination and inform the patient that some tests will need to be run.

The patient is quite anxious during the examination, and while she is comfortable having you speak openly with her mother about everything, she wants to ask some questions before inviting her mother to join the conversation. First, the patient is very uncomfortable and wants to know if there is anything that you can give her to help her to get the irritation to go away. Second, she wants to know if it is some kind of infection that will go away with antibiotics. Finally, she wants to know if this is a sexually transmitted disease.

Discussion

This patient has what can be termed vulvar ulceration. Whereas an erosion involves only the skin and epidermis, an ulceration has been defined as a disruption of the skin, epidermis, and dermis of the vulva [1]. This disruption is what causes such discomfort in patients. In determining the cause of vulvar ulcerations, approaches to the differential include using the appearance or morphology of the lesions to ascertain the underlying cause. However, determining whether or not the patient is sexually active (or if there has been an abuse) is crucial. While there is some overlap, the possible diagnoses for vulvar ulcers for those who are not sexually experienced are

Table 16.1 Diagnostic considerations of vulvar ulcers for women who are not sexually experienced (data from [1, 2])

Infectious etiologies
Viral:Epstein-Barr virus (EBV), cytomegalovirus (CMV), mumps, influenza
Bacterial:Salmonella, paratyphoid, staphylococcus, streptococcus, tuberculosis
Other:Candida, leishmaniasis, schistosomiasis, amoebiasis
Noninfectious etiologies:
Inflammatory:Autoimmune (e.g., Bechet's disease, Crohn's disease, psoriasis), bullous (e.g., bullous pemphigoid, Stevens-Johnson syndrome/toxic epidermolytic necrosis)
Others:Idiopathic or reactive aphthosis, trauma, medications (nonsteroidal anti-inflammatory drugs, fixed drug eruption), contact dermatitis, malignancy

Table 16.2 Diagnostic and clinical considerations of sexually transmitted infections that can cause vulvar ulcers (adapted from [1, 3])

Viral
Herpes simplex virus types 1 and 2 (HSV-1, HSV-2):multiple painful vesicular and/or ulcerative lesions can be present or absent
Human immunodeficiency virus:can see vesicular lesions in acute and early HIV infection
Bacterial
Haemophilus ducreyi (chancroid):painful genital ulcer and suppurative tender inguinal adenopathy
Chlamydia trachomatis serovars L1-3 (lymphogranuloma venereum): self-limited papule or ulcer at the site of infection; tender (usually unilateral) regional lymphadenopathy
Treponema pallidum (syphilis):painless lesion at the site of inoculation that ulcerates (chancre) and is associated with regional (usually bilateral) lymphadenopathy
Klebsiella granulomatis (granuloma inguinale or donovanosis):painless ulcerative lesions that can bleed, not associated with lymphadenopathy but psuedobuboes (subcutaneous granulomas) can be seen; frequent bacterial superinfection

important to consider (Table 16.1). Given that the workup of the acute episode in a patient that is not sexually experienced rarely reveals a cause, it is important to note that it is often likely secondary to idiopathic vulvar aphthosis, and symptomatic relief is the mainstay of treatment [2].

Although individuals with vulvar ulcers who are sexually active can have noninfectious causes of their lesions, they are most likely secondary to sexually transmitted infections with herpes and syphilis being most common depending on the population and location [3]. Table 16.2 represents the sexually transmitted infections that should be considered when seeing a patient with vulvar ulcers and their usual clinical manifestations. National data between 2007 and 2008 suggests prevalence rates of herpes simplex virus (HSV) type 2 of 16.5% among 15–49-year-old men and women in the United States, while prevalence rates of syphilis are much lower (0.08% of 18–49-year-olds from 2001 to 2004) [4]. These prevalence rates are driven by the lifelong latency of HSV as opposed to the definitive treatment of syphilis with antibiotics. Since 1988 there has been a decreasing trend of seroprevalence of HSV-2 [5]. Industrialized countries have also seen a decrease in HSV-1 at sexual debut prompting concern for increased numbers of adolescents who will be infected with HSV-1 genitally [6].

Both HSV-1 and HSV-2 can cause genital herpes and thus vulvar ulcers [7, 8]. Development of clinical signs and symptoms due to HSV genital infection begins after a brief incubation period (averaging just under a week but can be as long as 2 weeks). The virus replicates at the site of infection and travels via nerve fibers to the dorsal root ganglia where latency is established. Reactivation of the latent virus travels back along nerve fibers to the initial sites of infection [7]. While primary genital infection with HSV-1 is less likely to be symptomatic than HSV-2, the majority of primary genital HSV infections are asymptomatic. It is important to note, however, that asymptomatically infected individuals are potentially contagious and can transmit the virus to susceptible sexual partners [8, 9]. When symptoms are present, they can include local irritation (burning or itching) and vesicular lesions that can be unilateral but are more often bilateral and are in different stages (papules, vesicles, ulcerations, crusting, and eventual resolution). While the vesicles generally heal within 10 days, new vesicles can occur over 1 or 2 weeks, so it can take up to 3–4 weeks for complete resolution of all HSV lesions. The lesions are painful and can involve any part of the genitoanal area. The presence of the lesions can contribute to dysuria and subsequent urinary retention. Other symptoms that are reported in those with symptomatic primary infection include inguinal lymphadenopathy, fever, malaise, and headache. More serious complications include meningitis, neuralgias, and transverse myelitis [7–10]. There is evidence that primary genital infection with HSV is more likely symptomatic in persons without antibodies to either HSV-1 or HSV-2 [8]. Recurrent HSV can be asymptomatic (causing only viral shedding and risk of sexual transmission) or symptomatic (usually unilateral genital lesions are preceded by a prodrome of tingling or genital irritation). These lesions are generally less severe, do not necessarily look like classic herpes lesions, and can be mistaken for other genital lesions; thus, if a diagnosis of genital herpes has not yet been established, testing should be done.

There is a high index of suspicion for primary genital herpes in the young woman in this case. While this is not a new sexual partner, they recently stopped using condoms, which provide some protection against genital herpes [11, 12]; he could have had a new partner (and thus new infection, which could have been asymptomatic) since going to college, and she had unprotected sex with him within the last week. While she reports that when she and her partner started having sex he "got tested for everything," this rarely involves testing for HSV since screening without symptoms is not recommended. Additionally, the constellations of symptoms and signs that she presents with (flu-like illness, bilateral vulvar ulcerations, inguinal lymphadenopathy) are suggestive of primary genital herpes infection. Syphilis is unlikely given that it is more common in men who have sex with men and is associated with a single localized lesion or chancre. The lesions of primary syphilis are also less likely to be painful. The other possible sexually transmitted infections are less likely in an adolescent with one sexual partner but merit consideration. Chancroid is much more common in regions of Africa and the Caribbean, and the adenopathy is suppurative. Chancroid should be considered if there is no evidence of either HSV or syphilis on testing [3]. Similarly, granuloma inguinale is rarely seen in the United States, and the lesions are painless. The clinical hallmark of lymphogranuloma venereum is the tender lymphadenopathy rather than the genital lesions [3].

Nonsexually transmitted infections should be considered given that the patient's boyfriend was not feeling well. Reactive genital lesions caused by various nonsexually transmitted pathogens are referred to as Lipschutz lesions, particularly those associated with Epstein-Barr virus (EBV) [1, 13]. EBV is commonly seen in the college population. Genital ulcers may occur in 10–30% of individuals who have EBV and do not have to necessarily occur with more classic symptoms of EBV such as fever, rash, or pharyngitis [13]. However, her boyfriend does not have any symptoms suggesting EBV.

In considering noninfectious etiologies, autoimmune diseases are important to consider given the patient's mother's recent diagnosis of systemic lupus erythematosus. Bechet's disease, a systemic and multisystem vasculitis, must be considered. While genital lesions can be the initial presentation of the disease and are the second most common finding seen, this patient has no other clinical manifestations of Bechet's (recurrent oral ulcerations, recurrent genital lesions, eye lesions, and positive pathergy test), and the patient would need to be followed for this diagnosis over time [13]. Crohn's disease should also always be considered in an adolescent with genital ulcers. This chronicinflammatory bowel disease can have genital ulcers as an extraintestinal manifestation when gastrointestinal symptoms (diarrhea, blood in stool, weight loss) are absent; however, it is more common to see these genital lesions in patients with colonic involvement. This includes not only bloody stool and abdominal pain but also perianal lesions [1, 13]. This patient does not have any of these associated findings. The patient denies any trauma, medications that would cause vulvar ulcers, or lesions that would be consistent with aphthosis (recurrent ulcers, present orally and genitally).

While the young woman in the case likely has primary genital herpes infection, the clinical diagnosis is often unreliable; hence, it is important to establish a laboratory-confirmed diagnosis for prognostic and management purposes. Laboratory diagnosis can elucidate if the infection is due to HSV-1 or HSV-2. As mentioned previously, the two viruses can both cause genital ulcers, but clinically symptomatic recurrences with HSV-1 are less frequent. A clear, laboratory-supported diagnosis can help patients in decision-making around communication with future partners, suppressive therapy, and planning for future pregnancies. A negative test for HSV can also help patients avoid taking antivirals that are not effective or appropriate if they do not, in fact, have the infection and may warrant further diagnostic assessment [8].

While viral culture was once the gold standard for testing for genital HSV infection, it does not consistently detect HSV in patients with lesions that are close to healing. HSV PCR assays are more sensitive and less dependent on collection and the stage of the ulcer [8, 14]. This type of nucleic acid amplification test can clarify the HSV type and is increasingly available in labs [3, 8]. Since coinfections with other sexually transmitted infections are common, it is critical to test for other sexually transmitted infections—in this case syphilis (to rule it out as the cause of the vulvar ulceration), gonorrhea, chlamydia, and HIV. HIV testing is of particular concern given the importance of HSV in transmission of HIV [7].

While testing for HSV is critical when a patient presents with concerning genital lesions, general screening of asymptomatic patients is not recommended. Type-specific serologic assays (looking for HSV-1 and HSV-2 antibodies) exist but should not be used for screening. The serologic screening test for HSV-2 has low specificity; HSV-1 has been implicated in an increased number of genital herpes infections, but the antibody testing cannot pinpoint the site of HSV infection (the oral cavity versus the genital tract) [15]. The US Preventive Task Force and Centers for Disease Control and Prevention (CDC) do not recommend screening asymptomatic patients (specifically adolescents, adults, pregnant women, and those with no history of genital HSV infection) for genital HSV as the possible negative effects of anxiety and impact on relationships can be quite devastating [3, 15, 16]. Type-specific serology could be useful in clinical situations where there are recurrent genital symptoms with negative HSV PCR, clinical diagnosis of HSV that was not supported with laboratory findings, and patients who report that their sexual partners have genital HSV [3]. A recent response to the USPTF recommendation to avoid screening more widely in those without a history of lesions cautions that such recommendations might ignore the important role of the serologic tests in establishing diagnoses for those who are currently asymptomatic but have a history with recurrent lesions as well as the impact on management [17]. Determining viral type can help to manage the disease (different approach to HSV-1 which is associated with fewer recurrences) and inform partners if they are infected or not, as well as decrease stigma given the new strategies involving daily suppressive therapy that help to decrease transmission [17].

To address this patient's questions, immediate relief can be achieved with local measures such as sitz baths (warm and shallow water that can provide temporary relief and can also help with painful urination), barrier creams that help to avoid burning with urination, and over-the-counter pain medicines. Antiviral therapy (usually orally but can be given intravenously for extreme cases) that is started within 72 h of the onset of lesions shortens the amount of time with symptoms, encourages lesion resolution, and stops viral shedding. Treatment with any antiviral with activity against HSV (acyclovir, famciclovir) is effective, but valacyclovir is most commonly used because of its easy dosing schedule (1 g twice a day for 7–10 days) [8]. While antivirals do not eradicate or cure the infection, they do shorten the duration of and ameliorate symptoms. Additionally, in the past, patients were treated with antivirals for recurrences of genital HSV (episodic therapy) but not started on daily suppressive therapy to reduce recurrences, unless they had a certain number of genital HSV outbreaks per year. Now, any patients with genital HSV can start on suppressive therapy, even after the first episode. There is evidence that suppressive therapy lowers symptomatic recurrences, asymptomatic shedding of HSV, and transmission to sexual partners [8].

Patients diagnosed with genital herpes are not only diagnosed with a sexually transmitted infection but a chronic disease that needs to be managed rather than definitively treated. Patients can have a range of responses including extreme sadness, shame, and fear of rejection. These usually resolve with education and information. There are several resources available to providers and patients (www.ashasexualhealth.org). It is critical to review the involvement of sexual partner or inform future sexual partners as well as approaches to risk reduction for transmission to partners. Suppressive therapy, abstinence when active lesions are present, and condom use are all important approaches [8].

This patient was informed of the likelihood of primary genital HSV infection and started on valacyclovir. She informed her partner who was going to see his doctor to get serologic testing. The patient's symptoms had resolved within 72 h, and the HSV PCR was positive for HSV-2. The patient was offered suppressive antiviral therapy, but she chose to wait; she was given a prescription for episodic treatment if needed and was encouraged to have it at a nearby pharmacy or fill it to have in the home so that it could be started immediately at any signs of an outbreak. Since there was no way to know when her boyfriend first was infected and she believed he was not involved in other concurrent sexual relationships, they started using condoms again. She was made aware of the importance of discussing her genital herpes with future providers, especially if she ever plans to get pregnant given the possibility and impact of neonatal transmission.

Clinical Pearls and Pitfalls-Bulleted Teaching Summary Highlights

- In approaching young women with vulvar ulcers, it is important to determine whether or not they are sexually active to determine which diagnoses should be considered.
- In sexually active women, HSV and syphilis must be considered, but HSV is a more common cause of vulvar ulcers; both HSV-1 and HSV-2 can cause genital HSV.
- Primary infection that is symptomatic is easier to diagnose clinically, but establishing a clear diagnosis with HSV PCR assay can be important for anticipatory guidance and future management depending on the HSV type.
- Recurrent genital HSV infection can be confused with other clinical presentations of vulvar irritation, and thus if testing has not occurred in the past, it should be done at the time that the patient presents with lesions.
- Serologic testing for HSV subtypes should be reserved for specific clinical situations (recurrent vulvar ulcers without clear etiology, partner with genital HSV) and not used for general screening, particularly not in adolescents or pregnant women.
- There is no definitive cure for HSV as the virus lives and replicates in ganglion roots and can recur.
- Primary infection is best managed with antivirals to speed up recovery and decrease the severity and duration of symptoms.

- Recurrent infections (which are less common and less severe with HSV-1) can be managed episodically or with suppressive therapy to decrease symptoms, shedding, and transmission to partners.
- Supporting patients through the diagnosis of genital HSV and helping to answer questions regarding sexual health, managements during pregnancy, and future partners is an important aspect of genital HSV care.
- There are currently no effective preventive or treatment vaccines for HSV.

References

1. Lewis FM, Velangi SS. An overview of vulvar ulceration. Clin Obstet Gynecol. 2005;48(4):824–37.
2. Rosman IS, Berk DR, Bayliss SJ, et al. Acute genital ulcers in nonsexually active young girls: case series, review of the literature, and evaluation and management recommendations. Pediatr Derm. 2012;29(2):147–53.
3. Centers for Disease Control and Prevention. Sexually transmitted diseases treatment guidelines. MMWR Recomm Rep. 2015;64(RR-3):1–137.
4. Satterwhite CL, Torrone E, Meites E, et al. Sexually transmitted infections among US women and men: prevalence and incidence estimates, 2008. Sex Transm Dis. 2013;40(3):187–93.
5. Fanfair RN, Zaidi A, Taylor LD, et al. Trends in seroprevalence of herpes simplex virus type 2 among non-hispanic blacks and non-hispanic whites aged 14 to 49 years—United States, 1988 to 2010. Sex Transm Dis. 2014;40(100):860–4.
6. Bradley H, Markowitz LE, Gibson T, et al. Seroprevalence of herpes simplex virus types 1 and 2—United States, 1999-2010. J Infect Dis. 2014;209:325–33.
7. Stanberry LR. Genital and perinatal HSV infections. In: Stanberry LR, Rosenthal SL, editors. Sexually transmitted diseases: vaccines, prevention and control. 2nd ed. New York: Elsevier; 2013. p. 273–313.
8. Gnann JW, Whitley RJ. Genital herpes. NEJM. 2016;375:666–74.
9. Bernstein DI, Bellamy AR, Hook EW. Epidemiology, clinical presentation, and antibody response to primary infection with herpes simplex virus type 1 and type 2 in young women. Clin Infect Dis. 2013;56(3):344–51.
10. Whitley RJ, Kimberlin DW, Roizman B. Herpes simplex viruses. Clin Infect Dis. 1998;26:541–55.
11. Wald A, Langenberg AG, Link K, et al. Effect of condoms on reducing the transmission of herpes simplex virus type 2 from men to women. J Am Med Assoc. 2001;284(24):3100–6.
12. Wald A, Langenberg AG, Krantz E, et al. The relationship between condom use and herpes simplex virus acquisition. Ann Intern Med. 2005;143(10):707–13.
13. Sehgal VN, Pandhi D, Khurana A. Nonspecific genital ulcers. Clin Dermatol. 2014;32:259–74.
14. LeGoff J, Pete H, Belec L. Diagnosis of genital herpes simplex virus infection in the clinical library. Virology. 2014;11:83.
15. US Preventive Services Task Force Recommendation Statement. Serologic screening for genital herpes infection. JAMA. 2016;316(23):2525–30.
16. US Preventive Services Task Force Evidence Report. Serologic screening for genital herpes. JAMA. 2016;316(23):2531–43.
17. Hook EW. A recommendation against serologic screening for genital herpes infection—what now? JAMA. 2016;316(23):2493–4. http://www.ashasexualhealth.org/stdsstis/herpes/
18. Martin ET, Krantz E, Gottlieb SL, et al. A pooled analysis of the effect of condoms in preventing HSV-2 acquisition. Arch Intern Med. 2009;169(13):1233–40.

Suggested Educational Reading, References, and Policies

Centers for Disease Control and Prevention. Sexually Transmitted Diseases Treatment Guidelines. MMWR Recomm Rep. 2015;64(RR-3):1–137.
Gnann JW, Whitley RJ. Genital herpes. N Engl J Med. 2016;375:666–74.
US Preventive Services Task Force Evidence Report. Serologic screening for genital herpes. JAMA. 2016;316(23):2531–43.
US Preventive Services Task Force Recommendation Statement. Serologic screening for genital herpes infection. JAMA. 2016;316(23):2525–30.
www.ashasexualhealth.org

Chapter 17
Case of a Girl with a Positive Pregnancy Test

Bianca Stortini and Nathalie Fleming

Case

Emma, a previously healthy 16-year-old girl, comes to your office because of recurrent nausea. Her menstrual cycle has been irregular since her menarche (age 13). She has been in a new relationship with a 17-year-old boyfriend and sexually active with him for the past 6 months. They rely on condoms for contraception. Her parents are unaware that she is sexually active. Her nausea has worsened, and her periods are still irregular.

Once your evaluation is complete, you order a pregnancy test, which is positive. Emma is in shock. She never thought she could become pregnant. "But I still have my periods!"

She is worried and anxious. "What am I going to do?" "I don't know if this is what I want." "What are my options?" "Are there risks for me or my baby if I decide to go on with the pregnancy?" "What are my options to prevent this from happening again soon?"

B. Stortini, M.D. • N. Fleming, M.D., F.R.C.S.C. (✉)
Division of Gynecology, Department of Surgery, Children's Hospital of Eastern Ontario, Ottawa, ON, Canada

Department of Obstetrics, Gynecology and Newborn Care, The Ottawa Hospital, Ottawa, ON, Canada

Faculty of Medicine, University of Ottawa, Ottawa, ON, Canada
e-mail: nfleming@cheo.on.ca

H.J. Talib (ed.), *Adolescent Gynecology*,
https://doi.org/10.1007/978-3-319-66978-6_17

Discussion

Statistics

Teen Pregnancy

Like the majority of young girls who become pregnant, Emma's pregnancy was unplanned. In 2011, nearly half of the pregnancies in the United States (US) were unplanned in girls and women of reproductive age [1]. In 2011, the US teen *pregnancy rate* (15–19 years) was 52.4/1000 (The National Campaign to Prevent Teen and Unplanned Pregnancy 2016). In 2014, the teen *birth rate* was 24.2/1000, a decrease of 9% since 2013 and a decrease of 61% since 1991 [2]. The 2014 decline was observed in all races and origins (Fig. 17.1), but the Hispanic and the non-Hispanic black teens remain the one with the highest rates of pregnancies (38/1000 and 34.9/1000, respectively) [2]. The decline in teen pregnancy is primarily attributable to increased contraceptive use (86%) but also to the delay in sexual debut [3]. Although the 2014 US teen birth rate has been the lowest since 1960, it is still higher than the rate of other developed countries. In Canada, the teen *pregnancy rate* (15–19 years) was 28.2/1000 in 2010 [4].

However, it is important to note that not all teen pregnancies are unplanned. In fact, the Millennium Cohort Study suggested 15% of teens planned their pregnancy (Bradshaw 2006). Similarly, a Canadian study found that 15% of adolescents presenting to an abortion clinic had initially intended to conceive (Goltset al. 2003), while 33% of teens presenting to youth pregnancy clinic reported a desire to become pregnant (Kives and Jamieson 2001). Efforts to promote and offer effective contraception for this group of teens would not have prevented these pregnancies (Black et al. 2012).

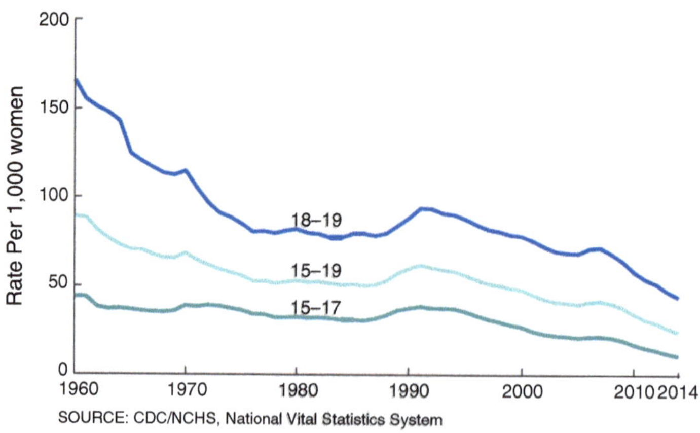

Fig. 17.1 Teen Birth Rates (US) [2]

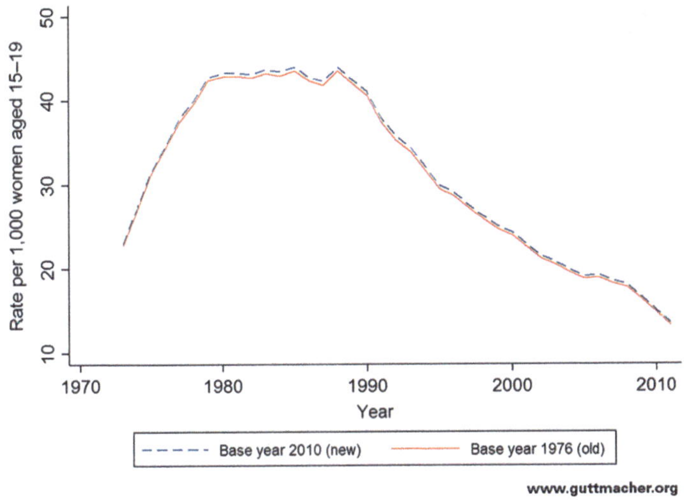

Fig. 17.2 US Abortion Rates (15–19 years) 1973–2011 (Kost and Isaac 2016)

Abortion

In 2011, 21% of all pregnancies in the USA ended in abortion [5]. In 2014, 12% of the US abortions were in teenagers: 8%, 3%, and <0.2% in the 18–19 years, 15–17 years, and <15 years age groups, respectively [5]. In 2011, the abortion rate in the 15–19 years was 13.5/1000 women, a significant decrease since its peak in 1988 (Fig. 17.2) (Kost and Isaac 2016).

Many reasons may explain this decline, including an increase in effective contraception utilization and a decrease in the unintended pregnancy rates [6].

In Canada, a decline was also seen in the abortion rate to teens (age 15–19) reaching 14.7/1000 women in 2010 compared to 19.4 in 2001 [4].

Adoption

Adoption rates have also seen a steady and continuous decline since the 1960s. Less than 5% of US pregnant teens chose adoption [7]. This important reduction is most likely explained by the legalization of abortion and greater social acceptance of nonmarital childbearing and family support programs. Also, the fall in teen pregnancy rates over the last 15 years is likely a contributor [7].

Risk Factors

There are many risk factors for a teen to become pregnant. Young women living in poverty, experiencing violence, and having lower educational attainment are particularly at risk. [8]. Teens with earlier sexual debut and more lifetime sexual partners are also associated with increased risk of pregnancy [9]. Other risks include girls who are part of ethnic minority groups, as well as those with mental health problems [10].

In addition, teens who use drugs and alcohol, have low self-esteem, and experience significant peer pressure to engage in sexual activity are at significant risk. Finally, youth who lack access to contraception or do not correctly or consistently use reliable methods of contraception will have a higher likelihood of experiencing an unintended pregnancy (Black et al. 2012).

Conversely, close family relationships, religious beliefs, knowledge of sexuality, strong academic performance, and involvement in extracurricular activities appear to be protective against early sexual activity (Black et al. 2012), hence unintended pregnancy.

Presenting Symptoms of Teen Pregnancy

Teens are highly fecund and have a 90% likelihood of becoming pregnant within a year without using contraception [3].

They can present with a variety of symptoms such as abdominal pain, nausea, vomiting, vaginal bleeding, amenorrhea, and irregular periods [10]. One should have a low threshold for pregnancy testing in this age group.

In addition, it is important to ensure that the teen is not a victim of sexual abuse or sexual exploitation, especially in the preteen and early teen years [11].

Pregnancy Options

Every teen should have access to counseling regarding their pregnancy options [8]. It is important to discuss every option in a clear, concise, and nonjudgmental manner, with complete up-to-date information provided on all the available options to the patient and other concerned persons [12, 13]. Three options are available [12, 13] :

1. Parenting: Carrying the pregnancy to delivery and raising the baby
2. Adoption: Carrying the pregnancy to delivery and placing the baby for adoption
3. Termination of pregnancy

Every healthcare provider (HCP) should be familiar with the laws in their state or country and available services in their community to provide the best counseling to their patients.

Decision-Making in Teens

Taking a decision about the future of the pregnancy can be a difficult moment for the pregnant teen. It is possible that they may not have all the necessary cognitive abilities, due to normal development process, to make a rational decision (Loke and Lam 2014). They frequently turn to their partner and also their mother for support (Loke and Lam 2014). To make their decision, teens take into account multiple factors, such as their relationship with their boyfriend, family advice/support, practical considerations, their personal values, and their views on adoption (Loke and Lam 2014). Bender elaborated a model of decision-making in an unplanned pregnancy. The five stages include acknowledging the pregnancy, formulation of alternative outcomes, consideration of options, commitment to one choice, and finally adhering to the decision. Ambivalence is an important but normal process in teens [14].

Parenting

Being pregnant in the teenage years involves risks for the young mother, and these risks can be potentiated by multiple social aspects frequently encountered in teen pregnancy. Generally, teen pregnancies have higher maternal, obstetrical, and neonatal risks, those being higher in younger girls (≤15 years) [8].

Pregnant teens are more likely than their nonpregnant peers to have lower educational attainment, to drop out of school, and to have a lower socioeconomic status which can perpetuate the cycle of poverty [8, 10]. Furthermore, their children are also more likely to have lower educational attainment, to grow up in a single mother household, to be involved in alcohol and drugs, and to become pregnant as a teen themselves [8].

Indeed, poverty, lower educational level, and inadequate family support contribute to the adverse health outcomes in the pregnant mother and her child [11].

In addition, stigmatization of teenage mothers is frequently seen. Indeed, 40% of teen moms feel stigmatized by their pregnancy. Some are more likely to suffer such as those who are unmarried, are socially isolated, have aspirations to finish college, and experience verbal abuse and family criticism [10].

Even though there may be several negative consequences, other protective factors have been associated with improved outcomes in teen mothers: optimal social support, completing the education before getting pregnant, being part of programs for teen mothers, and continuing school without a repeat pregnancy in the 24 months after a pregnancy [11]. Indeed, family factors are important to optimize the outcomes for the mother and her child. These include early child care provided by the family of the baby, support that allows the teen mother to complete school, lively and adequate interaction between the child and father, and stable relationships [11]. Paternal involvement is important, as there are multiple benefits for the child [10].

Prenatal Care

Many studies have described that teens delay accessing prenatal care services [8]. Reasons vary but include ambivalence toward their pregnancy options, late diagnosis, desire to hide the pregnancy, fear of apprehension of their child, being victims of violence, and being unaware of the importance of prenatal care. Other reasons include concerns with judgmental attitudes of healthcare providers and financial barriers [8]. However, prenatal care for teens is of utmost importance as a lack or delay in care is associated with adverse maternal, obstetrical, and neonatal outcomes [8]. In addition, multidisciplinary teen-focused prenatal care leads to better outcomes than traditional prenatal care, such as reduction in preterm birth (PTB), low birth weight (LBW) and neonatal intensive care unit (NICU) admission, increase in spontaneous vaginal delivery, and reduction in operative delivery rates [8]. Furthermore, these specialized programs have the potential to lead to significant healthcare cost savings by reducing these complications.

There are specifics elements that should be considered in teen pregnancy (Table 17.1), including the adverse perinatal outcomes (Table 17.2).

Table 17.1 Elements to Consider in Teen Pregnancy [8, 10, 15, Magee et al. 2014]

Elements to consider	Facts	Adverse outcomes	Prevention and treatment
Sexually transmitted infections	Less likely to use condoms Prevalence of chlamydia at initial visit 11.1–31% High recurrence rate during the pregnancy (22.1%) Concomitant infections	PTB PPROM Chorioamnionitis Postpartum infection Vertical transmission/ infection in neonate	Education Encouragement to use condom Screening upon presentation for prenatal care, third trimester, and postpartum Treatment and test of cure (as per national guidelines)
Bacterial vaginosis	Teens should be considered high risk, i.e., inherently high risk of PPROM, PTL, and PTB	PTL PTB PPROM	Screening upon presentation for prenatal care, third trimester, and postpartum Treatment (as per national guidelines)
Smoking, substance abuse, and alcohol abuse	Higher rates of smoking and substance abuse than adults Pregnancy is a powerful incentive to cut down or stop	SA PTL PROM Placenta previa Placental abruption IUGR LBW IUFD Maternal hypertension Congenital anomalies Neurobehavioral effects on baby NAS ADHD (long term)	Education Encouragement toward reduction of smoking, substance abuse, and alcohol consumption Cessation programs Routine and repeat screening

(continued)

Table 17.1 (continued)

Elements to consider	Facts	Adverse outcomes	Prevention and treatment
Violence and coercion	Increased risk of violence (1.8 times) IPV in pregnant teens is between 26 and 31% At risk of sexual coercion	Late prenatal care LBW PTB IUFD Postpartum depression	Routine and repeat screening Questions about all types of violence (sexual, physical, psychological)
Mood disorders	16–44% depression during pregnancy 50% teen moms experience depressive symptoms in early postpartum High prevalence of anxiety	Postpartum depression (47%) Increase risk of repeat pregnancies PTB SGA Unresponsive mothering Behavioral and cognitive problems in children	Routine and repeat screening for mood disorders every trimester and postpartum Perinatal mental health consultation
Anemia and nutritional care	50–66% pregnant teens are anemic Poor weight gain	LBW	Nutritional assessment Prenatal vitamins, other macro/micronutrient supplementation (ex: iron supplement), and food supplementation
Hypertensive disorders	Conflicting evidence	Maternal: CNS, cardiorespiratory, hematological, renal and hepatic complications Fetal: abnormal FHR, IUGR, oligohydramnios, abnormal dopplers, placenta abruption, IUFD	Usual care as for the adult population

ADHD attention-deficit hyperactivity disorder, *CNS* central nervous system, *FHR* fetal heart rate, *IPV* intimate partner violence, *IUFD* intrauterine fetal death, *IUGR* intrauterine growth restriction, *LBW* low birth weight, *NAS* neonatal abstinence syndrome, *PPROM* premature preterm rupture of membranes, *PROM* premature rupture of membranes, *PTB* preterm birth, *PTL* preterm labor, *SA* spontaneous abortion, *SGA* small for gestational age

Table 17.2 Risk and Prevention of Adverse Perinatal Outcomes [8, 10]

Adverse outcomes	Risk	Prevention
Congenital anomalies		Anatomic ultrasound at 16–20 weeks
CNS (anencephaly, spina bifida, hydrocephaly, microcephaly)	OR 1.08	
GI anomalies (gastroschisis, omphalocele)	OR 1.86	
MSK anomalies (cleft lip, cleft palate, polydactyly, syndactyly)	OR 1.06	

(continued)

Table 17.2 (continued)

Adverse outcomes	Risk	Prevention
PTB		Accurate dating scan Screen and treat STI and bacterial vaginosis Frequent prenatal visit in second and third trimester Screen for substance use and violence
<37 weeks	OR 1.76	
<32 weeks (very)	OR 2.4	
<28 weeks (extremely)	OR 2.48	
BW		Frequent prenatal visit in second and third trimester Ultrasound for growth and well-being at 32–34 weeks Nutritional assessment and support
LBW (<2500 g)	OR 1.37	
Very LBW (<1550 g)	OR 1.47	
IUGR	OR 1.21	Ultrasound for growth and well-being at 32–34 weeks
SGA	OR 1.14	
Stillbirths	OR 1.31	
NICU admissions	aRR 1.08	
Neonatal deaths	OR 1.15	

aRR ajusted relative risk, *BW* birth weight, *CNS* central nervous system, *GI* gastrointestinal, *IUGR* intrauterine growth restriction, *LBW* low birth weight, *MSK* musculoskeletal, *OR* odd ratio, *PTB* preterm birth, *SGA* small for gestational age, *STI* sexually transmitted infections

Adoption

Multiple factors and influences have been associated with the choice of adoption in teen pregnancy. Indeed, teens who choose adoption tend to be white, come from better socioeconomic status and from a relatively small family, are still in school, and have high educational and vocational goals. In addition, they have favorable attitudes about adoption and recognize that they have a number of alternatives to early child-rearing [7].

Furthermore, girls with high educational and vocational goals are more likely to postpone sexual activity, to use contraception, and to choose either adoption or abortion as their final decision compared with teens that do not have these objectives. In the past, white women have been more likely to relinquish their child for adoption than black and Hispanic women. In the recent decades, white women tend to follow the trends of women of other races, contributing to the decline in adoption [7].

Mothers of teenagers and birth fathers also have an important influence on the decision of adoption. Mothers of young women who attended at least 1 year of college were three times more likely to advocate for adoption, compared with those who did not complete high school. Additionally, the birth father's preference for adoption is the most powerful predictor of consistency to choose this option [7].

Donnelly and Voydanoff completed a longitudinal study on 113 pregnant or newly postpartum teens examining the consequences of parenting ($n = 87$) compared to placing for adoption ($n = 26$) over a 24-month period after childbirth [16].

Teens who chose to relinquish their baby for adoption were likely to experience more regret and sorrow than those who chose to parent. However, they did not experience psychological difficulties over the first 2 years postpartum, and there was no difference between the levels of depression and personal efficacy between women who decide to parent compared with those who gave their child in adoption [16].

Even if pregnant teens rarely choose adoption, they should always have the opportunity to discuss this option throughout the pregnancy [12, 13]. To make appropriate referrals, the HCP should be familiar with the medical, legal, counseling, and social services resources available to facilitate adoption in their state [12].

Abortion

"When a woman experiences an unplanned, abnormal or risky pregnancy and wishes to terminate, she should have access to evidence-based, safe abortion care, especially given that safe abortion protects the lives of women" [6]. Multiple laws surround abortion care. Providers who take care of teens need to be aware of these laws, as they change from state to state and between countries [6]. Interestingly, most pregnant teens choose to consult a parent in their decision to have an abortion, regardless of their state's law status [17].

Similar to the delay in obtaining prenatal care, teens obtain abortions later in their pregnancy than adults [17]. Unfortunately, restrictive laws contribute to the delay, as well as other barriers, such as distance, gestational age limits, and costs. Consequently, the later the teens seek abortion care, the more costly, less accessible, and less safe it is [17].

There appears to be good outcome in girls who choose abortion, such as better socioeconomic status, higher educational goals and achievement, higher self-esteem, greater feelings of being in control of their situation, low level of anxiety, and better able to plan their future [17].

Repeat Teen Pregnancy

Unfortunately, teen pregnancy is often a cycle: after one pregnancy, there is often a second one. Rapid repeat pregnancy (RRP) is defined as a pregnancy within 2 years of the previous pregnancy [3] and occurs in 25–35% of teen mothers [8]. About two-thirds of these pregnancies are unintended (Table 17.3). Consequently, teens are also at an increased risk of repeat abortion, which is more likely to occur in the second trimester [3].

Repeat pregnancies in teens have been linked to low educational achievement, increased dependence on governmental support, increase in infant's mortality, and low birth weight [11].

There are multiple ways to intervene to prevent or delay the next pregnancy in a teenager [11]. First, it is important to determine the educational objectives of the teen

Table 17.3 Risk Factors for Rapid Repeat Pregnancy [3, 11]

Teen factors	Social factors	Protective factors
Early resumption of intercourse postpartum	Poverty	Use of LARC
Nonusage of LARC	Married/living with male partner	Living alone or with parent
Young age	Teen and/or mother with low level of education	Attending school
Back to school >6 months after delivery	Major child care assistance	
Previous intended pregnancy	Poor family support	
Prior poor obstetrical outcomes (miscarriage, stillbirths)	Not living with both parents in the household as a teen	
Previous abortion	Peers who are teen parents	
Depression		
Lack of aspiration, vocation		
IPV		

LARC long-acting reversible contraception, *IPV* intimate partner violence

and emphasize the importance of completing high school. Thus, referring the teen to programs that enable her to return to school can be beneficial. Furthermore, the HCP can help provide motivation to postpone a second pregnancy. Finally, contraceptive counseling should be initiated during pregnancy with emphasis on long-acting reversible contraception (LARC) as the optimal contraceptive choice.

Indeed, LARC methods are effective in reducing RRP in teenagers by up to 35% versus their peers using other methods or no method [3]. Also, the use of LARC decreases the risk of repeat abortion, especially if initiated around the time of the initial abortion [3]. Finally, the use of LARC methods has a greater impact on decreasing repeat pregnancy than comprehensive social support and counseling [3].

Several medical societies, such as The American College of Obstetricians and Gynecologists, the Society of Obstetricians and Gynaecologists of Canada, and the American Academy of Pediatrics, have issued recommendations advocating for the use of LARC as first-line method for contraception in teens [13, 18, 19].

Back to the Case

Emma informed her boyfriend that she was pregnant. He was also in shock. She received an informative pregnancy options counseling from her HCP. After several days, she disclosed her pregnancy to her mother, as well as her worries about her pregnancy options. Emma was surprised to find out how supportive her mother was regarding her news. Emma was ambivalent between parenting and having an abortion.

Her boyfriend was supportive and took part in the decision process, without coercion. Emma decided to continue her pregnancy, and parent her child. She was referred to a multidisciplinary teen-focused center for her prenatal care. Emma and her boyfriend were satisfied, happy, and comfortable with their decision.

Clinical Pearls and Pitfalls

- Teen pregnancy remains a public health concern, and continued efforts are needed to reduce the teen pregnancy rate.
- Not all teen pregnancies are unintended.
- A low threshold for pregnancy testing is necessary in this age group, regardless of the sexual history.
- Poverty and lower educational attainment are worldwide risk factors for teen pregnancy.
- Every pregnant teen should have access to a clear, up-to-date, and nonjudgmental counseling regarding the different options available.
- Become a parent, have an abortion, or give the baby up for adoption are the three options for the pregnant teens.
- The HCP should be familiar with the laws in their state or country and available services in their community for the various pregnancy options.
- The young woman's mother and partner are the most helpful support to help her decision-making.
- Multidisciplinary teen-focused prenatal care has been demonstrated to lead to better pregnancy outcomes.
- Rapid repeat pregnancy is defined as a pregnancy within 2 years of a previous pregnancy, and it occurs in 25–35% of teen mothers.
- LARC methods should be first-line contraceptives offered to teens who are at risk of unintended or repeat pregnancy.

References

1. Guttmacher Institute. Guttmacher Institute. 2016. Retrieved 2016 from Guttmacher Institute. https://www.guttmacher.org.
2. Hamilton BE, Martin JA, Osterman MJ, Curtin SC, Mathews T. National vital statistics reports-reports births: final data for 2014. 2015. Retrieved 1 June 2016 from Centers for Disease Control and Prevention. http://www.cdc.gov/nchs/nvss/births.htm.
3. Baldwin MK, Edelman AB. The effect of long-acting reversible contraception on rapid repeat pregnancy in adolescent: a review. J Adolesc Health. 2013;52(4 Suppl):S47–53.
4. Mc Kay A. Trends in Canadian national and provincial/territorial teen pregnancy rates: 2001-2010. Can J Hum Sexuality. 2012;21:161–75.
5. Guttmacher Institute. Induced Abortion in the United States. n.d. Retrieved 06-08, 2016 from Guttmacher Institute. https://www.guttmacher.org/fact-sheet/induced-abortion-united-states.
6. Schreiber CA, Traxler S. State of family planning. Clin Obstet Gynecol. 2015;58(2):392–408.

7. Miller BC, Coyl DD. Adolescent pregnancy and childbearing in relation to infant adoption in the United States. Adopt Q. 2000;4(1):3–25.
8. Fleming N, O'Driscoll T, Becker G, Spitzer RF. Adolescent pregnancy guidelines. J Obstet Gynaecol Can. 2015;37(8):S1–S20.
9. Cavazos-Regh PA, Krauss MJ, Spitznagel EL, Schootman M, Cottler LB, Bierut LJ. Associations between multiple pregnancies and health risk behaviors among U.S. adolescents. J Adolesc Health. 2010;47(6):600–3.
10. McCarthy FP, O'Brien U, Kenny LC. The management of teenage pregnancy. BMJ. 2014; 349:1–6.
11. Pinzon JL, Jones VF. Care of adolescent parents and their children. Pediatrics. 2012;130(t6):e1743–56.
12. American Academy of Pediatrics. Counselling the adolescent about pregnancy options. Pediatrics. 1998;101(5):938–40.
13. The American College of Obstetricians and Gynecologists. Committee Spinion #539: adolescent and long-acting reversible contraception: implants and intrauterine devices. *Obstet Gynecol.* 2012;*120*(4):983–8.
14. Bender SS. Three cases of adolescent childbearing decision-making: the importance of ambivalence. Adolescence. 2008;43(172):861–79.
15. Wong S, Ordean A, Kahan M. Substance use in pregnancy. J Obstet Gynaecol Can. 2011;33(4):367–84.
16. Donnelly BW, Voydanoff P. Parenting versus placing for adoption: consequences for adolescent mothers. Fam Relat. 1996;45(4):427–34.
17. Davis AR, Beasley AD. Abortion in adolescents: epidemiology, confidentiality and methods. Curr Opin Obstet Gynecol. 2009;21(5):390–5.
18. American Academy of Pediatrics. Policy statement. Contraception for adolescents. *Pediatrics.* 2014;*134*(4):e1244–56.
19. The Society of Obstetricians and Gynaecologists of Canada. Canadian Contraception Consensus (Part 3 of 4): Chapter 7 - Intrauterine contraception. *J Obstet Gynaecol Can.* 2016;*38*(2):182–200.
20. Jones J. Who adopts? Characteristics of women and men who have adopted children. 2009. Retrieved July 9, 2016 from Centers for Disease Control and Prevention. http://www.cdc.gov/nchs/data/databriefs/db12.pdf.

Recommended Reading

American Academy of Pediatrics. Counselling the adolescent about pregnancy options. Pediatrics. 1998;101(5):938–40.

American Academy of Pediatrics. Policy statement. Contraception for adolescents. *Pediatrics.* 2014;*134*(4):e1244–56.

Fleming N, O'Driscoll T, Becker G, Spitzer RF. Adolescent pregnancy guidelines. J Obstet Gynaecol Can. 2015;37(8):S1–S20.

Guttmacher Institute. https://www.guttmacher.org.

The American College of Obstetricians and Gynecologists. Committee Opinion #539: Adolescent and long-acting reversible contraception: implants and intrauterine devices. *Obstet Gynecol.* 2012;*120*(4):983–8.

The American College of Obstetricians and Gynecologists. Pregnancy choices: raising the baby, adoption, and abortion. 2013, February. Retrieved November 29, 2016, from The American Congress of Obstetricians and Gynecologists: https://www.acog.org/-/media/For-Patients/faq168.pdf? dmc=1&ts=20161129T1805434425.

Chapter 18
Case of a Girl Seeking Birth Control

Jennifer L. Northridge and Sofya Maslyanskaya

The Case

AB is a 17-year-old sexually active girl with migraines with aura who presents for contraceptive management. Her menarche was at 12 years of age. She has regular monthly periods lasting 7 days and describes them as heavy. She reports that during the first 2 days of her menses, she has to change a super absorbent pad every 2 h because the pads are soaked with clots. She reports that she has never been pregnant and has never been diagnosed with any sexually transmitted infections (STIs). When she visited her pediatrician 3 months ago, she was started on depot medroxyprogesterone acetate injection (DMPA) for contraception as well as daily iron pills for treatment of mild iron deficiency anemia (Fig. 18.1). Since starting DMPA, her menses have been lighter with spotting for the past month. She states that she does not want to continue taking DMPA because she is worried that she may be gaining weight and is bothered by the unpredictable uterine bleeding.

AB is followed by a pediatric neurologist for migraine headaches with aura that are well controlled with nortriptyline. She has no other medical problems, is not taking any other medications, and has no history of prior surgeries. Family history is significant for migraines with aura for her mother. There is no family history of bleeding disorders or anemia.

Upon physical examination, AB is found to have a normal blood pressure 113/66 mmHg and a body mass index (BMI) of 27 kg/m^2. Examination of the heart, lungs, and abdomen are within normal limits. Breasts are Tanner stage 5 without

J.L. Northridge, M.D.
Division of Adolescent Medicine, Joseph M Sanzari Children's Hospital, The Pediatric Hospital for Hackensack University Medical Center, Hackensack, NJ, USA

S. Maslyanskaya, M.D. (✉)
Division of Adolescent Medicine, Children's Hospital at Montefiore, The Pediatric Hospital for Albert Einstein College of Medicine, Bronx, NY, USA
e-mail: smaslyan@montefiore.org

H.J. Talib (ed.), *Adolescent Gynecology*,
https://doi.org/10.1007/978-3-319-66978-6_18

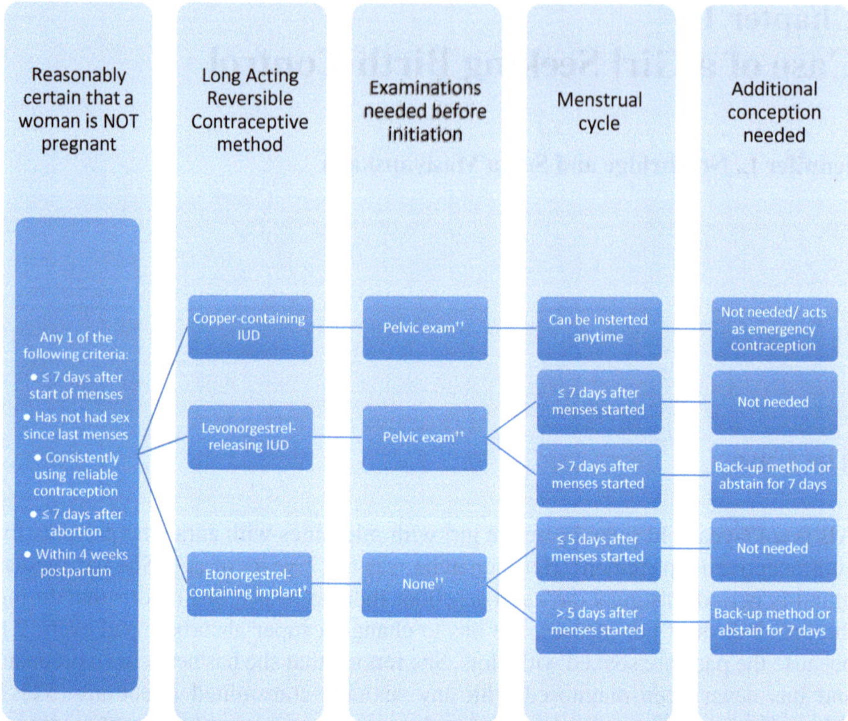

† *For implants*, if a health care provider is uncertain whether the woman might be pregnant, the benefits of starting the implant likely exceed any risk and the women should follow-up with a pregnancy test in 2–4 weeks.

††Additionally, providers can consider a urine pregnancy test; however, they should be aware of the limitations of the accuracy of the test based upon the timing of last sex [1].

Fig. 18.1 When to start using long-acting reversible contraception (LARC), including copper-containing intrauterine devices (IUDs), levonorgestrel-releasing IUDs, and implants

masses, and pubic hair is shaved in Tanner stage 5 distribution. On external genital examination, no vulvar lesions or vaginal discharge are noted.

Laboratory testing 3 months prior to the visit was significant for a microcytic, hypochromic anemia with a hemoglobin 11.2 gm/dL, negative urine nucleic acid amplification testing for gonorrhea and chlamydia, and negative serum human immunodeficiency virus (HIV) antibody testing.

AB's Questions and Concerns Elicited During the Visit

1. *Can I take the pill?*
2. *What other contraceptives would you recommend for me?*
3. *If I decide on the IUD, do I have to have anesthesia for the IUD insertion?*
4. *Can I get an IUD today?*

Can I Take the Pill?

Prior to the initiation of any contraceptive method, it is essential to review the adolescent patient's medical history to assess which contraceptive methods would carry unacceptable health risks. In particular, physicians should ask if there is a history of migraines with aura or clotting disorders to determine if the adolescent has an elevated thromboembolic risk. Other medical conditions that predispose a patient to thrombotic events, including cancer, systemic lupus erythematosus with positive antiphospholipid antibodies, and complicated valvular heart disease, should be elicited during the medical history. On physical examination, it is essential to obtain a blood pressure if considering estrogen-containing methods such as "the pill," a common phrase referring to combined oral contraceptives (COCs). In addition, if inserting an intrauterine device (IUD), a patient requires a bimanual examination and cervical inspection to ensure that she does not have cervicitis or pelvic inflammatory disease [1]. The Centers for Disease Control and Prevention (CDC) has published and periodically updates the US Medical Eligibility Criteria for Contraceptive Use, adapted from the World Health Organization (WHO) *Medical Eligibility Criteria for Contraceptive Use* [2]. This report provides evidence-based guidelines for the safe use of contraceptive methods for women with various medical conditions and characteristics, including venous thromboembolism and migraines with aura. An accompanying abbreviated decision-making tool "Summary Chart" is arranged by contraceptive method, including IUDs, implants, DMPA, progestin-only pills (POPs), and COCs, and provides clinical guidance for providers to help counsel women about contraceptive method choice and safety [2, 3].

Based on the US Medical Eligibility for Contraceptive Use, AB's history of migraines with aura is a category "4" or unacceptable health risk for use of estrogen-containing contraceptives, including COCs [2]. Therefore, her provider must counsel AB that initiation of "the pill" has unacceptable health risks and is not an appropriate option for her. In general, adolescent girls have a very low incidence of thrombosis (1–10 per 100,000 per year) [4]. The thrombotic risk from COCs (reported relative risk of 3–5) is often weighed against the thrombotic risk of unplanned pregnancy (reported relative risk of 4.3–10) [4]. In the case of AB, however, migraines with aura is a risk factor for ischemic stroke [5], and this risk is further increased in conjunction with combined hormonal contraception use. After explaining the unacceptably high risks to AB, a non-estrogen-containing contraceptive alternative should be recommended for her.

What Other Contraceptives Would You Recommend for Me?

In order to provide high-quality counseling to an adolescent requesting contraception, health-care practitioners must provide information about the relative effectiveness of the method, method use, health risks and medical contraindications, side effects, and non-contraceptive benefits of each available method, so that she can make an informed choice. After determining which contraceptive methods are safe for her to use, a menstrual history might aid in individualization of the best contraceptive method that has additional benefits of reduced menstrual bleeding or improvement in dysmenorrhea, if these are concerns for the adolescent.

It is also helpful to obtain insight into the adolescent's reproductive life plan, including experiences with previous contraceptive methods, including the reasons for discontinuation, if applicable. Of note, the experiences of an adolescent's friends and family members are important to ascertain, as they influence family planning decisions of adolescents. For example, AB does not want to continue using DMPA because of the associated unpredictable vaginal bleeding; therefore, etonogestrel implant may not be the method best suited for this adolescent, given its similar side effect of unpredictable vaginal bleeding. Further, since previous studies have demonstrated that DMPA is more likely to be associated with weight gain compared to other contraceptive methods such as COCs [6], discontinuation of DMPA is reasonable and respects the adolescent's reproductive right to choose her contraceptive method. One important aspect of promoting adherence to contraceptive methods is investigation of which side effects are tolerable and which benefits are most desirable for each patient.

Counseling should start with most efficacious contraceptive methods, namely, long-acting reversible contraceptives (LARCs), including copper and levonorgestrel IUDs and subdermal etonogestrel implants [7]. Studies have shown that with this tiered counseling approach, adolescents are more likely to choose a LARC method [8]. The American Academy of Pediatrics recommends LARC methods as first-line contraceptive options for adolescents given their efficacy, safety, and ease of use [9]. Previous studies involving adolescents have shown that LARC methods have higher continuation and satisfaction rates compared to COCs [10]. Further, the improved access to LARC methods and increased use in adolescents may decrease pregnancy, abortions, and birth rates in this age group [10]. During counseling, we recommend emphasizing the importance of dual methods using a condom at every sexual encounter to decrease the risk of STI acquisition. Finally, it is important to ask questions about the adolescent's relationship and screen for intimate partner violence and reproductive coercion, as this may influence whether or not partner-independent methods are preferred [11, 12].

Medication Interactions

Prior to initiating contraception, it is important to check for any medication interactions. Specifically, there are medications that can decrease contraceptive effectiveness by inducing cytochrome P4503A (CYP3A), including rifampin and antiepileptic medications including topiramate, oxcarbazepine, and phenobarbital. Additionally, other medications have significant medication interactions with hormonal contraceptives, including the antiretroviral fosamprenavir and lamotrigine when used as monotherapy [2]. Many medications commonly prescribed to adolescents including selective serotonin reuptake inhibitors (SSRIs) and antifungals have no medication interactions with COC, DMPA, IUDs, or implants. See Table 18.1 for interactions between contraceptives and medications commonly prescribed to adolescents. For AB, there are no significant medication interactions with any contraceptive method.

Long-Acting Reversible Contraception

LARC methods, including the intrauterine devices and the birth control implant, are the most effective forms of reversible birth control currently available. Both types of IUDs and contraceptive implants are highly effective at preventing pregnancy, with fewer than 1 in 100 women who use them becoming pregnant [13]. Previous studies have found that women using IUDs and contraceptive implants were 20 times less likely to have an unintentional pregnancy than women using COCs, the patch, or the ring [14]. In one study, adolescents and young adults who used COCs, the contraceptive patch, or ring had higher rates of unintended pregnancy compared to older women, due to lower adherence to these methods by adolescents [14]. In comparison, LARC is a user-independent method with very low failure rates regardless of age [13]. Finally, LARCs are reversible and demonstrate a rapid return to fertility after removal [15–17].

Implant

The subdermal contraceptive implant is a flexible rod, the size of a matchstick that is inserted subdermally in the upper arm [18]. It releases etonogestrel, a progestin, and protects against pregnancy for up to 3 years. The current implant on the market is Nexplanon®. It differs from its predecessor Implanon® by having the additional benefit of being radiopaque [9]. The mechanism of action is prevention of ovulation via thickening of the cervical mucus making it more difficult for sperm to enter the uterus and thinning of the endometrial lining so that a fertilized egg is less likely to successfully implant [18].

Intrauterine Device

Today, four IUDs are approved for use in the United States: a copper-releasing device (ParaGard®) and three hormone-releasing devices (Mirena®, Skyla®, and Liletta®) [9]. All four of these IUDs have monofilaments that minimize the risk of bacterial transmission as compared to the multifilament threads utilized in the Dalkon Shield, an IUD that was recalled in 1975 given its association with pelvic inflammatory disease [19].

Table 18.1 Potential drug interactions with contraceptive medications

	Medication	LNG IUD	Copper IUD	ENG implant	DMPA	Combined pill, patch, ring
Antiretroviral medication	Non-nucleoside reverse transcriptase inhibitors/ efavirenz	No known interaction between ARV therapy and IUD use. IUD insertion has some theoretic risks if the woman is not clinically well or not receiving ARV therapy although benefits generally outweigh these infectious risks		Theoretically could decrease contraceptive effectiveness, consider another method or dual contraceptive use	No restriction	Theoretically could decrease contraceptive effectiveness, consider another method or dual contraceptive use
	Protease inhibitor/ fosamprenavir	No known interaction between ARV therapy and IUD use. IUD insertion has some theoretic risks if the woman is not clinically well or not receiving ARV therapy although benefits generally outweigh these infectious risks		Theoretically could decrease level and effectiveness of fosamprenavir, consider another method	No restriction	Risks usually outweigh benefits, as may decrease levels and effectiveness of fosamprenavir
	Ritonavir-boosted protease inhibitors (ritonavir-boosted atazanavir, darunavir, fosamprenavir, saquinavir, or tipranavir)	No known interaction between ARV therapy and IUD use. IUD insertion has some theoretic risks if the woman is not clinically well or not receiving ARV therapy although benefits generally outweigh these infectious risks		Theoretically could decrease contraceptive effectiveness, consider another method or dual contraceptive use	No restriction	Theoretically could decrease contraceptive effectiveness, consider another method or dual contraceptive use

Antiepileptic medication	Oxcarbazepine, phenobarbital, phenytoin, carbamazepine, topiramate, primidone	No restriction	No restriction	Theoretically could decrease contraceptive effectiveness, consider another method or dual contraceptive use	No restriction	Risks of pregnancy usually outweigh benefits, as may decrease contraceptive effectiveness
	Lamotrigine	No restriction	No restriction	No restriction	No restriction	Risks usually outweigh benefits when lamotrigine taken as monotherapy as ethinyl estradiol decreases lamotrigine levels
Antibiotic	Rifampin or rifabutin	No restriction	No restriction	Theoretically could decrease contraceptive effectiveness, consider another method or dual contraceptive use	No restriction	Risks of pregnancy usually outweigh benefits as may decrease contraceptive effectiveness
Supplement	St John's wart	No restriction	No restriction	Theoretically could decrease contraceptive effectiveness, consider another method or dual contraceptive use	No restriction	Theoretically could decrease contraceptive effectiveness, consider another method or dual contraceptive use

(continued)

Table 18.1 (continued)

	Medication	LNG IUD	Copper IUD	ENG implant	DMPA	Combined pill, patch, ring
Immunosuppressant	Mycophenolate mofetil	No restriction	No restriction	Theoretically could decrease contraceptive effectiveness, consider another method or dual contraceptive use		Theoretically could decrease contraceptive effectiveness, consider another method or dual contraceptive use
	Cyclosporine	No restriction	No restriction	Consider monitoring cyclosporine levels given theoretical drug interaction with progestin-only methods		Hormonal contraceptives may increase cyclosporine levels—monitor blood levels closely
	Sirolimus	No restriction	No restriction	Consider monitoring sirolimus levels given theoretical drug interaction with progestin-only methods		Hormonal contraceptives may increase sirolimus levels—monitor blood levels closely

Data from the Centers for Disease Control and Prevention's Medical Eligibility Criteria [2], the American Academy of Pediatrics' Contraception for Adolescents [9], and additional references [29–31]

ENG implant etonogestrel implant, *LNG IUD* levonorgestrel intrauterine device, *DMPA* depot medroxyprogesterone acetate, *ARV* antiretroviral

The copper-releasing IUD is a T-shaped polyethylene device with 380 mm^2 of copper. The main mechanism of action is by the release of copper ions which interfere with sperm mobility. It is approved to provide contraception for up to 10 years and may also be used as emergency contraception within 5 days of unprotected intercourse [20]. The Mirena® IUD is a radiopaque T-shaped device with 52 mg of levonorgestrel and has been approved for up to 5 years [19]. The Liletta® IUD also contains 52 mg of levonorgestrel. The Federal Drug Administration (FDA) has currently approved its use for up to 3 years, but studies are ongoing to assess if it is effective for an extended duration of up to 5 years [21]. Finally, Skyla® is the only IUD with FDA approval for use in nulliparous adolescents and young women. It is slightly smaller than the Mirena® IUD, contains only 13.5 mg of levonorgestrel, and is approved for up to 3 years of use [22]. The main mechanism of action of these three levonorgestrel-releasing systems is to thicken the cervical mucus, therefore creating a barrier to sperm entering the uterus, and additionally to thin the endometrial lining, therefore making it less likely that a fertilized egg will implant [19].

If I Decide on the IUD, Do I Have to Have Anesthesia for the IUD Insertion?

Many adolescents have significant misconceptions and anxiety about the IUD insertion procedure, so it is important to proactively counsel them. First, it is important to explain that having an IUD inserted involves a pelvic examination. If possible, it is often helpful for patients who have never undergone a pelvic examination before to be shown a speculum. Further, anticipatory guidance should be provided that a pelvic examination should not hurt, but may feel uncomfortable. Sterile technique is used to minimize the risk of infection. General anesthesia is not indicated for the overwhelming majority of adolescents, with the exception of some patients with moderate to severe intellectual disability. There is limited evidence that a lidocaine paracervical block may reduce pain during IUD insertion [23]. Misoprostol and nonsteroidal anti-inflammatories may be offered, although studies published to date have not found that these methods decrease pain perception. In general, adolescents are able to tolerate the procedure well without any pain medication or sedation [24, 25]. The IUD strings are cut a few centimeters past the cervix and thus should not bother patients or their partners [26].

Can I Get an IUD Today?

After extensive counseling, AB decides a levonorgestrel IUD for contraception, given its non-contraceptive benefit of treating menorrhagia [19]. AB presented to her visit 12 weeks after her DMPA injection and thus was within the time window of its effectiveness for pregnancy prevention. Therefore, AB is a candidate for having an IUD inserted immediately, given the reasonable certainty that she is not pregnant. If there is any possibility of an early, undetected pregnancy, as in a case of a young girl who was not on reliable contraception who had unprotected intercourse 7 days ago, the risk of having an IUD inserted in a pregnant girl would outweigh the benefit. In this situation, an adolescent should be provided with another contraceptive method until it can be established with reasonable certainty that she is not pregnant and an IUD may be safely inserted. If a woman has had unprotected intercourse in the last 5 days, consider offering emergency contraception if pregnancy is not desired, such as a copper IUD or emergency contraceptive pills. Figure 18.1 provides additional information about quick-starting LARCs, including levonorgestrel and copper IUDs and etonogestrel implants [1].

Following Up with AB

AB returns to see her provider 6 weeks later. Overall, she is satisfied with her levonorgestrel IUD, except that she is bothered by unscheduled spotting which lasts approximately a week between her menses. She reports that she knows that she was counseled to expect changes in bleeding patterns with the levonorgestrel IUD, yet she is concerned because she has a new partner and they have had unprotected sex without a condom. She denies any fever or chills, abdominal or pelvic pain, pain during sex, vaginal discharge, dysuria, or any other urinary symptoms. Upon physical examination, AB has a normal vulva without lesions, normal cervix without friability, no vaginal discharge, and the IUD string is visualized protruding from the cervical os. There is no cervical motion tenderness and no adnexal tenderness or masses palpated on bimanual examination. She consents to chlamydia and gonorrhea nucleic acid amplification testing.

AB should be reassured that given her normal examination, her unscheduled spotting is likely due to the levonorgestrel IUD and is expected to resolve 3–6 months after insertion. Anticipatory guidance should be provided that over time the bleeding will improve with the possibility of amenorrhea or oligomenorrhea by 24 months [19]. She may be offered naproxen 500 mg twice daily for 5 days to decrease the bleeding associated with her levonorgestrel IUD [27, 28].

Clinical Pearls and Pitfalls

- Confidentiality must be assured for adolescents obtaining reproductive and sexual health services including contraception. Can consult Guttmacher Institute's "An overview of minors' consent law" (2016) to obtain state-specific laws regarding minor consent to contraception.

- Prior to prescribing any contraception method, review a patient's medical history and consult the Centers for Disease Control and Prevention's "Summary Chart of U.S. Medical Eligibility Criteria for Contraceptive Use" (2016), which assesses the safety of different contraceptive methods by medical condition.
- Ensure no medication interactions with patient's current medications and desired contraceptive method. Table 18.1 lists common medication interactions in adolescents.
- Long-acting reversible contraception including copper and levonorgestrel IUDs and subdermal etonogestrel implants are first-line contraceptive options for adolescents (American Academy of Pediatrics, Policy statement: Contraception for adolescents, 2014).
- The Centers for Disease Control and Prevention's "Effectiveness of family planning methods" (2010) is a helpful tool to provide comprehensive contraceptive counseling starting with the most efficacious long-acting reversible contraceptive methods.
- Effective contraceptive counseling should be individualized according to the adolescent's reproductive life plan, previous contraceptive method use, and preferences regarding which side effects are tolerable and desired. Some of the more common benefits and side effects are discussed in the American Academy of Pediatrics' "Policy statement: Contraception for adolescents" (2014).
- To determine if a patient can start a contraceptive method and what medical evaluations are required prior to initiation, providers can consult "U.S. selected practice guidelines for contraceptive use, 2016." Additionally a guide to quick starting an IUD or implant is provided in Fig. 18.1.
- Follow-up care for patients with different contraceptive methods including guidance on how to manage patients with IUDs who develop pelvic inflammatory disease and management of common side effects is included in the "U.S. selected practice guidelines for contraceptive use, 2016."

References

1. Curtis KM, Jatlaoui TC, Tepper NK, et al. U.S. selected practice recommendations for contraceptive use, 2016. MMWR. 2016;65(RR-04):1–66. 10.15585/mmwr.rr6504a1.
2. Curtis KM, Tepper NK, Jatlaoui TC, et al. U.S. medical eligibility criteria for contraceptive use, 2016. MMWR. 2016;65(RR-03):1–104. 10.15585/mmwr.rr6503a1.
3. Centers for Disease Control and Prevention. Summary chart of U.S. medical eligibility criteria for contraceptive use. 2016. Available via CDC. http://www.cdc.gov/reproductivehealth/contraception/pdf/summary-chart-us-medical-eligibility-criteria_508tagged.pdf. Accessed 29 July 2016.
4. Trenor CC, Chung RJ, Michelson AD, et al. Hormonal contraception and thrombotic risk: a multidisciplinary approach. Pediatrics. 2011;127(2):347–57. https://doi.org/10.1542/peds.2010-2221.
5. Spector JT, Kahn SR, Jones MR, et al. Migraine headache and ischemic stroke risk: an updated meta-analysis. Am J Med. 2010;123(7):612–24. https://doi.org/10.1016/j.amjmed.2009.12.021.

6. Beksinska ME, Smit JA, Kleinschmidt I, et al. Prospective study of weight change in new adolescent users of DMPA, NET-EN, COCs, non-users and discontinuers of hormonal contraception. Contraception. 2010;81(1):30–4. https://doi.org/10.1016/j.contraception.2009.07.007.
7. Centers for Disease Control and Prevention. Providing quality family planning services: recommendations of CDC and the U.S. Office of Population Affairs. MMWR. 2014;63(RR-04):1–54.
8. Secura GM, Madden T, McNicholas C, et al. Provision of no-cost, long-acting contraception and teenage pregnancy. N Engl J Med. 2014;371(14):1316–23. https://doi.org/10.1056/NEJMoa1400506.
9. American Academy of Pediatrics. Contraception for adolescents. Pediatrics. 2014;134(4):1257–81. https://doi.org/10.1542/peds.2014-2300.
10. Peipert JF, Zhao Q, Allsworth JE, et al. Continuation and satisfaction of reversible contraception. Obstet Gynecol. 2011;117(5):1105–13. https://doi.org/10.1097/AOG.0b013e31821188ad.
11. American College of Obstetricians and Gynecologists. ACOG committee opinion no. 518: intimate partner violence. Obstet Gynecol. 2012;119:412–7. https://doi.org/10.1097/AOG.0b013e318249ff74.
12. American College of Obstetricians and Gynecologists. ACOG committee opinion no. 554: reproductive and sexual coercion. Obstet Gynecol. 2013;121:411–5. https://doi.org/10.1097/01.AOG.0000426427.79586.3b.
13. Trussell J. Contraceptive efficacy. In: Hatcher RA, Trussell J, Stewart F, et al., editors. Contraceptive technology. 18th ed. New York: Ardent Media, Inc.; 2004.
14. Winner B, Peipert JF, Zhao Q, et al. Effectiveness of long-acting reversible contraception. N Engl J Med. 2012;366:1998–2007. https://doi.org/10.1056/NEJMoa1110855.
15. Funk S, Miller MM, Mishell DR, et al. Safety and efficacy of Implanon, a single-rod implantable contraceptive containing etonogestrel. Contraception. 2005;71(5):319–26.
16. Hova GG, Skjeldestada FE, Hilstadb T. Use of IUD and subsequent fertility – follow-up after participation in a randomized clinical trial. Contraception. 2007;75(2):88–92.
17. Stoddard AM, Xu H, Madden T, et al. Fertility after intrauterine device removal: a pilot study. Eur J Contracept Reprod Health Care. 2015;20(3):223–30. https://doi.org/10.3109/13625187.2015.1010639.
18. Darney P, Patel A, Rosen K, et al. Safety and efficacy of a single-rod etonogestrel implant (Implanon): results from 11 international clinical trials. Contraception. 2009;91(5):1646–53. https://doi.org/10.1016/j.fertnstert.2008.02.140.
19. Beatty MN, Blumenthal PD. The levonorgestrel-releasing intrauterine system: safety, efficacy, and patient acceptability. Ther Clin Risk Manag. 2009;5:561–74.
20. American College of Obstetricians and Gynecologists. Practice bulletin 121: long-acting reversible contraception: implants and intrauterine devices. Obstet Gynecol. 2011;118:184–96.
21. Eisenberg DL, Schreiber CA, Turok DK, et al. Three-year efficacy and safety of a new 52-mg levonorgestrel-releasing intrauterine system. Contraception. 2015;92(1):10–6. https://doi.org/10.1016/j.contraception.2015.04.006.
22. Nelson A, Apter D, Hauck B, et al. Two low-dose levonorgestrel intrauterine contraceptive systems: a randomized controlled trial. Obstet Gynecol. 2013;122:1205–13. https://doi.org/10.1097/AOG.0000000000000019.
23. Lopez LM, Bernholc A, Zeng Y, et al. Interventions for pain with intrauterine device insertion. Cochrane Database Syst Rev. 2015;(7):CD007373. doi:https://doi.org/10.1002/14651858.CD007373.pub3.
24. Hubacher D, Reyes V, Lillo S, et al. Pain from copper intrauterine device insertion: randomized trial of prophylactic ibuprofen. Am J Obstet Gynecol. 2006;195(5):1272–7.
25. Sääv I, Aronsson A, Marions L, et al. Cervical priming with sublingual misoprostol prior to insertion of an intrauterine device in nulliparous women: a randomized controlled trial. Hum Reprod. 2007;22(10):2647–52.
26. Johnson BA. Insertion and removal of intrauterine devices. Am Fam Physician. 2005;71(1):95–101.
27. Friedlander E, Kaneshiro B. Therapeutic options for unscheduled bleeding associated with long-acting reversible contraception. Obstet Gynecol Clin North Am. 2015;42(4):593–603. https://doi.org/10.1016/j.ogc.2015.07.004.

28. Madden T, Proehl S, Allsworth JE, et al. Naproxen or estradiol for bleeding and spotting with the levonorgestrel intrauterine system: a randomized controlled trial. Am J Obstet Gynecol. 2012;206(129):e1–8. https://doi.org/10.1016/j.ajog.2011.09.021.
29. Krajewski CM, Geetha D, Gomez-Lobo V. Contraceptive options for women with a history of solid-organ transplantation. Transplantation. 2013;95(10):1183–6. https://doi.org/10.1097/TP.0b013e31827c64de.
30. Sucato GS, Murray PJ. Developmental and reproductive health issues in adolescent solid organ transplant recipients. Semin Pediatr Surg. 2006;15(3):170–8.
31. Maddox DD, Rahman Z. Etonogestrel (Implanon), another treatment option for contraception. Drug Forecast. 2008;33(6):337–47.

Recommended Reading

American Academy of Pediatrics. Policy statement: contraception for adolescents. Pediatrics. 2014;134(4):1244–56. https://doi.org/10.1542/peds.2014-2299.

American College of Obstetricians and Gynecologists. ACOG Committee Opinion No. 642: increasing access to contraceptive implants and intrauterine devices to reduce unintended pregnancy. Obstet Gynecol. 2015;126(412-417):44–8.

Centers for Disease Control and Prevention. Effectiveness of family planning methods. 2010. Available at https://www.cdc.gov/reproductivehealth/unintendedpregnancy/pdf/contraceptive_methods_508.pdf. Accessed 20 July 2016.

Centers for Disease Control and Prevention. Summary chart of U.S. medical eligibility criteria for contraceptive use. 2016. Available at http://www.cdc.gov/reproductivehealth/contraception/pdf/summary-chart-us-medical-eligibility-criteria_508tagged.pdf. Accessed 29 July 2016.

Curtis KM, Jatlaoui TC, Tepper NK, et al. U.S. selected practice recommendations for contraceptive use, 2016. MMWR. 2016;65(RR-04):1–66. 10.15585/mmwr.rr6504a1.

Guttmacher Institute. An overview of minors' consent law as of March 1, 2016. State Policies in Brief. 2016. Available at https://www.guttmacher.org/sites/default/files/pdfs/spibs/spib_OMCL.pdf. Accessed 2 Aug 2016.

Chapter 19
Case of a Girl with Condom Failure

Karen Browner-Elhanan

A 17-year-old girl presents to your office 4 days after the condom slipped off during sexual intercourse with her boyfriend. She has been sexually active with him for about 6 months; she has used condoms "properly" every sexual encounter previous to that and has never been pregnant. She has never been tested for sexually transmitted infections. Her mother is very anxious about the possibility that she may already be pregnant, as they read online that you should take emergency contraceptive pills within 3 days after unprotected intercourse, and she remembers you telling her that when she saw you for her annual examination. At the time of the examination, you had counseled about contraceptive options, including long-acting reversible contraceptives and emergency contraception, but the patient had declined birth control as she had never been sexually active at the time and stated that she was not planning on becoming sexually active in the near future. For that reason, you had not given her a prescription for emergency contraception.

She has no desire to become pregnant as is planning to go away to college next fall. She is an "A" student and is very active in high school choir. The patient and her mother had been discussing making an appointment for a long-acting reversible contraceptive when she disclosed to her mother about the recent unprotected intercourse upon her return from visiting her boyfriend in another state. As they had been staying at a remote location where he was working for the summer, there was no medical clinic or pharmacy accessible to them.

The patient states she feels well, and her past medical history is unremarkable except for obesity (BMI is 30) and some mild gastroesophageal reflux disease, for which she is taking omeprazole for the past few weeks. Her last menstrual period was 2 weeks ago, and her periods come monthly since age 12. She does not smoke. She uses over-the-counter topical medications for her acne, and other over-the-counter

K. Browner-Elhanan, M.D. (✉)
Pediatrics-Adolescent Medicine, Renown Children's Hospital, Reno, NV, USA
e-mail: drkj@optimum.net

H.J. Talib (ed.), *Adolescent Gynecology*,
https://doi.org/10.1007/978-3-319-66978-6_19

medications include only occasional paracetamol for occasional headaches. Her boyfriend is the one who provides the condoms as they are routinely dispensed at his school.

Her mother is asking if it is too late for emergency contraception of any kind. She is concerned about unwanted pregnancy and also sexually transmitted infections. Both the mother and daughter would like to know if she can start birth control immediately after taking care of "this issue." They are also concerned that her weight would make hormonal contraception less effective and "not an option."

The adolescent in this case is in need of emergency contraception for unprotected sexual intercourse 4 days prior to her visit to your office. Her mother has accompanied her, is supportive of her decision to see you, and acknowledges her need for a visit today and birth control. Despite recent statistics indicating a decline in teen pregnancy rates in the USA, teen pregnancy is still an undesired outcome of teen behavior in many cases. Many teens hide their sexual activity from adults, and thus their contraceptive use may be sabotaged [1]. The current rate of decrease in teen pregnancy is due mostly to increased, and earlier, education about contraceptive use, including education about long-acting contraceptives and emergency contraception and only minimally due to increased abstinence rates, according to recent studies [2]. About half of 15- to 19-year-old females state they have had sexual intercourse "ever," with 10% or more reporting they have been forced to have sex. Presently, more than 80% of pregnancies in adolescents are unintended and result from contraceptive nonuse or inappropriate use. The most commonly used method of birth control by teenagers is the condom, followed by oral contraceptive use [3]. Both of these methods have large risks of misuse or failure [4]. Hence, the concerns of your patient and her mother are reasonable.

Adolescent pregnancies, especially unplanned ones, have higher complication risks, including ectopic implantation, placenta previa, pregnancy-induced hypertension, and premature delivery, even with early and proper prenatal care, which may be difficult for adolescents to access. Adolescent mothers are less likely to graduate from school and more likely to live in poverty. The children of adolescents are more likely to have poor health outcomes, including low birth weight and higher rates of infant mortality, as well as lower educational achievement in the long run [5].

Emergency contraception is the only method designed to prevent pregnancy after intercourse. Providers ideally educate teens about contraceptive options, including emergency contraception and its availability prior to the need for it. This patient was educated but did not receive a prescription to have on hand or accessibility to immediate care. Medical literature has shown that women, especially teenagers, are most likely to use emergency contraception when they have it on hand [6]. Indications for the use of emergency contraception include unprotected vaginal intercourse, whether consensual or due to sexual assault, as well as missed doses of regular hormonal contraception. These indications include missing three doses in a row of an active hormonal contraceptive pill, having a contraceptive vaginal ring out for more than 3 h in a week when it should have be in, or having the patch off for more than 24 h in a "patch on week." Condom breakage or slippage, as in this scenario, is an indication for emergency contraception [6].

This patient's last menstrual period was about 2 weeks prior to the encounter, putting her at relatively high risk for pregnancy to occur. As she does not desire to become pregnant at this time, emergency contraception should be prescribed. The concern that "it may be too late" is appropriate, but the best response to her mother's fears is that hormonal emergency contraception is *most* effective when used within the first 24 h after unprotected intercourse or contraceptive failure. It can, however, be used within 120 h of unprotected intercourse to reduce the risk of pregnancy [6]. Hormonal emergency contraception is useful even with other birth control methods, and its effectiveness does not depend on the other methods (which previously failed). The patient can be prescribed the emergency contraception today and may be a candidate for LARCs (implant or intrauterine device) or oral contraceptives by quick start in addition. Emergency contraception which may be recommended includes the FDA-approved levonorgestrel and ulipristal acetate, off-label use of combination oral contraceptives ("Yuzpe" method), or insertion of a copper IUD.

In February of 2007, the FDA approved nonprescription access to Plan B for those 18 years of age and older. In 2009, the age limit was changed to 17 years of age and older, but this change did not actually happen until April 2013, when the US district courts ordered the FDA to lift a ban on the age restriction which had been put in place on over-the-counter availability of levonorgestrel-based emergency contraception. Two months later, the FDA allowed a one-pill formulation ("Plan B One-Step") to be available without age restrictions in the USA. The FDA granted Plan B One-Step 3 years of exclusive right to sell the product. Other products are now available on pharmacy shelves. The availability of the one-step generic brands to under 17 year old patients varies by state [7]. Two-pill formulations of levonorgestrel-based emergency contraception remain behind the counter and are not sold without a prescription to anyone under 17 years of age.

In August 2012, it became required by law that all FDA-approved contraceptive methods be covered by insurance without extra costs; most insurers will cover all costs of prescription emergency contraception. The table provided by the Guttmacher Institute indicates updated emergency contraception policies by state [7] (www.guttmacher.org).

The progestin-only regimens of emergency contraception contain levonorgestrel, which was first FDA approved in 1999. It is currently marketed under a number of different names, including Plan B (and One-Step), Take Action, and Next Choice. The regimen originally consisted of two pills containing levonorgestrel 0.75 mg, with directions to take second pill 12 h after the first pill. The one-step formulation, now used, is 1.5 mg taken at once. Package labeling indicates use within 72 h of intercourse, but the provider recommendations that it may be used up to 120 h after intercourse are supported by studies showing that pregnancy is prevented [8, 9]. Current retail cost is approximately $40.

No pregnancy testing or physical examination is required prior to use of this method [8]. The only contraindication to the progestin-only regimen is known pregnancy. There is no concern for teratogenicity, but there is an obvious lack of utility if the patient is already pregnant. Nausea and vomiting may occur, but the only common adverse side effect is heavy menstrual bleeding at the time of menses. No serious adverse side effects have been found. If vomiting does occur, an antiemetic is recommended, and the dose should be repeated. Patients should have a pregnancy test if they do not have a normal period within 3 weeks. This patient, especially if she is to be started on contraception by a quick start method afterward, should definitely have a pregnancy test within 3 weeks.

The mechanism of action of hormonal emergency contraception includes inhibition of ovulation, disruption of follicular development, and interference of the maturation of the corpus luteum. There are conflicting studies about the effect on endometrial histology affecting implantation of an already fertilized egg. Neither progestin-only or combined hormonal pills interrupt established pregnancies, nor have they been linked to teratogenic effects [8].

Combined oral contraceptive pills have not been labeled for emergency contraception but have been declared safe and effective within 72 h of unprotected intercourse to be used as such. Their use ("Yuzpe method," first developed in 1974) requires a prescription. This method should not be used if there are contraindications to estrogen use and involves taking two doses of pills, each containing a minimum of 100 μg of ethinyl estradiol and a minimum of 500 μg of levonorgestrel. There is the highest risk of nausea and vomiting compared to other methods of emergency contraception with this method.

As nausea and vomiting may occur in 50% of users, an antiemetic is recommended about an hour before administration of the dosage. The dose should also be repeated or switched to levonorgestrel, if vomiting occurs. Fatigue, breast tenderness, headache, abdominal pain, and dizziness may also occur.

Efficacy of the progestin-only method (1.1% pregnancy rate) compared to Yuzpe method (3.2%) is greater, especially if timing is indicative of a higher risk of pregnancy (midcycle). With either of these methods of emergency contraception in general, emergency contraception will lower the chance of pregnancy by ¾ in adolescent females having unprotected sex in the middle of their cycle. So, if 100 adolescent females have unprotected intercourse in the middle of their cycles and 8 will become pregnant without emergency contraception, with it, only 2 will become pregnant at that time with either of these methods [8, 9].

Another extremely effective emergency contraceptive product now used, especially in overweight patients (although it becomes less effective with BMI over 35), is a second-generation selective progesterone receptor modular. A single pill of ulipristal acetate 30 mg, a progesterone agonist/antagonist, was approved by the FDA in 2010 as emergency contraception. Indicated up to 120 h after unprotected sexual intercourse, it works as well on day 5 as on day 1 after intercourse. This medication is available by prescription only and is a pregnancy category X drug as fetal loss is a risk during the first trimester.

Pregnancy should be excluded before use but does not necessarily require an office visit if a patient cannot come to the office. A patient's menstrual history should be reviewed, and she can report the results before a prescription is called in.

The mechanism of action includes inhibition of follicular development and rupture and LH surge with a decrease of endometrial thickness causing a direct effect on implantation. It also increases endometrial bleeding. Similar to other methods, the dose must be repeated if vomiting occurs within 3 h of original dosing.

Ulipristal lowers the pregnancy rate by 85%, which is not affected by timing of the dose. A pregnancy test is indicated if a period does not occur more than 7 days later than expected after taking the medication, and a patient must be told to return for evaluation if severe abdominal pain occurs within a few weeks after administration, as ectopic pregnancy may occur.

Studies have frequently shown that hormonal contraception is in fact less effective at preventing pregnancy in overweight women. This is also true when used as emergency contraception. Ulipristal is more effective than progestin-only methods in mildly obese women with BMI under 35, but in more obese women, copper IUD is preferred, if it is an option [10]. The patient in this vignette should have a pregnancy test in your office and may have been offered and prescribed ulipristal today without concern for her obesity or length of time since unprotected sex affecting its efficacy; however, ulipristal should be avoided in drugs increasing gastric pH such as H2 antagonists and proton pump inhibitors.

The best option for women with a BMI of over 35 is the copper intrauterine device as the most effective emergency contraception and can be placed up to 120 h after unprotected intercourse as such and is 99.9% effective. Copper IUD is also favorable to ulipristal if the patient is on epileptic or antiretroviral drugs.

Pregnancy should be excluded prior to placement. Cooper IUD as emergency contraception has not been discussed extensively in AAP policy statements or discussions as there are few pediatricians placing IUDs. The IUD may be difficult to obtain within this period of time, but it will last after placement for 10 years. Adverse effects include mild abdominal pain at placement, intermittent spotting, and heavier periods and dysmenorrhea occasionally. Contraindications to the copper IUD include, besides suspected pregnancy, severe uterine distortion, active pelvic infection, and copper allergy or Wilson's disease. Other types of IUDs are not effective as emergency contraception at all [11–13].

During the emergency contraceptive visit and follow-up, it should be emphasized that emergency contraception used routinely to prevent pregnancy is not as effective as other methods. STI testing and treatment for the patient are important as a part of visit and subsequent follow-up, as well as a discussion for ongoing contraception. Oral contraceptive pills and long-acting reversible methods of contraception should be quickly started on follow-up visit, without waiting for menses. Studies have shown that effective hormonal contraception is most effective 5 7 days after emergency hormonal contraception, as prior to that they may compete for progesterone receptors. Copper IUD would be an effective method of long-lasting contraception as well as a method of emergency contraception at the present visit, with a skilled provider.

References

1. Eisenberg ME, Bernat DH, Bearinger LH, Resnick MD. Support for comprehensive sexuality education: perspectives from parents of school-age youth. J Adolesc Health. 2008;42(4):352–9.
2. Lindberg L, Santelli J, Desai S. Understanding the decline in adolescent fertility in the United States 2007-2012. J Adolesc Health. 2016;59:577–83.
3. Cwiak C, Howard B, Hsieh J, Riccioti N, Sucato GS. Sexual and contraceptive behaviors amongst adolescents requesting emergency contraception. J Pediatr Adolesc Gynecol. 2016;29:643–7.
4. Lopez LM, Grimes, DA, Gallo, MF, Stockton LL, Schultz KF, "Skin patch and vaginal ring versus oral contraceptives for contraception", Cochrane Database Syst Rev. 2013;(4):CD003552.
5. Thompson G, Canadian Pediatric Society, Adolescent Health Committee. Meeting the needs of adolescent parents and their children. Paediatr Child Health. 2016;5:273.
6. American Academy of Pediatrics Committee on Adolescents. Emergency contraception. Pediatrics. 2012;130(6):1174–82.
7. The Guttmacher Institute for Reproductive Health. "Emergency contraception" table of geographic regions. www.guttmacher.org. Last updated 1 Nov 2016.
8. Practice bulletin 152: "Emergency Contraception". J Obstet Gynecol. 2015;126(3):e1–11.
9. Fok WK, Blumenthal PD. Update on emergency contraception. Curr Opin Obstet Gynecol. 2016;28(6):522–9.
10. Emergency Contraception in overweight women: an IUD is preferable. Prescrire Int. 2014;23(155):300–1.
11. Simmons KB, Edelman AB. Contraception and sexual health in obese women. Best Pract Res Clin Obstet Gynecol. 2015;29(4):466–78.
12. Physicians for Reproductive Health. http://prh.org/teen.
13. Royal College of Obstetricians and Gynecologists, Faculty of Sexual & Reproductive Healthcare (FSRH). Statement on quickstarting hormonal contraception. in FSRH guideline "Emergency contraception", copyright 29 May 2017.

Chapter 20
Case of a Girl with Obesity Seeking Birth Control

Jessica Rieder, Courtney Sims, and Elissa Gross

Case

A 17-year-old Hispanic girl presents to the clinic for contraceptive management. She has a past medical history significant for obesity, dyslipidemia, prehypertension, and prediabetes.

The patient is sexually active and interested in hormonal contraception. She reports that coitarche occurred at 15 years of age and she has had four male lifetime partners. She reports that she never uses condoms and was treated for chlamydia last year. She has been with her current partner for the past 4 months. Menarche was at age 12. She has monthly periods, which last 5–6 days with moderate flow, and she has mild dysmenorrhea, which improves with the use of ibuprofen. Her last menstrual period was 2 weeks ago. She states that her partner is 20 years old and wants children now. She would prefer to be engaged first and complete her education but also wants a baby especially with her current partner because she is confident they are going to stay together.

She is currently taking no medications for her dyslipidemia, prehypertension, or prediabetes, although she has tried to lose weight by skipping meals. She has poor sleep hygiene, regularly skips breakfast and lunch, drinks at least 3–4 sugary beverages per day, and does not exercise. She is unhappy with the way she looks and wants to

J. Rieder, M.D., M.S. (✉)
Division of Adolescent Medicine, The Pediatric Hospital for Albert Einstein College of Medicine, Children's Hospital at Montefiore, Bronx, NY, USA
e-mail: JRIEDER@montefiore.org

C. Sims
Department of Pediatrics, The Pediatric Hospital for Albert Einstein College of Medicine, Children's Hospital at Montefiore, Bronx, NY, USA

E. Gross
Division of Hospital Medicine, The Pediatric Hospital for Albert Einstein College of Medicine, Children's Hospital at Montefiore, Bronx, NY, USA

H.J. Talib (ed.), *Adolescent Gynecology*,
https://doi.org/10.1007/978-3-319-66978-6_20

lose weight. She is considering bariatric surgery to help her to lose weight. She has no other significant past medical history. Family history is positive for hypertension in her mother and type 2 diabetes mellitus in her maternal grandmother. She denies toxic habits.

On physical examination, the patient is a well-appearing young woman with obesity. Her weight is 121.3 kg, her height is 165.3 cm, and her BMI is 44. Her BP is 127/82 and her pulse is 73. Her head and neck exams are within normal limits. Her heart and lung exams are normal. Her abdomen is obese and with abdominal striae but otherwise without masses or organomegaly. Her skin exam is significant for acanthosis nigricans at her posterior neck and in both axillae. She is Tanner stage 5 for both breast and pubic hair development. Recent bloodwork demonstrates a total cholesterol of 205 mg/dL, HDL cholesterol of 32 mg/dL, and a HbA1c of 6.0%.

Question: Of the different contraception options available to this patient, which choice would be best?

Discussion

Over the last 30 years, childhood obesity has more than doubled in children and quadrupled in adolescents [1], with severe forms of obesity increasingly prevalent, particularly among adolescents and non-Hispanic blacks [2]. Special attention should be paid to preventing unintended pregnancy in girls with obesity because pregnancy in obese women and girls increases the risk for gestational diabetes, hypertensive disorders, thromboembolic complications, operative delivery, late stillbirth, birth injury, having their infants admitted to NICU, and the persistence of obesity and the development of its comorbidities later in life [3]. Despite these risks, until recently, contraceptive clinical trials have largely excluded overweight or obese women, and there is limited evidence regarding contraceptive effectiveness and safety for this population [4].

There are several issues to consider when choosing a contraceptive method for an adolescent girl with obesity. First, the increased risks for cardiovascular disease and diabetes and the increased risks for persisting obesity in adulthood are important considerations when prescribing hormonal contraceptives. Secondly, there is evidence that increasing obesity may decrease the efficacy of some contraceptive modalities. Thirdly, despite higher risks for pregnancy-related complications, overweight or obese females have been shown to be less likely to use contraception than their normal-weight peers, and it is important to discern reasons, including the inability to negotiate contraceptive use with their partners when considering different contraceptive options. A final consideration relates to providing effective contraception for obese adolescents who need emergency contraception or are considering bariatric surgery.

Contraceptive Safety

Obesity in adolescence is associated with both short- and long-term health consequences: up to 70% of obese youth having at least one risk factor for cardiovascular disease, such as high cholesterol or hypertension and a high prevalence of prediabetes, increase their future risk for the development of diabetes. Further, obesity in adolescents is associated with a greater likelihood of having obesity in adulthood with the increased risk of adult health problems such as heart disease, type 2 diabetes, stroke, osteoarthritis, and several forms of cancer.

The fifth edition of the Medical Eligibility Criteria (MEC) for Contraceptive Use published by the World Health Organization (WHO) and the US Medical Eligibility Criteria (MEC) for Contraceptive Use, 2010, adapted from the 2014 edition of the WHO MEC, is an important resource for guiding contraceptive management in medically complex teens, including those with obesity and its associated comorbidities [5, 6]. A category 1 assignment indicates that there are no restrictions for the use of the contraceptive method. For category 2, the advantages of using the method generally outweigh the theoretical or proven risks. For category 3, the theoretical or proven risks usually outweigh the advantages of using the method, and for category 4, the health risks are unacceptable if the contraceptive method is used [6]. While there are risks associated with the use of progestin-only, estrogen-containing, implantable, and intrauterine device (IUD) contraceptives, the use of these contraceptives are much safer than being obese and pregnant [7].

According to the US MEC for Contraceptive Use 2010 guidelines, adolescents with obesity (BMI $\geq$ 30 kg/m^2) and no other comorbidities can safely use progestin-only contraceptives, including the implants and both the levonorgestrel and copper IUDs without restriction (category 1) (see Table 20.1) [6]. Depot medroxyprogesterone acetate (DMPA) use among adolescents less than the age of 18 years, however, may affect peak bone mass levels, and the extent to which bone mineral density (BMD) is regained or the risk for future fracture risk increases is unknown (category 2) [6]. As mentioned above, obesity increases risk for cardiovascular disease, and adolescents with multiple risk factors for cardiovascular disease including diabetes, hypertension, past history of a deep vein thrombosis (DVT) or pulmonary embolism (PE), a known thrombogenic mutation such as factor V Leiden deficiency, and known hyperlipidemias can safely use the copper IUD without restriction (category 1). Adolescents who have adequately controlled hypertension, a family history of a first-degree relative with a DVT or PE, and a superficial venous thrombosis can also safely use progestin-only contraceptives, including the implants and the levonorgestrel IUD without restriction (category 1). The use of progestin-only contraceptives, including the implants and the levonorgestrel IUD, generally outweighs the risks (category 2) if adolescents with obesity also have inadequately managed hypertension, a history of DVT/PE, a known thrombogenic mutation, a known hyperlipidemia, or diabetes.

For all adolescents and women with obesity, the advantages of using estrogen-containing contraceptives (pill, patch, ring) generally outweigh the theoretical or

Table 20.1 Contraceptive management guide for adolescents with obesity and common comorbidities

Condition	COC/P/R	POP	DMPA	Implants	LNG-IUD	Cu-IUD
Age	Menarche to	Menarche to	Menarche to	Menarche to	Menarche to	Menarche to
	<40 years = 1	<18 years = 1	<18 years = 2	<18 years = 1	<20 years = 2	<20 years = 2
	≥40 years = 2	18–45 years = 1	18–45 years = 1	18–45 years = 1	≥20 years = 1	≥20 years = 1
Obesity						
(a) ≥30 kg/m² BMI	2	1	1	1	1	1
(b) Menarche to <18 years and ≥30 kg/m² BMI	1	1	2	1	1	1
Multiple risk factors for arterial cardiovascular disease (smoking, diabetes, and HTN)	3–4	2	3	2	2	1
Adequately controlled HTN/ uncontrolled HTN	3/4	1/2	2/3	1/2	1/2	1
History DVT or PE/acute DVT	3–4/4	2	2	2	2	1/2
Known hyperlipidemias	2/3	2	2	2	2	1
Diabetes	2	2	2	2	2	1
Bariatric surgery						
(a) Restrictive procedures: decrease storage capacity of the stomach	1	1	1	1	1	1
(b) Malabsorptive procedures: decrease absorption of nutrients and calories	COCs:3 P/R: 1	3	1	1	1	1

Adapted from the Centers for Disease Control and Prevention (CDC). US Medical Eligibility Criteria for Contraceptive Use, 2010 [6]

COC combined oral contraceptives, *P* patch, *R* ring, *POP* progestin-only contraceptives, *DMPA* depot medroxyprogesterone acetate, *LNG-IUD* levonorgestrel IUD, *Cu-IUD* copper IUD

proven risks (category 2) (see Table 20.1) [6]. This assessment is based on the data that demonstrate that obese women who use combined oral contraceptives (COCs) are more likely than obese women who do not use COCs to experience VTE and this risk has been found to be additive in users of estrogen-containing contraceptives.

Women who use COCs have not been shown to have a higher risk of acute myocardial infarction or stroke than do obese nonusers. Further, adolescents with known dyslipidemias without other known cardiovascular risk factors can generally use estrogen-containing contraceptives, although the increased levels of total cholesterol, low-density lipoprotein (LDL), and triglycerides, as well as decreased levels of high-density lipoprotein (HDL), are known risk factors for cardiovascular disease. Similarly, blood pressure should be checked in adolescent girls with obesity as both obesity and COCs contribute to elevations in blood pressure. Combined oral contraceptives have no effect on long-term diabetic control and thus can be safely used in adolescents with well-controlled type 1 or type 2 diabetes mellitus (category 2). They should not be offered however to diabetic adolescents with poor metabolic control or have hypertension, nephropathy, or retinopathy [6].

Other comorbid conditions that need to be considered are nonalcoholic steatohepatitis (NASH) and polycystic ovarian syndrome. The effect of hormonal contraception on the progression of NASH is not well documented, and the use of hormonal contraception in obese adolescents with PCOS will be reviewed elsewhere.

Contraceptives and Continued Weight Gain

The potential for weight gain is another consideration when choosing a contraceptive for youth with obesity. The use of DMPA is associated with weight gain, and this weight gain is exacerbated for girls with obesity at the initiation of DMPA use. In a study of 450 adolescent girls aged 12–18 years, Bonny et al. demonstrated that adolescents with obesity who initiated DMPA were more likely ($p < 0.001$) to gain weight (mean weight gain of 9.4 kg) than adolescents with obesity who used either combined oral contraceptives (COCs) (0.2 kg) or no method (3.1 kg) [7]. They were also more likely to gain weight than adolescents who did not have obesity and initiated DMPA use. In contrast, there has been no associated demonstration of the use of estrogen-containing contraceptives and weight gain. A causal relationship between the use of these contraceptives and weight gain was not supported from the available evidence from a large systematic review of 49 trials evaluating the use of COCs or the patch [8].

Contraceptive Efficacy

The inherent effectiveness of some hormonal contraceptives may be diminished in obese adolescents. Higher metabolic rates, increased clearance of drugs metabolized in the liver, increased circulating blood volume, and higher drug sequestration in adipose tissue may result in decreased serum drug levels and inadequate contraceptive efficacy in obese adolescents [9]. Contraceptive failure rates with COC and the patch may be higher in adolescents with obesity; however, the failure rates are lower than those associated with barrier methods. While Westhoff et al. demonstrated that obese woman had lower maximum values of ethinyl estradiol than normal-weight women (85.7 vs. 129.5 pg/mL, $p < 0.01$), the lower concentration did not significantly impact follicular activity, and ovulation was still suppressed [10]. Dinger et al., however, found that among more than 55,000 US women, the COC failure rate was slightly higher in women with a BMI ≥ 35 kg/m^2 compared with women with BMI <35 (adjusted HR 1.5 (95% CI 1.3–1.8)) and risk of COC failure increases among overweight women as the COC estrogen dose decreases [11]. Studies evaluating the efficacy of the Ortho Evra contraceptive patch have included more overweight and obese women than other methods. A 2002 multi-centered, open-labeled study found that contraceptive failure may have been increased among obese women weighing more than 90 kg [12]. Small studies evaluating the effectiveness of the estrogen-progestin pill, patch, or vaginal ring have demonstrated no differences in contraceptive failure for these methods in overweight or obese women relative to normal-weight women with therapeutic hormone levels and adequate suppression of follicular development in obese women using the ring [12, 13].

The intrauterine device (IUD), contraceptive implant, and DMPA are all effective methods of contraception for adolescents with obesity. A copper- or levonorgestrel-releasing IUD is the best contraceptive option for obese adolescents. The Contraceptive CHOICE Project, a large prospective cohort study including thousands of women, with 27% and 35% of subjects meeting criteria for overweight and obesity, respectively, demonstrated overall failure rates of less than 1 pregnancy per 100 woman-years regardless of BMI [14]. The implant has also been found to be highly effective in obese women. Mornar et al. demonstrated that while obese women with the implant had lower concentration of plasma hormones compared to their nonobese counterparts, these differences did not reach statistical significance and there were no pregnancies in women who weighed ≥70 kg [15]. Despite its association with weight gain, DMPA has been shown to be an effective contraceptive method for obese women with no pregnancies documented in over 16,000 woman-cycles of DMPA use [16].

Contraceptive Use

Obese adolescents are less likely to use contraception than their normal-weight counterparts, even though they do not differ in their frequency of sexual intercourse or their number of partners [3]. Additionally, obese adolescents are less likely to use a pill for their contraception choice, while their rates of condom, IUD, injectable, and withdrawal method remain the same as their normal-weight counterparts [3]. These differences may be due to several factors. Obese adolescents have been shown to have lower self-esteem [17]. Lower self-esteem has been associated with earlier initiation of sexual intercourse and riskier behavior [18]. Obese adolescents with low self-esteem may not feel comfortable asking a physician for sexual health education and discussing appropriate contraception use. Physicians, who may lack time and may not feel comfortable counseling adolescents about sexual health, may provide poor health education on appropriate contraceptive choices in this high-risk group [19, 20]. It is important to be aware that differences exist between adolescents that are obese and their normal-weight counterparts with regard to their contraception use. Time should be taken to address both weight status and proper and appropriate contraception use given that both areas have significant impact on adolescent health (see Table 20.2).

Other Considerations: Bariatric Surgery and Emergency Contraception

Adolescents considering bariatric surgery need highly effective and safe contraception prior to undergoing any procedures. Oral contraceptives are not recommended (category 3) because of the increased risk for DVT/PE in the postoperative period and the potential for decreased effectiveness of oral medications associated with bariatric procedures involving a malabsorptive component [5]. All other non-oral contraceptive methods are acceptable alternatives, although long-acting reversible contraceptives are recommended because of the increased fecundity associated with weight loss.

While the fifth edition of the WHO MEC for Contraceptive Use has recently recommended that obese women can use levonorgestrel, ulipristal acetate (UPA), or combined oral contraceptive (COC) regimens for emergency contraceptive pills (ECPs) without restriction (MEC category 1), ECPs may be less effective among women with BMI ≥ 30 kg/m^2 compared to women with a BMI < 25 kg/m^2 [5]. Copper IUD insertion is a safe emergency contraception option which may be more effective for obese patients [5].

Recommendations

For our 17-year-old patient with obesity, prehypertension, dyslipidemia, prediabetes, and significant challenges related to negotiating contraceptive use, we recommend either the copper- or levonorgestrel-releasing (Mirena or Skyla) IUD or the etonogestrel implant for highly effective and safe contraception. The use of potentially less effective estrogen-containing contraceptives such as the pill or patch increases her risk for pregnancy-related complications related to her hypertension and prediabetes if she were to become pregnant, and they also place her at increased risk for future cardiovascular disease. If the patient were uncomfortable choosing one of the long-acting reversible contraceptive options, she can be offered a COC

Table 20.2 An example of contraceptive counseling for the adolescent with obesity, comorbidities, and difficulties negotiating contraception

Provider: So, I know we have talked about many things during this visit but I also wanted to discuss birth control with you today. How do you feel about that? And, just a reminder, you are 17 and almost an adult, but some patient's still worry that their parents will find out. We keep all our discussions about sex and reproduction confidential, but since you are 17, we will not share any of your healthcare information. Ok, back to birth control. What do you think?	*Patient*: I don't know. My boyfriend wants to have a baby but I want to finish school first and I would also like to at least be engaged first
Provider: Finishing school is very important. Have you talked to your boyfriend about your concerns?	*Patient*: Yes, but he keeps saying that he wants a baby now
Provider: The choice of whether you get pregnant is good to discuss with your partner, but the decision of what to do with your body is up to you. You know that right? No one can force you to do anything with your body that you do not want to do.	*Patient*: I know. He's not forcing me but I just don't know what to do. He doesn't want to wear a condom
Provider: Because of the other health concerns we have discussed today—the risk for high blood pressure and your abnormal risks for high cholesterol and diabetes—I would encourage you to use condoms and another form of birth control. Have you heard of the IUD and implant?	*Patient*: I think so. I'm really scared I'll get pregnant
Provider: Ok. Both of these methods are the safest and most effective forms of birth control for you. Also once inserted, you do not need to do anything more until you want to take them out. So, your boyfriend does not even have to know about them until you are ready to tell him.	*Patient*: Really?!
Provider: Yes! The IUD stands for intrauterine device and is used mostly to prevent sperm from fertilizing the egg. There are two types, but a small "T-shaped" device made of flexible plastic is inserted into your uterus. The copper IUD releases copper into the uterus and can last up to 10–12 years, and the Mirena releases a hormone called levonorgestrel and can last up to 6 years. The Skyla, a smaller, slightly lower-dose version of the Mirena, lasts up to 3 years (show model).	*Patient*: It goes inside me?! Does it hurt?
Provider: It can be a little uncomfortable at first and cause some cramping but after that, you usually do not feel it. It is a great option because it is a birth control that can last for years without you having to do anything.	*Patient*: Hmm… but what if I change my mind?
Provider: Then, the IUD can be removed. Simple as that.	*Patient*: What are my other options?
Provider: There is also the implant that I mentioned. It is a thin, flexible rod that is the size of a match that is inserted in your upper arm and can last up to 4 years (show model). It also works by releasing a hormone, progestin. I will let you know, however, that the implant can change your period. Some women stop having their period all together, some have longer and heavier periods, and some women spot.	*Patient*: Oh, I don't like that. I can't imagine having heavier periods. Oh no!

(continued)

Table 20.2 (continued)

Provider: It doesn't happen to every woman but you need to know that it may happen to you.	*Patient*: What about the pill?
Provider: The pill is an option but I would not recommend it for you. There are concerns that the pill may not be effective for women whose weight is in the range that yours is. Also, the fact that you have high blood pressure and high cholesterol increases your risk for blood clots in your legs or lungs while on the pill and may increase your risk for future heart disease. There is also the patch, which is changed once a week, but again, it may not be as effective and may have similar risks.	*Patient*: Hmm…there is a lot to think about! I just don't want to get pregnant right now. Maybe I should just think about it for a little while?
Provider: That is up to you, but the longer you go without a form of birth control, with a partner who isn't using condoms, the higher risk you are of becoming pregnant. Tell me your concerns about each one so we can talk about it.	*Patient*: That sounds good. The IUD just sounds scary
Provider: It's really not. I can show you a quick video online of how it works (show video).	*Patient*: Oh, that's not so bad. I want the one that lasts for the shorter time

Table 20.3 Contraceptive counseling pearls

• Make sure that concerns about confidentiality are addressed
• Be direct and honest about healthcare options and concerns
• Speak frankly and concretely
• Use models, pictures, and videos to assist your discussion
• Encourage positive life goals and aspirations
• Make sure to look out for signs of dating violence or sexual abuse

with a lower ethinyl estradiol dose (20–30 μg), the patch, or the ring, although she needs to be apprised of the potential safety and efficacy issues associated with these methods. DMPA, although an effective option, is less appealing given its association with continued weight gain. Importantly, this patient may suffer from low self-esteem and is at an increased risk for high-risk sex behaviors. It is imperative that she receives counseling related to the effective use of contraception and barrier contraceptive use to prevent unwanted pregnancy and the acquisition of STIs (see Tables 20.2 and 20.3). The patient would also benefit from knowing her emergency contraceptive options and the importance of highly effective contraception should she be interested in pursuing bariatric surgery. The patient should be counseled that Plan B or ella may not be as effective as the copper-releasing or levonorgestrel-releasing IUD for emergency contraception and these options will provide highly effective contraception to prevent pregnancy prior to and following bariatric surgery should she pursue this weight loss option in the future.

References

1. Ogden CL, et al. Prevalence of overweight and obesity in the United States, 1999-2004. JAMA. 2006;295(13):1549–55.
2. Skinner A, Skelton JA. Prevalence and trends in obesity and severe obesity among children in the United States, 1999-2012. JAMA Pediatr. 2014. https://doi.org/10.1001/jamapediatrics.2014.21.
3. Chang T, et al. Sexual behavior and contraceptive use among 18-19-year-old adolescent women by weight status: a longitudinal analysis. J Pediatr. 2015;167:586–92.
4. Lopez LM, et al. Hormonal contraceptives for contraception in overweight or obese women. Cochrane Database Syst Rev. 2013;(4):CD008452.
5. WHO medical eligibility for contraceptive use. 5th ed. Available at http://apps.who.int/iris/bitstream/10665/181468/1/9789241549158_eng.pdf?ua=1. Accessed on 07/10/2016.
6. Centers for Disease Control and Prevention (CDC). U.S. medical eligibility criteria for contraceptive use. MMWR Recomm Rep. 2010;59(RR04):1–6.
7. Bonny AE, et al. Weight gain in obese and nonobese adolescent girls initiating depot medroxyprogesterone, oral contraceptive pills, or no hormonal contraceptive method. Arch Pediatr Adolesc Med. 2006;160(1):40–5.
8. Gallo MF, et al. Combination contraceptives; effects on weight. Cochrane Database Syst Rev. 2014;(1):CD003987.
9. Greydanus DE, et al (2009). Concepts of Contraception for adolescents with obesity: pathways of judicial moderation. pediatrics faculty publications. Paper 137. Available at: http://uknowledge.uky.edu/pediatrics_facpub/137. Accessed on 7/10/2016.
10. Westhoff C, et al. Pharmacokinetics of a combined oral contraceptive in obese and normal-weight women. Contraception. 2010;81(6):474.
11. Dinger J, et al. Effectiveness of oral contraceptive pills in a large U.S. cohort comparing progestogen and regimen. Obstet Gynecol. 2011;117(1):33.
12. Zieman M, et al. Contraceptive efficacy and cycle control with the Ortho Evra/Evra transdermal system: the analysis of pooled data. Fertil Steril. 2002;77(2 Suppl 2):S13.
13. Dragoman M, et al. Contraceptive vaginal ring effectiveness is maintained during 6 weeks of use: a prospective study of normal BMI and obese women. Contraception. 2013;87(4):432–6. Epub 2012 Dec 10.
14. Xu H, et al. Contraceptive failure rates of etonogestrel subdermal implants in overweight and obese women. Obstet Gynecol. 2012;120(1):21.
15. Mornar S, et al. Pharmacokinetics of the etonogestrel contraceptive implant in obese women. Obstet Gynecol. 2012;207(2):110.e1.
16. Segall-Gutierrez P, et al. Follicular development and ovulation in extremely obese women receiving depo-medroxyprogesterone acetate subcutaneously. Contraception. 2010;81(6):487.
17. Griffiths LJ, et al. Self-esteem and quality of life in obese children and adolescents: a systematic review. Int J Pediatr Obes. 2010;5:282–304.
18. Ethier KA, et al. Self-esteem, emotional distress and sexual behavior among adolescent females: inter-relationships and temporal effects. J Adolesc Health. 2006;38(3):268–74.
19. Alexander SC, et al. Sexuality talk during adolescent health maintenance visits. JAMA Pediatr. 2014;168:163–9.
20. O'Brien SH, et al. Identification, evaluation, and management of obesity in an academic primary care center. Pediatrics. 2004;114:e154–9.

Chapter 21
Case of a Girl on Psychotropic Medications Seeking Birth Control

Jean Someshwar and Rollyn M. Ornstein

Julie is a 17-year-old young woman who comes to a follow-up appointment after starting combined oral contraceptive pills (COCs) for dysmenorrhea around 1 year ago. She had come to clinic frequently at the start of the last school year and was eventually diagnosed with depression for which she was placed on sertraline. Her mother accompanies Julie to clinic today and appears distraught. She explains that since Julie was last seen, she has been having worsening behavioral issues at school and at home and was diagnosed with bipolar disorder. Her symptoms were so severe that she was recently hospitalized in a mental health facility and was discharged home on quetiapine in addition to sertraline. Her mother is now concerned regarding the possibility of medication interactions between quetiapine, sertraline, and the COC.

Speaking with Julie independently, she says that she was hearing voices prior to her hospitalization but that is improving with her new medication. She admits that when she was ill, she would forget to take her COC but now is taking it regularly. She has had multiple sexual partners in the past year but is currently sexually active with one male partner, who uses condoms inconsistently. She admits that she has had some recent conflict with her partner because it is hard for her to "get in the mood" for sex, but is quick to describe the relationship with her boyfriend as "supportive" and "good," and says she feels safe and not coerced into sexual activity against her will. She states that her relationship with her parents is "difficult" and does not want to reveal her current sexual activity to her family.

J. Someshwar, M.D.
Division of Adolescent and Young Adult Medicine, Children's National Health System, George Washington University, Washington, DC, USA

R.M. Ornstein, M.D. (✉)
Division of Adolescent Medicine and Eating Disorders, Penn State Hershey Children's Hospital, Hershey, PA, USA
e-mail: rornstein@pennstatehealth.psu.edu

H.J. Talib (ed.), *Adolescent Gynecology*,
https://doi.org/10.1007/978-3-319-66978-6_21

Julie does not want to stop her COC, because she feels that she is having less cramping with her periods and also does not want to become pregnant. She asks whether there are medication interactions between COC and quetiapine or sertraline or any other medications that her psychiatrist might prescribe. She wants your opinion about contraceptive choice. She also wonders if it is normal that she is less interested in sex than her partner.

Discussion

Mental health disorders commonly emerge during childhood and adolescence and, per the World Health Organization, represent one of the leading causes of disability worldwide [1]. Recent epidemiological studies demonstrate that around 25% of youth will have a diagnosed mental disorder in the past year, with the most common condition being anxiety disorder, followed by behavior disorders such as attention-deficit hyperactivity disorder, mood disorders including dysthymia and depression, and substance use disorders [2]. As the prevalence of mental health disorders in adolescents is significant, pediatric and adolescent providers should have familiarity with medications used in mental health treatment. As an example, atypical antipsychotic medications have been increasingly prescribed over the last two decades, particularly in youth [3].

Adolescents with mental health disorders have a high risk for unintended pregnancies compared to the general population, which poses challenges for their reproductive health care [4]. Several studies have investigated links between mental health symptoms and high-risk behaviors, including risky sexual health practices. Women with serious mental illness have been shown to have high rates of lifetime sexual partners, increased prevalence of sexually transmitted infections, and infrequent use of contraception [4, 5]. Primary care providers are often a critical point of contact for their patients with mental health disorders and may be required to provide guidance on the suitability of various contraceptive options, including COC, in conjunction with psychotropic medications. We will review the potential interactions, risks, side effects, and benefits of the COC when simultaneously used with medications for mental health disorders. Additionally, we will review possible teratogenicity of psychotropic medications that may occur as a consequence of ineffective or absent contraception in the sexually active female and discuss alternative options for contraception in this population.

Although there is some concern among patients and providers about COC causing or exacerbating symptoms of depression, studies show that the use of COC, as well as other forms of hormonal contraception, does not increase depressive symptoms compared to baseline in reproductive-age women with major depression and bipolar disorder [6–8]. In fact, a protective effect was noted in a recent study of depressive symptoms in patients using COC, with decreased symptoms and fewer suicide attempts in patients on hormonal contraception compared with all other women. In this same study, women on progestin-only methods, including long-acting

Table 21.1 Antipsychotic medications and effects on serum prolactin (Adapted from Clinical Pediatric and Adolescent Gynecology, Psychiatric disorders and reproductive health)

Medication	Effect on serum prolactin
Risperidone	Significant elevation
Haloperidol	Significant elevation
Olanzapine	Moderate elevation
Ziprasidone	Moderate elevation
Quetiapine	Relative sparing
Clozapine	Relative sparing
Aripiprazole	Relative sparing

reversible contraception (LARC), also reported lower levels of depressive symptoms, but no significant findings were noted regarding the prevalence of suicidality [7]. With that said, it is important to consider interactions between COC and medications used to treat depression and bipolar disorder.

Selective serotonin reuptake inhibitors (SSRIs) are the most commonly prescribed medications for anxiety and depression. Neither SSRIs nor benzodiazepines, which are anxiolytic medications, are associated with clinically significant pharmacokinetic interactions with COC [9]. Antiepileptic and atypical antipsychotic medications, which are frequently used as adjunctive therapy in the treatment of mental health disorders, do have several notable interactions with COC [9]. Specifically, COC lowers the circulating levels of both valproate and lamotrigine, potentially decreasing the effectiveness of these mood stabilizers. Particularly, lamotrigine levels can be decreased significantly by up to 60% of previous levels [10]. However, this only applies to situations where lamotrigine is used as monotherapy. If lamotrigine and valproate are used concurrently, along with COC, there are no interactions [9]. Conversely, when taken with COC, the atypical antipsychotic clozapine, mainly used in the treatment of schizophrenia, may have significant increases in blood levels to three times greater than baseline, leading to clinical side effects including hypotension, sedation, tremor, and nausea. Other antiepileptic medications, such as carbamazepine and topiramate, as well as the non-prescription medication St. John's Wort, commonly used for dysthymia, enhance metabolism of COC by induction of the cytochrome P450 system, which may lead to a reduction in its efficacy in pregnancy prevention [9].

Antipsychotics are known to be associated with varying degrees of hyperprolactinemia, which may occur due to blockage of the inhibitory effects of dopamine on prolactin (see Table 21.1). When the serum prolactin level is elevated to 60 ng/mL or greater, amenorrhea may ensue through suppression of gonadotropin-releasing hormone and thereby luteinizing hormone and follicle-stimulating hormone, which leads to hypogonadotropic hypogonadism and often decreased libido. Galactorrhea can also occur through direct action of prolactin on breast tissue. As there are variations in sensitivity to hyperprolactinemia, not all patients develop these symptoms. There may be an age effect with respect to development of hyperprolactinemia in women, with younger age associated with higher prolactin levels. Antidepressants, including monoamine oxidase inhibitors, tricyclics, and SSRIs, may also be associated with a modest increase in serum prolactin, although it is less likely to be clinically significant. The induction of hyperprolactinemia is primarily through serotonergic pathways; however, sertraline is the most potent dopamine reuptake inhibitor, and the most frequent cause of increased prolactin, among the SSRIs. There is limited data on the effect of antidepressants on prolactin secretion [11].

Many antipsychotics are associated with weight gain and thus contribute to metabolic and endocrine derangements, including insulin resistance [12]. Valproate is also associated with weight gain, as well as polycystic ovary syndrome. This may be secondary to its inhibition of the cytochrome P450 enzymes, leading to increases in androgen concentration and decreases in sex hormone-binding globulin (SHBG). There may also be direct effects on ovarian production of androgens. Duration of valproate treatment and free testosterone levels have been found to be significantly associated, suggesting a possible cumulative effect of valproate on androgen production [12, 13].

In some women, sexual side effects, e.g., lowered libido and decreased signs of sexual arousal, can be seen with COC use, likely due to increases in SHBG which lower levels of serum-free testosterone. SSRI use may be associated with decreased libido as well. Several studies suggest a relationship between estrogen and serotonin transporter expression with the binding affinity of serotonin receptors being affected, thereby leading to a decrease in sexual desire and/or functioning [14].

The most serious adverse effect associated with COC use in the general population is increased risk of vascular thrombosis. Some studies have suggested that patients on antipsychotic drugs might also be at increased risk of venous thromboembolism, with patients on an atypical antipsychotic such as quetiapine being at the highest risk [15]. There does not seem to be an additive effect for patients on COC simultaneously with antipsychotic drugs, however [16].

Benefits may exist for COC use in patients with schizophrenia as there are postulated positive effects of estrogen on cognitive functioning. Women with schizophrenia tend to present later than men, which is felt to be due to a protective effect of estrogen. Further, women may have more severe symptoms of schizophrenia during low-estrogen phases of their menstrual cycle. This has led to investigations using estrogen as a therapeutic agent for schizophrenia itself [17]. However, this may be less relevant in younger patients.

Drawbacks to the use of COC in patients with significant mental health issues might include difficulty with compliance, particularly during times of exacerbation of psychiatric symptoms. Patients may have distortions of risk around contraception or may have a belief that they are unable to become pregnant on their psychotropic medications [18]. Furthermore, symptoms of stress and depression, substance abuse, and impulsivity may all lead to a high rate of unprotected intercourse and subsequent risk for unintended pregnancy if inconsistently compliant with COC.

If adolescents and young women with depression or bipolar disorder are not being effectively contracepted, there are also concerns for the teratogenicity of certain medications used in treatment. One such medication, valproate, has been associated with major malformations, including neural tube defects, long-term adverse

Table 21.2 Psychotropic medications and interactions with combined oral contraceptives

Medication	Interaction with COC
SSRI	No significant interaction
Carbamazepine	Decreased efficacy of COC
Lamotrigine	Decreased lamotrigine levels
Topiramate	Decreased efficacy of COC
Clozapine	Increased clozapine levels
Benzodiazepines	No significant interaction

neurocognitive effects, and cardiac abnormalities. However, a recent retrospective review showed that only 30% of reproductive-age females who were prescribed valproate for a mental health disorder were on any form of hormonal contraception and provider counseling regarding teratogenicity of valproate was documented in only 13% of potentially affected patients [19]. Other medications used in mental health treatment which may be associated with major congenital malformations include lithium and carbamazepine, which can cause cardiac defects, and benzodiazepines, which may be linked to an increased incidence of cleft lip or palate [20]. Counseling regarding LARC, e.g., intrauterine devices and contraceptive implants, as a more reliable alternative option for pregnancy prevention, would be advised in patients for whom COC compliance is difficult [4, 5].

When counseling the adolescent patient with a mental health disorder about contraception, there may be individual factors around patient beliefs, goals, and preferences that impact decisions around contraceptive method choice. It is important to note that there may be significant interactions between certain psychotropic medications and hormonal methods of contraception (Table 21.2). LARC methods, which include the intrauterine device and the implantable rod, are increasingly being used by adolescent females in the US [21]. As LARC offers highly effective birth control without the need for frequent personal attention or health visits, these methods may be optimal for patients with mental health disorders that may interfere with medication compliance. Certainly, imparting the most accurate information around potential risks, benefits, and side effects of all options to patients on psychotropic medications allows for an informed patient choice.

- Psychotropic medications may interact with the combined oral contraceptive, leading to increased or decreased levels of medications causing changes in efficacy or side effects.
- Effectiveness of the combined oral contraceptive may decrease with concomitant use of certain psychotropic medications, e.g. carbamazepine and topiramate.
- SSRIs are not known to significantly interact with COCs pharmacologically.
- Long-acting reversible contraceptives may be a preferred contraceptive method in patients on psychotropic medications for greater efficacy in pregnancy prevention and avoidance of pharmacologic interactions.
- Ineffective contraception in patients on psychotropic medications may lead to teratogenic side effects in the event of unintended pregnancy.

References

1. Murray CJ, et al. Disability-adjusted life years (DALYS) for 291 diseases and injuries in 21 regions, 1991-2010: a systematic analysis for the Global Burden of Disease study 2010. Lancet. 2012;380(9859):2197–223.
2. Merikangas KR, et al. Epidemiology of mental disorders in children and adolescents. Dialogues Clin Neurosci. 2009;11(1):7–20.
3. Burcu M, et al. Atypical antipsychotic use among medicaid-insured children and adolescents: duration, safety, and monitoring implications. J Child Adolesc Psychopharmacol. 2014;24(3):112–9.
4. Hall KS, et al. The risk of unintended pregnancy among young women with mental health symptoms. Soc Sci Med. 2014;90:62–71.
5. Hall KS, et al. Role of young women's depression and stress symptoms in their weekly use and nonuse of contraceptive methods. J Adolesc Health. 2013;53(2):241–8.
6. Young EA, et al. Influences of hormone-based contraception on depressive symptoms in premenopausal women with major depression. Psychoneuroendocrinology. 2007;32:843–53.
7. Keyes KM, et al. Association of hormonal contraceptive use with reduced levels of depressive symptoms: a national study of sexually active women in the United States. Am J Epidemiol. 2013;178(9):1378–88.
8. Pagano HP, et al. Safety of hormonal contraception and intrauterine devices among women with depressive and bipolar disorders: a systematic review. Contraception. 2016;94:641–9. doi:https://doi.org/10.1016/jcontraception.2016.06.012.
9. Curtis KM, et al. U.S. Medical Eligibility criteria for contraceptive use, 2016. MMWR Recomm Rep. 2016;65(RR-3):1–104. doi:https://doi.org/10.15585/mmwr.rr6503a1.
10. Herzog A, et al. Valproate and lamotrigine level variation with menstrual cycle phase and oral contraceptive use. Neurology. 2009;72(10):911–4.
11. LaTorre D, Falorni A. Pharmalogical causes of hyperprolactinemia. Ther Clin Risk Manag. 2007;3(5):929–51.
12. Correll CU, Carlson HE. Endocrine and metabolic adverse effects of psychotropic medications in children and adolescents. J Am Acad Child Adolesc Psychiatry. 2006;45:771–91.
13. Rasgon NL, Altshuler LL, Fairbanks I, et al. Reproductive function and risk for PCOS in women treated for bipolar disorder. Bipolar Disord. 2005;7:246–59.
14. Bishop JR, et al. The association of serotonin transporter genotypes and selective serotonin reuptake inhibitor (SSRI) associated sexual side effects: possible relationship to oral contraceptives. Hum Psychopharmacol. 2009;24(3). https://doi.org/https://doi.org/10.1002/hup 1006.
15. Parker C, Coupland C, Hippisley-Cox J. Antipsychotic drugs and risk of venous thromboembolism: nested case-control study. BMJ. 2010;341:c4245.
16. Zornberg GL, Jick H. Antipsychotic drug use and risk of first-time idiopathic venous thromboembolism: a case-control study. Lancet. 2000;356(9237):1219.
17. Bergemann N, et al. Estrogen and comprehension of metaphoric speech in women suffering from schizophrenia: results of a double-blind, placebo-controlled trial. Schizophr Bull. 2008;34(6):1172–81.
18. Hall KS, et al. Contraception and mental health: a commentary on the evidence and principles for practice. Am J Obstet Gynecol. 2015;212(6):740–6.
19. Gotlib D, et al. Guideline adherence for mentally ill reproductive aged women with valproic acid: a retrospective chart review. J Clin Psychiatry. 2016;77(4):527–34.
20. ACOG Practice Bulletin: clinical management guidelines for Obstetrician-Gynecologists. 2008;111(4):1001–20.
21. Finer LB, et al. Changes in use of contraceptive methods in the US, 2007-2009. Fertil Steril. 2012;98(4):893–7.

Suggested Reading

AACAP Practice Parameter for the use of psychotropic medication in children and adolescents. J Am Acad Child Adolesc Psychiatry 2006

ACOG Practice Bulletin: Clinical management guidelines for obstetrician-gynecologists. 2008;111(4):1001–20.

World Health Organization. Medical eligibility criteria for contraceptive use. 5th ed. Available at: http://www.who.int/reproductive-health/publications/mec. Accessed 8 June 2016.

Part IV
Special Populations of Adolescents

Chapter 22
Gynecologic Care and Contraception in the Medically Complex Adolescent

Amanda M. Jacobs

Case

A 17-year-old Hispanic girl presents to her general pediatrician for contraceptive and gynecological evaluation. She was diagnosed with systemic lupus erythematosus (SLE) 1 year ago after presenting with arthritis and Raynaud's syndrome with autoantibodies and antiphospholipid antibodies. Her renal function deteriorated following the diagnosis. A renal biopsy evaluating SLE-related renal complications revealed active class IV lupus nephritis with segmental glomerulosclerosis. Her rheumatologist recommended starting cyclophosphamide for her nephritis. During her evaluation prior to starting cyclophosphamide, a medication with teratogenic effects, she was screened for pregnancy risk. She disclosed that she was sexually active with one male partner. She was referred to her pediatrician for contraceptive and gynecologic care. Her medication regimen includes prednisone, hydroxychloroquine, enalapril, famotidine, and iron.

Her menstrual history is significant for regular menses lasting 7 days. However her menses became more frequent in the last 4 months, occurring on and off every 2–3 weeks. Her last menstrual period occurred 3 weeks prior to presentation at her pediatrician's office. Her menses are associated with menstrual cramps but no nausea, emesis, diarrhea, constipation, fatigue, or headaches. Her menses are not subjectively heavy, occurring without clots or soiling of clothes or sheets. Menarche occurred at age 13 years.

Upon obtaining a sexual history, she discloses that she identifies as heterosexual with two total lifetime partners. Onset of sexual activity occurred at age 15 years. She has been with her current partner for 9 months. She has never been pregnant or

A.M. Jacobs, M.D. (✉)
Division of Adolescent Medicine, Department of Pediatrics,
Children's Hospital at Montefiore, Albert Einstein College of Medicine,
Bronx, NY, USA
e-mail: Amanda.mcnear.jacobs@gmail.com

H.J. Talib (ed.), *Adolescent Gynecology*,
https://doi.org/10.1007/978-3-319-66978-6_22

used non-condom contraception. She was diagnosed with asymptomatic chlamydia once 1 year ago, for which she and her partner were treated. She reports using condoms about 60% of the time; however, she did not use a condom during her last sex 2 weeks ago.

On exam, vital signs were as follows: BP 120/67, pulse 91, respiratory rate 12, and temperature 98.0 °F. In general, she was well appearing with a normal heart, lung, and abdomen exam. Her genital exam was significant for Tanner stage 5 for pubic hair. She has a normal-appearing introitus, urethral meatus, and perineum without lesions. On bimanual exam, she had an anteverted uterus with no cervical motion or adnexal tenderness. Her ovaries were not palpable bilaterally. Her cervix did not have an ectropion, erythema, or friability.

Discussion

Several questions come up as the pediatrician is evaluating this patient for gynecologic care and contraception.

1. What routine gynecologic care should this patient receive?
2. What contraceptive options are effective and safe with this chronic illness and the medications needed to manage it?

Routine Pap Smear Screening in the Immune Suppressed Patient

Systemic lupus erythematosus (SLE) is a condition involving immune dysregulation, and as such patients with SLE have some degree of immune suppression. Additionally, managing this illness often requires administering medications that further suppress immune function. Women and adolescent girls with immune suppression for any reason require special gynecologic care. The American Congress of Obstetricians and Gynecologists (ACOG) recommends initiating Pap smear screening in healthy young women at age 21 years [1]. However, adolescent girls and young women who are immune suppressed require earlier initiation and more frequent Pap smear screening [1, 2].

The goal of Pap smear screening is to detect precancerous and cancerous lesions of the cervix due to the human papillomavirus (HPV) infection. The prevalence of HPV infection is highest in sexually active adolescents and gradually declines with age [3]. This decline is largely due to immune system clearance of the virus [4]. However, sexually active adolescent girls and young women with compromised immune systems are likely to have impaired clearance of HPV infection. This leads to a higher prevalence of persistent cervical HPV infections and precancerous and cancerous cervical lesions. These findings have been supported in the scientific literature in adult women with HIV, SLE, inflammatory bowel disease, and organ transplants [5–8].

HPV infection and precancerous cervical lesions have been well studied in adolescents with HIV. The current recommendation is to initiate screening of immune-suppressed adolescent girls or young women after the onset of sexual activity, every 6 months in the first year, and then yearly thereafter regardless of their age. However, there are no scientific studies or major society recommendations to guide the age at initiation and frequency of Pap smear screening in females younger than 21 years with immune compromise resulting from mechanisms other than HIV. ACOG suggests that it is reasonable to utilize the recommendations for HIV-infected persons until further studies provide scientific evidence to guide our management. Conditions with non-HIV-related immune compromise may include organ or bone marrow transplantation, SLE, and inflammatory bowel disease. The adolescent with SLE discussed above is immune supressed and has been sexually active for 2 years. According to these guidelines, she should have a Pap smear now and annually going forward.

Routine Sexually Transmitted Infection Screening and Prevention in Girls with Immune Suppression

Immune-compromised adolescent girls and young women require regular sexually transmitted infection (STI) screening, as do all sexually active adolescents, as part of routine gynecologic care. Adolescents and adults under the age of 25 years have the highest prevalence of STIs of any age group. This is the rationale for regular screening in this age group. Some immune-compromised patients, like those with HIV, have even higher rates of STIs as compared to healthy patients [9]. Moreover, many STIs are commonly asymptomatic. For these reasons, it is important to ensure regular STI screening in adolescents and young adults with immune compromise.

Recommendations exist for screening STIs in patients with HIV. However there are no guidelines for screening patients with other immune-compromising conditions. Since immune compromise is the basis for these unique recommendations in those with HIV, it is reasonable to screen all persons with immune compromise according to these guidelines. The CDC recommends annual screening of all sexually active persons with HIV with site-specific nucleic acid amplification tests for gonorrhea and chlamydia at each site of exposure, as well as screening for trichomonas vaginalis and syphilis [10]. In the case of adolescents with immune compromise without HIV, it is reasonable to also screen annually for HIV. The CDC recommends screening more frequently (biannually) based on high-risk behavior if the patient is in a high-prevalence area. The patient discussed above deserves a conversation about her exposure to the different types of intercourse (anal, oral and vaginal). Swabs for nucleic acid amplification tests for Gonorrhea and Chlamydia can be obtained from any site where she has had sex. A vaginal swab is similarly sensitive when testing for Gonorrhea and Chlamydia as compared to a cervical swab or urine sample. The most accurate method to detect Trichomonas is also with a nucleic acid amplification test (vaginal/cervical swab or urine).

The prevention of STIs should also be considered when providing gynecologic care. In addition to risk reduction behavior counseling, vaccination against HPV should also be employed. Since the HPV vaccine is not a live vaccine, there are no contraindications for its use in immune-compromised individuals. However, studies in persons with cancer or who have organ transplants showed reduced immune responses to all vaccines and as a result had lower vaccine efficacy. This has also been shown with the HPV vaccine [11, 12]. On the other hand, people with immune compromise are also at increased risk for persistent HPV infection and precancerous cervical lesions resulting from HPV. Therefore there are no recommendations to delay or alter the vaccine schedule for HPV as is recommended by the CDC [2, 13].

Contraceptive Contraindications for the Medically Complex Adolescent and Young Woman

It is important for providers who care for adolescents with chronic medical conditions to address pregnancy risk and contraception. Many women with chronic illnesses are as likely to become pregnant as their healthy counterparts. For example, women following organ transplantation had higher rates of pregnancy than those who did not have organ transplantation [14]. In addition, pregnancy in women with chronic illness can carry an increased risk of worsening disease or danger to the fetus. There are safe contraceptive choices for most women with chronic illnesses. When comparing the risk of getting pregnant and the risks of pregnancy to the health of the mother and fetus to the risk of contraception, the benefits of contraception outweigh the risks, especially in the case of those with chronic illnesses.

Barrier methods, like condoms, prevent sexually transmitted infections as well as pregnancy. However, they have low actual use contraceptive efficacy when used alone. Therefore condoms should be encouraged but only in conjunction with a more efficacious method, like a hormonal contraceptive or a copper intrauterine device (IUD). Due to the complexity of non-condom contraceptive methods in chronic illness, the remainder of this chapter will discuss these methods only.

When caring for adolescents and young women with chronic medical conditions, there are often multiple concerns with how their illness and medications interact with contraception, and the risk of pregnancy to their health and that of the fetus. This case illustrates some common contraindications and concerns. Both the Centers for Disease Control and Prevention (CDC) and the World Health Organization publish and regularly update safety recommendations for all available non-condom contraceptive methods for use in many different chronic illnesses for your reference [15, 16]. These recommendations are free and easily accessible on the Internet. These safety recommendations can help guide the provider in their contraceptive counseling and provision in many different circumstances.

One of the most common concerns with hormonal contraception in persons with chronic illness, and in particular this case, is the risk of thrombosis. Estrogen is known to increase the risk of thrombosis slightly in healthy persons. When considering contraception in persons with conditions that carry an increased risk of thrombosis, contraceptive counseling may present challenges. Contraceptive methods that contain estrogen include the combined oral contraceptive pill (COC), the contraceptive patch, and the vaginal ring. The estrogen in these contraceptive methods stimulates protein synthesis in the liver, increasing all of the liver's manufactured proteins, including clotting factors. This is the mechanism by which estrogen increases the risk of thrombosis in all women.

Several studies show that women with SLE do not have an increased risk of thrombosis with any contraceptive method as compared to women without SLE [17, 18]. However, women with SLE and antiphospholipid antibody syndrome do have an increased risk of thrombosis with estrogen-containing contraceptives [19, 20]. Therefore adolescent girls and young women with SLE and antiphospholipid antibody syndrome should be counseled to avoid estrogen-containing contraception. Other conditions that increase the risk of thrombosis and are contraindicated with estrogen-containing contraceptives include thrombogenic mutations, nephrotic syndrome, less than 21-days postpartum, prolonged immobilization, valvular disease, malignancy, and migraines with aura (see Table 22.1).

There are other concerns when using estrogen-containing contraceptives in adolescents and women with chronic illness. Included in these are estrogen's ability to increase blood pressure when used in persons with hypertension and interference with contraceptive metabolism when used in persons with liver disease. There are no contraceptive concerns with renal disease in general as seen in this case (except for the increased risk with thrombosis in nephrotic syndrome). Progestin-only-containing contraceptives and non-hormonal contraceptives have been studied extensively and have not been found to increase the incidence of thrombosis. These methods include the progestin-only pills (POPs), the depot medroxyprogesterone acetate injection (DMPA), the contraceptive implant, and the progestin and copper IUDs. All of these methods can be offered to people with an increased risk of thrombosis without contributing to this risk.

In the case discussed above, estrogen containing contraceptives (COC, patch, vaginal rign) are contraindicated. However the remaining contraceptive methods are safe with her medical issues and medications.

Contraceptive Efficacy and Teratogenic Medications

Several concerns arise with the use of non-condom contraception and medications used to treat this patient's renal disease/SLE. In particular, several of her medications are known teratogens. Cyclophosphamide and enalapril are classified as pregnancy safety category D (positive evidence of human fetal risk), and hydroxychloroquine is classified as a pregnancy category C (animal studies show

Table 22.1 Contraceptive contraindications with chronic illness and medications

Conditions with contraceptive contraindications	COCs, patch, vaginal ring	POPs	DMPA	Implant	Progestin IUD	Copper IUD
Risk of thrombosis						
Antiphospholipid antibody syndrome	X					
History of thrombosis and high risk for recurrence	X					
History of thrombosis and lowrisk for recurrence	RX					
Acute thrombosis	X					
Family history of thrombosis						
Major surgery with prolonged immobilization	X					
Migraines with aura	X					
Smoking under age 35						
Multiple risk factors for cardiovascular disease (diabetes, hypertension, smoking)			RX			
Hypertension, poorly controlled	X					
Thrombogenic mutations	X					
History of stroke or ischemic heart disease	X					
History of endocarditis	X					
Pulmonary hypertension	X					
High risk for atrial fibrillation	X					
Severe hyperlipidemia	RX		RX			
Cancer	RX					
Nephrotic Syndrome	X					
Risk for osteopenia: prolonged steroid use, chronic kidney disease, anorexia nervosa, primary ovarian insufficiency			RX			
Poorly controlled diabetes			RX			
Gall bladder disease	RX					
Malabsorption due to inflammatory bowel disease or bariatric surgery	RX for COC	RX				
Acute or flare of viral hepatitis	X					
Cirrhosis	X	RX	RX	RX		
Hepatocellular adenoma or hepatoma	X	RX	RX	RX		

(continued)

Table 22.1 (continued)

Conditions with contraceptive contraindications	COCs, patch, vaginal ring	POPs	DMPA	Implant	Progestin IUD	Copper IUD
Complicated organ transplant	X					
Severe thrombocytopenia			RX			RX
Diabetes with complications	RX		RX			
Distorted uterine cavity					X	X
Pelvic inflammatory disease or STI[a]					X	X
AIDS[a]					RX	RX
Medications interactions						
Increase metabolism of contraceptive with reduced efficacy	RX	RX				
Rifampin						
Anticonvulsants (phenytoin, carbamazepine, barbiturates, primidone, topiramate, oxcarbazepine, lamotrigine)	RX	RX				
Ritonavir-boosted protease inhibitors	RX	RX				
Reduced efficacy: St John's Wort	RX					
May increase plasma levels of medication: cyclosporine, sirolimus	RX	RX	RX	RX	RX	

COCs combined oral contraceptive pill, *POP* progestin only pill, *DMPA* depot medroxyprogesterone acetate injection, *IUD* intrauterine device
X absolute contraindication, *RX* relative contraindication
[a]Contraindication is for insertion only, not continuation of IUD with pelvic inflammatory disease or STIs

adverse fetal effects, but there are no controlled human studies) (see Table 22.2). Administration of a teratogenic medication should always warrant consideration of pregnancy risk. All sexually active adolescents and women are at risk for unplanned pregnancy, even when using a contraceptive method. In fact, 43% of adult women with unplanned pregnancies were using a contraceptive method (either inconsistently or incorrectly) when becoming pregnant [21]. This is also true for women taking known teratogenic medications. One study showed that 40% of women taking a teratogenic medication and COCs were taking their COC in a suboptimal frequency, threatening the efficacy [22]. As such, a contraceptive method with high efficacy and low user-dependent use error should be offered as a first-line method for adolescents and women taking teratogenic medications.

Efficacy should also factor strongly into contraceptive counseling in chronic illnesses where the risk of pregnancy would severely affect the health of the woman

Table 22.2 Teratogenic medications.

Pregnancy safety category X: positive evidence of serious fetal abnormalities in animals, humans, or both	Pregnancy safety category D: positive evidence of human fetal risk	Pregnancy safety category C: animal studies show adverse fetal effects but there are no controlled human studies
Acitretin	Amikacin	Angiotensin converting enzyme inhibitors and angiotensin receptor blockers: first trimester
Atorvastatin	Angiotensin converting enzyme inhibitors and angiotensin receptor blockers: second and third trimester	Amlodipine
Diethylstilbestrol	Carbamazepine	Caffeine
Finasteride	Cyclophosphamide	Capreomycin
Leflunomide	Fluconazole	Cyclosporine
Methotrexate	Kanamycin	Fluoroquinolones
Methylene blue	Lithium	Hydroxychloroquine
Misoprostol	Methimazole	Gabapentin
Simvastatin	Mycophenolate	Minoxidil
Testosterone, danazol	Paramethadione	Prednisone
Thalidomide	Penicillamine	Selective serotonin reuptake inhibitors
Warfarin	Phenobarbitol	Tramadol
	Phenytoin	Triamterene
	Retinoids (topical and systemic)	Trimethoprim
	Streptomycin	Trazadone
	Sulfa drugs	Vitamin K
	Tetracycline	
	Topiramate	
	Valproate	

or fetus. These conditions include SLE, valvular heart disease, type I and II diabetes mellitus, seizure disorder, thrombogenic mutations, hypertension, bariatric surgery or organ transplantation in the past 2 years, HIV/AIDS, and sickle cell disease.

While perfect-use efficacy rates for hormonal contraception are around 99%, these are not the actual efficacy rates seen in women without reminders and who are not enrolled in scientific studies. Actual-use efficacy rates are actually much lower [23, 24]. For example, the actual-use efficacy rates for the oral contraceptive pill in adult women is 91%. Actual-use efficacy rates are similarly lower for the contraceptive patch and ring. There are no data describing actual efficacy rates in adolescents. Contraceptive methods which remove administration errors and adherence issues have actual-use efficacy rates which are the same as perfect-use efficacy rates. For example, the efficacy rates for intrauterine devices and the contraceptive implant are higher than 99%. While national data have not calculated efficacy rates for progestin-only pills, they are likely to be lower than COCs due to the rapid drop in serum levels after 24 h of ingestion. These pharmacokinetics allow for a rapid time to ovulation when forgetting to take the POP every 24 h. This makes it essential that POP users administer their pills every 24 h, which is an uncommon feat. For this reason, it is likely that POPs have low efficacy and should not be considered a first-line contraceptive method for any adolescent or young woman.

Continuation rates are an additional consideration when discussing contraceptive efficacy. Continuation rates in adolescents for some contraceptive methods are low. For example, many adolescents stop their contraceptive method unintentionally when forgetting to refill their prescription or return for the DMPA administration in a timely fashion. In a study of adolescent's contraceptive continuation rates, both the progestin and copper intrauterine device and the contraceptive implant had continuation rates that were more than twice that of any other hormonal method (81% for the progestin IUD, 76% copper IUD, 82% contraceptive implant, 47% for depot medroxyprogesterone acetate, 47% COC, 41% contraceptive patch, and 31% vaginal ring) [25]. In summary, the contraceptive implant and the progestin and copper IUDs have the highest efficacy rates and continuation rates. For these reasons, these methods should be offered as first-line contraception for anyone, but especially those who are taking teratogenic medications.

Contraceptives and Medication Interactions

Some medications used to treat chronic illnesses directly interfere with COCs, the contraceptive patch, vaginal ring, and POPs. The most commonly used medications that pose this interference do so by accelerating metabolism of the contraceptive through increasing liver microsomal enzyme activity, thus reducing the efficacy of the contraceptive. This is true with many anticonvulsants, rifampin, griseofulvin, and certain antiretroviral medications (CDC MEC). In the event that COC use is necessary, a low-dose COC should be avoided. A pill formulation with a minimum of 30 μg of ethinyl estradiol should be used along with consistent condom use. Herbal supplements such as St. John's wort can also increase the metabolism of these contraceptive methods. While the antibiotic rifampin can reduce the efficacy of these contraceptive methods, there is no evidence that other antibiotics affect the efficacy of any contraceptive method. Additionally, the efficacy of other contraceptive methods like DMPA, all intrauterine devices, and the contraceptive implant is not affected by any medication interactions. In contrast, contraceptive methods like COCs, the contraceptive patch, vaginal ring, and POPs can increase serum levels of medications used in chronic illnesses, increasing the risk of toxicity of these medications. This can be seen with the use of lamotrigine, tacrolimus, cyclosporine, and sirolimus.

Other important medication interactions need to be considered when starting contraceptives with adolescents and young women who are taking medications for chronic illnesses. In this case, the patient is taking prednisone, which has known adverse effects on bone mineral density. In addition, DMPA has the effect of temporarily reducing bone mineral accrual during the adolescent and young adult time period. Using DMPA and prednisone simultaneously has cumulative adverse effects on bone density and should be avoided. Reductions in bone mineral density or accrual has not been shown in other contraceptive methods, including the progesterone-only methods like the contraceptive implant, the progestin IUD, or the progestin-only pills (POPs).

There are several contraceptives that also have non-contraceptive benefits including improved acne, dysmenorrhea, hirsutism, anemia, and lighter and shorter menses. In addition, some contraceptive methods can even improve some chronic illnesses. This can be seen with DMPA and seizure disorder as well as DMPA and sickle cell disease. Some conditions are not affected by any contraceptive methods. These include uncomplicated organ transplant, SLE without antiphospholipid antibody syndrome, migraines without aura, well-controlled hypertension, chronic or carrier of viral hepatitis, and the administration of nucleoside and non-nucleoside reverse transcriptase inhibitors for HIV.

Summary

Gynecologic care for adolescents and young women with immune-compromising conditions needs to employ earlier and more frequent Pap smear screening than those who are healthy, in addition to regular STI screening. Contraceptive method selection can be complicated in adolescents and young women with chronic illnesses. Use of the CDC Medical Eligibility Chart can help guide safety concerns with many chronic illnesses and medications that affect contraceptive efficacy or safety. Contraceptive method efficacy should also be considered with conditions where pregnancy can adversely impact the health of the adolescent, woman, or fetus or with the use of teratogenic medications. In general, the contraceptive implant and all IUDs have the highest efficacy and continuation rates and the lowest interactions with medications and chronic illnesses as compared to other contraceptive methods.

Clinical Pearls and Pitfalls

- For immune-compromised patients, the recommended screening after onset of sexual activity includes:
  - Annual: gonorrhea and chlamydia nucleic acid amplification test at each site of exposure; urine, vaginal, or cervical trichomonas vaginalis by nucleic acid amplification; syphilis serology; and HIV test
  - Twice in the first year after onset of sexual activity and then annually thereafter: Pap smear

- Recommended sexually transmitted infection prevention: HPV vaccine series as per ACIP guidelines.
- Intrauterine devices and the contraceptive implant have high efficacy and continuation rates and are infrequently contraindicated for use in persons with chronic illness, who are taking teratogenic medications or have medication interactions with contraceptive methods.

References

1. ACOG Practice Bulletin Number 157: cervical cancer screening and prevention. Obstet Gynecol. 2016;127(1):e1–20.
2. Panel on Opportunistic Infections in HIV-Infected Adults and Adolescents. Guidelines for the prevention and treatment of opportunistic infections in HIV-infected adults and adolescents: recommendations from the Centers for Disease Control and Prevention, the National Institutes of Health, and the HIV Medicine Association of the Infectious Diseases Society of America. http://aidsinfo.nih.gov/contentfiles/lvguidelines/adult_oi.pdf. Accessed 14 May 2016.
3. Centers for Disease Control and Prevention. Sexually transmitted disease surveillance 2009. Atlanta: U.S. Department of Health and Human Services; 2010.
4. Ho GYF, Bierman R, Beardsley L, Chang CJ, Burk RD. Natural history of cervicovaginal papillomavirus infection in young women. N Engl J Med. 1998;338(7):423.
5. Klumb EM, Araújo ML Jr, Jesus GR, et al. Is higher prevalence of cervical intraepithelial neoplasia in women with lupus due to immunosuppression? J Clin Rheumatol. 2010;16:153.
6. Origoni M, Stefani C, Dell'Antonio G, et al. Cervical Human Papillomavirus in transplanted Italian women: a long-term prospective follow-up study. J Clin Virol. 2011;51(4):250–4.
7. Ellerbrock TV, Chiasson MA, Bush TJ, et al. Incidence of cervical squamous intraepithelial lesions in HIV-infected women. JAMA. 2000;283(8):1031.
8. Kane S, Khatibi B, Reddy D. Higher incidence of abnormal pap smears in women with inflammatory bowel disease. Am J Gastroenterol. 2007;103(3):631–6.
9. Phipps W, Stanley H, Kohn R, Stansell J, Klausner JD. Syphilis, chlamydia, and gonorrhea screening in HIV-infected patients in primary care, San Francisco, California, 2003. AIDS Patient Care STDS. 2005;19(8):495.
10. CDC, Health Resources and Services Administration, National Institutes of Health, American Academy of HIV Medicine, Association of Nurses in AIDS Care, International Association of Providers of AIDS Care, the National Minority AIDS Council, and Urban Coalition for HIV/AIDS Prevention Services. Recommendations for HIV prevention with adults and adolescents with HIV in the United States, 2014. http://stacks.cdc.gov/view/cdc/26062.
11. Kumar D, Unger ER, Panicker G, Medvedev P, Wilson L, Humar A. Immunogenicity of quadrivalent human papillomavirus vaccine in organ transplant recipients. Am J Transplant. 2013;13(9):2411–7. Epub 2013 Jul 9.
12. Markowitz LE, Dunne EF, Saraiya M, Lawson HW, Chesson H, Unger ER, Centers for Disease Control and Prevention (CDC), Advisory Committee on Immunization Practices (ACIP). Quadrivalent human papillomavirus vaccine: recommendations of the Advisory Committee on Immunization Practices (ACIP). MMWR Recomm Rep. 2007;56(RR-2):1.
13. Robinson CL, Advisory Committee on Immunization Practices (ACIP), ACIP Child/Adolescent Immunization Work Group. Advisory Committee on Immunization Practices recommended immunization schedules for persons aged 0 through 18 years – United States, 2016. MMWR Morb Mortal Wkly Rep. 2016;65(4):86–7.
14. Guazzelli CAF, Torloni MR, Sanches TF, et al. Contraceptive counseling and use among 197 female kidney transplant recipients. Transplantation. 2008;86:669.

15. Medical eligibility criteria for contraceptive use. 4th ed. World Health Organization. 2015. http://www.who.int/reproductivehealth/publications/family_planning/MEC-5/en/. Accessed 25 April 2016.
16. U.S. Medical Eligibility Criteria for contraceptive use, 2010: adapted from the World Health Organization medical eligibility criteria for contraceptive use. 4th ed. http://www.cdc.gov/reproductivehealth/unintendedpregnancy/usmec.htm. Accessed 25 April 2016.
17. Petri M, Kim MY, Kalunian KC, et al. Combined oral contraceptives in women with systemic lupus erythematosus. N Engl J Med. 2005;353:2550–8.
18. Sanchez-Guerrero J, Uribe AG, Jimenez-Santana L, et al. A trial of contraceptive methods in women with systemic lupus erythematosus. N Engl J Med. 2005;353:2539–49.
19. Choojitarom K, Verasertniyom O, Totemchokchyakarn K, et al. Lupus nephritis and Raynaud's phenomenon are significant risk factors for vascular thrombosis in SLE patients with positive antiphospholipid antibodies. Clin Rheumatol. 2008;27:345–51.
20. Wahl DG, Guillemin F, de Maistre E, et al. Risk for venous thrombosis related to antiphospholipid antibodies in systemic lupus erythematosus–a meta-analysis. Lupus. 1997;6:467–73.
21. Finer LB, Zolna MR. Declines in unintended pregnancy in the United States, 2008–2011. N Engl J Med. 2016;374(9):843–85.
22. Steinkellner A, Chen W, Denison SE. Adherence to oral contraception in women on Category X medications. Am J Med. 2010;123(10):929.
23. Hatcher RA. Contraceptive technology. 20th ed. Bridging the Gap Communications; 2011.
24. Trussell J. Contraceptive failure in the United States. Contraception. 2011;83:397.
25. Rosenstock JR, Peipert JF, Madden T, Zhao Q, Secura GM. Continuation of reversible contraception in teenagers and young women. Obstet Gynecol. 2012;120(6):1298–305.

Suggested Educational Reading, References, and Policies

The American Congress of Obstetricians and Gynecologists. Practice Bulletin Number 157: cervical cancer screening and prevention. Obstet Gynecol. 2016;127(1):e1–20.
Medical eligibility criteria for contraceptive use. 5th Edition. World Health Organization. http://www.who.int/reproductivehealth/publications/family_planning/MEC-5/en/.
U.S. Medical Eligibility Criteria for contraceptive use. http://www.cdc.gov/reproductivehealth/unintendedpregnancy/usmec.htm.
2015 Sexually transmitted diseases treatment guidelines. Centers for Disease Control and Prevention. http://www.cdc.gov/std/tg2015/

Chapter 23
Case of a Girl with Cancer Seeking Fertility Counseling

Priscilla Rahmer, Catherine Benedict, and Jonathan D. Fish

Case

An 18 year-old girl has been experiencing right leg pain with a progressively worsening limp for the last 2 months. She initially presented to her pediatrician 3 weeks ago, where an X-ray revealed a lesion extending from the proximal right femoral metaphysis to the midshaft with an associated sunburst pattern of periosteal reaction (Fig. 23.1a). A subsequent MRI ordered by an oncologic orthopedic surgeon revealed a right femoral mass with a soft tissue component (Fig. 23.1b). An open biopsy confirmed a diagnosis of Ewing sarcoma. An evaluation for metastatic disease was negative.

The young woman is otherwise healthy, with no significant past medical history. She has never been hospitalized nor had surgery. She has not been taking any medications, vitamins, or supplements. She lives at home with her parents and two younger siblings. There is no family history of childhood cancers. She is sexually active with one partner, and they use condoms for birth control. She experienced menarche at 13 years of age. Although her menses were irregular in frequency, intensity, and duration for the first 2 years, she has had regular, monthly menses for

P. Rahmer, F.N.P.
Pediatric Hematology/Oncology and Stem Cell Transplantation, Steven and Alexandra Cohen Children's Medical Center of New York, New Hyde Park, NY, USA

C. Benedict, Ph.D.
Department of Medicine, Zucker School of Medicine at Hofstra/Northwell, Hempstead, NY, USA

J.D. Fish, M.D. (✉)
Pediatric Hematology/Oncology and Stem Cell Transplantation, Steven and Alexandra Cohen Children's Medical Center of New York, New Hyde Park, NY, USA

Zucker School of Medicine at Hofstra/Northwell, Hempstead, NY, USA
e-mail: jfish1@northwell.edu

H.J. Talib (ed.), *Adolescent Gynecology*,
https://doi.org/10.1007/978-3-319-66978-6_23

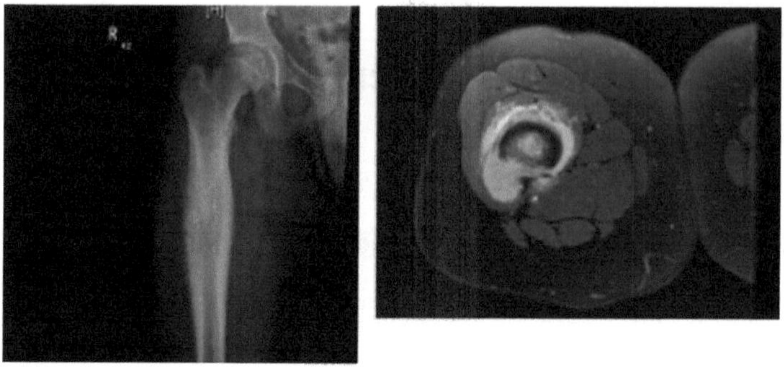

Fig. 23.1 Imaging of femur. (**a**) X-ray. (**b**) MRI

the last 3 years that have occurred every 28 days and last for 5 days. She has never used any form of tobacco and does not drink alcohol, although she has been smoking marijuana one–two times per week.

Her pediatric oncologist discussed her diagnosis, prognosis, and the treatment plan in detail. She learned that there is a 75% chance that she will be cured, meaning the cancer will go away, stay away, and never come back. In order to accomplish that, she will receive 12 weeks of neoadjuvant chemotherapy given in six two-week cycles and then will have surgery to remove the tumor. Following surgery, she will receive an additional 22 weeks of adjuvant chemotherapy in 11 two-week cycles. In total, she will be treated for ~36 weeks and will receive:

- 375 mg/m^2 doxorubicin
- 3500 mg/m^2 etoposide
- 27 mg/m^2 vincristine
- 8400 mg/m^2 of cyclophosphamide
- 63 g/m^2 of ifosfamide

The plan is to start treatment as soon as possible.

After learning the treatment plan, the patient and her parents ask several questions about the potential impact of the cancer treatment on her fertility, including:

1. Will the treatment affect her ability to have children?
2. If there is a chance that the treatment will make her infertile, is there anything that can be done before treatment to preserve her fertility?
3. If she were to have biological children in the future, are there any additional risks to them?

Discussion

With an overall cure rate exceeding 80%, most adolescents and young adults (AYA) diagnosed with cancer will live many decades after their diagnosis. This remarkable success has been achieved mostly through the refinement of cancer treatments comprised of chemotherapy, radiation, and surgery. Despite the excellent oncologic prognosis, long-term survivors experience a high burden of morbidity from the late effects of cancer treatment. Over 70% experience at least one chronic disease as a consequence of cancer therapy [1, 2], and mortality among survivors greatly exceeds that of their peers [3]. With over 400,000 survivors of childhood cancer living in the United States, the health of this prevalent and medically complex patient population is a public health concern.

Among the late effects of cancer therapy, the possibility of infertility is among the most distressing aspects of survivorship for AYA, especially young women [4]. In 1975, a radiation oncologist named Giulio D'Angio coined the motto of survivorship "cure is not enough" [5]. To that end, it is imperative that young women such as the adolescent in the vignette receive accurate counseling as to the potential impact of their cancer treatment on fertility and be offered the opportunity to undergo fertility preservation techniques if fertility is threatened.

The Impact of Cancer Therapy on Fertility

Cancer treatment can affect female fertility by impacting the function of the ovaries, fallopian tubes, uterus, vagina, or hypothalamic-pituitary axis. While ovarian function can be affected by chemotherapy, radiation, or surgery, the uterus, vagina, and hypothalamic-pituitary axis are primarily at risk only from radiation and surgery. For the young woman in the vignette, there is no plan to radiate the pelvis nor would any surgery impact the reproductive structures. The greatest risk to her fertility is therefore the potential impact of chemotherapy on her ovaries.

Of the chemotherapeutics commonly used to treat childhood cancer, the group with by far the greatest impact on ovarian function is the alkylating agents. The risk for ovarian dysfunction is directly proportional to the cumulative lifetime alkylator dose, as measured in mg/m^2 (i.e., the dose based on the m^2 at the time it is delivered). The best studied alkylator in terms of its impact on ovarian function is cyclophosphamide. In order to better assess the impact of alkylator therapy on a given patient's fertility, each alkylator can be given a cyclophosphamide equivalence score as reported by Green et al. [6]. Common alkylators and their cyclophosphamide equivalence are shown in Table 23.1.

Ovarian dysfunction after cancer therapy can manifest in two forms:

1. Acute ovarian failure (AOF) occurs when women lose ovarian function during cancer treatment or soon after the completion of treatment.
2. Premature ovarian insufficiency (POI) occurs when women maintain ovarian function after cancer treatment but experience menopause before the age of 40.

Women less than 20 years of age who receive >7.5 g/m^2 of cyclophosphamide equivalents are at the highest risk for ovarian dysfunction. For the young woman in the vignette, the treatment protocol she has been presented with contains 8400 mg/m^2 cyclophosphamide + 63,000 mg/m^2 ifosfamide, for a total cyclophosphamide equivalence of 23,772 mg/m^2. She is thus at increased risk for ovarian dysfunction after the completion of treatment.

Table 23.1 Common alkylating agents and their cyclophosphamide equivalence

Cyclophosphamide	1
Ifosfamide	0.244
Procarbazine	0.857
Busulfan	8.823
Chlorambucil	14.286
BCNU	15
CCNU	16
Melphalan	40
Thiotepa	50
Nitrogen mustard	100

Data from Green DM, Nolan VG, Goodman PJ, et al. Pediatr Blood Cancer 2014;61:53–67

Table 23.2 Methods of fertility preservation in order of preference

Prepubertal girls	1. Ovarian tissue cryopreservation 2. Oophoropexy for girls receiving pelvic radiation
Postpubertal adolescents	1. Oocyte cryopreservation 2. Embryo cryopreservation for women who have identified a male partner 3. Ovarian tissue cryopreservation if unable to harvest oocytes 4. Oophoropexy for women receiving pelvic radiation
Young adult women	1. Embryo cryopreservation for women who have identified a male partner 2. Oocyte cryopreservation if embryo cryopreservation is not feasible 3. Ovarian tissue cryopreservation if unable to harvest oocytes 4. Oophoropexy for females receiving pelvic radiation

Methods of Fertility Preservation

For women at risk for ovarian dysfunction after cancer therapy, there are several approaches available for fertility preservation [7] (Table 23.2).

Embryo cryopreservation is the oldest and most successfully form of fertility preservation. It involves harvesting oocytes from the woman, collecting sperm from a male partner and generating embryos through in vitro fertilization (IVF). These embryos can then be safely and effectively cryopreserved for future use. Embryo cryopreservation has proven effective, with cancer survivors experiencing a 30% rate of live births versus 32% for patients who never had cancer [8]. Nonetheless, for AYA in particular, there are potential barriers to this approach. First, it requires that the young woman have an identified male partner with whom she wants to have biologic children. Second, oocyte harvesting requires time and ovarian stimulation, which may be challenging if there is a sense of urgency to begin cancer treatment. Newer methods of ovarian stimulation can be undertaken independent of menstrual cycle, which reduces the risk of delaying cancer treatment and allows for cancer therapy to start the day after oocyte harvest.

In addition to embryo cryopreservation, *oocyte cryopreservation* is considered an established method of fertility preservation by the American Society of Clinical Oncology (ASCO) [9]. It is the preferred method of fertility preservation for post-pubertal girls for whom embryo cryopreservation is not feasible. With oocyte cryo-preservation, there is no need for female patients to identify a male partner. Oocyte cryopreservation should be started prior to initiation of cytotoxic therapy. Similar to embryo cryopreservation, oocyte cryopreservation requires time and ovarian stimulation.

For prepubertal girls or AYA in whom oocyte harvesting is not feasible, *ovarian tissue cryopreservation* is the only alternative. In ovarian tissue cryopreservation, ovarian cortical tissue is collected, cryopreserved, and transplanted after completion of cancer treatment. Ovarian tissue may be transplanted into the pelvis (orthoptic transplant) or outside the pelvic region in the abdominal wall or forearm (hetero-topic transplant). Live births have been reported using this method in postpubertal females [10]. As this method of fertility preservation remains experimental, it should only be performed as part of an IRB-approved study at an institution with sufficient expertise and resources.

For women who will receive ovarian-threatening radiation, *oophoropexy (ovarian transposition)* may reduce the risk of ovarian dysfunction posttreatment. In this process, ovaries are surgically moved away from the radiation field and secured in an area that will not receive radiation. They can be placed outside the pelvis or moved high above the pelvic brim. Oophoropexy is clearly not beneficial for patients receiving total body irradiation or for those who will receive higher doses of alkylating agents. The procedure is minimally invasive and can be performed laparascopically.

Ovarian suppression during cancer therapy is more controversial with conflicting results from studies. The theory behind this technique is that oocytes are more susceptible to the impact of chemotherapeutics while they are dividing. Thus, GnRH agonists (GnRHa) are administered to completely suppress ovulation. The 2013 ASCO guidelines for fertility preservation have deemed GnRHa an ineffective method of fertility preservation, although there are ongoing studies that will help elucidate whether they can play a role.

For the young woman in the vignette, the best options for fertility preservation would be embryo or oocyte cryopreservation. Given her age, it is unlikely that embryo cryopreservation would be feasible, making oocyte harvest prior to starting therapy the preferred method.

Although oocytes can be safely cryopreserved, remaining ovarian tissue remains susceptible to the effects of the alkylators. There is the real possibility that the young woman in the vignette will experience acute ovarian failure immediately after completing cancer therapy or that she will experience premature menopause [11]. She should be informed of the symptoms of menopause and that hormone replacement may alleviate those symptoms.

Pregnancy Outcomes After Cancer Therapy

Multiple studies have examined pregnancy outcomes among survivors of childhood cancer. Women who received uterine or vaginal radiation have an increased risk for having a baby that is small for gestation age and for premature birth. Outside of those risks, however, it seems that the children of survivors of childhood cancer do not carry an increased risk of congenital anomalies nor a markedly increased risk for cancer (other than those with familial cancer syndromes) [12]. As such, the patient in the vignette can be counseled that any children she successfully carries to term should have similar risks to the general population.

Patient Decision-Making About Fertility Preservation

For patients and their parents, fertility decisions are often wrought with uncertainty as there is no right or wrong answer. Patients weigh the pros and cons of fertility preservation against taking a "wait and see" approach but are only guided by inexact estimates of infertility risk and likelihood of fertility preservation success. When counseling patients, it is important they understand that there is a failure rate and that cryopreserved oocytes do not guarantee fertility. Choosing to pursue fertility preservation adds to the physical and emotional toll of the cancer diagnosis and pending treatment. Many AYA have never considered how important it is for them to have a biologically related child (as opposed to alternative family building such as adoption), how comfortable they would be using assisted reproductive technology, or their religious, cultural, and ethical beliefs about fertility preservation. At a time of high emotional distress, patients must determine their personal values and priorities while also considering the opinions and recommendations of clinicians and family members.

Financial considerations are often a significant factor influencing decision-making, particularly as families may be facing substantial cancer-related costs or breaks in employment. Prior to starting the process of oocyte cryopreservation, it is important to counsel AYA that most fertility preservation techniques are not covered by health insurance. The cost is prohibitive for many patients, though significant differences in reproductive health-care coverage and access to fertility-related procedures exist internationally. While there are philanthropic organizations that can help defray the costs, much of cost is likely to fall to the family. Costs may include bills associated with the medication and procedure for egg retrieval, co-pays for office visits, storage fees of the frozen oocytes, as well as future costs for the use of frozen oocytes using assisted reproductive technology.

Addressing Fertility in Practice

When fertility issues are addressed prior to treatment, AYA have more positive experiences, less regret, higher levels of life satisfaction, and higher overall quality of life posttreatment irrespective of whether or not they pursued fertility preservation [13]. Special care should be taken to ensure patients' questions and concerns are being adequately addressed and to make referrals to a reproductive endocrinologist or fertility specialist whenever possible. Feeling ignored or dismissed can deter AYA from asking further questions leading to silent worrying.

It is important for providers to assess AYA fertility concerns regardless of treatment gonadotoxity as patients may worry unnecessarily due to a lack of information. Providers and parents often underestimate the degree to which younger patients are concerned about fertility, as these young women may prefer to avoid the issue altogether as a mechanism to manage anxiety and distress. AYA may express a lack of concern due to incorrect or unlikely assumptions about the promise and success of reproductive technology (or expected advances in technology). Likewise, AYA may assume they can rely on alternative family-building strategies in the future, such as adoption, without recognizing the high costs associated with these options. Having developmentally appropriate discussions that include patients to the extent they feel comfortable is optimal. Providers may need to balance their discussions about the realistic infertility risks with the need to allow for hope and optimism. Although parents may want to protect their children from information they deem too upsetting or be present during patient-provider discussions to control what is said, this is often counter to adolescents' desires and not received well.

Informational materials are often helpful to aid clinical discussions. Not surprisingly, adolescents tend to prefer online educational materials and support, whereas parents prefer informational booklets. Resources are available online including educational pamphlets to give patients and/or parents, provider pocket guides (including links to smartphone apps freely available for download), and fertility decision tree tools from trusted organizations including the Oncofertility Consortium, LIVESTRONG Fertility, and SaveMyFertility.org. Providers may also access online databases to find a fertility specialist in the area and fertility preservation locations through the American Society for Reproductive Medicine (www.reproductivefacts.org) and Alliance for Fertility Preservation (www.allianceforfertilitypreservation.org). The Oncofertility Consortium has published a fertility values clarification tool for adolescent females diagnosed with cancer including instructions and guidelines for providers (available free for download). It is critical to provide AYA with information about alternative family-building methods, such as adoption or using assisted reproductive technology with an egg donor or gestational carrier, to foster an understanding that having a biological child is not the only option. Due to prevalent assumptions about heterosexuality in the context of sexual and reproductive health care, it is important for providers to be conscious of the unique needs of lesbian, gay, and bisexual adolescents and how to be inclusive and respectful during clinical encounters [14].

Psychosocial Effects of Infertility and Fertility-Related Distress

The importance of having comprehensive fertility discussions is highlighted by the significant and long-lasting effects that AYA cancer survivors experience when faced with confirmed or uncertain infertility. After treatment, female survivors report that fertility is one of the most distressing aspects of survivorship, and feelings of regret and discontent can persist even when motherhood is achieved through adoption or stepparenting [15]. The perception of impaired fertility alone can affect female survivors' self-concept and esteem and lead to worries surrounding dating, disclosure, rejection from partners (or future partners), peer relationships, and fulfilling future roles related to womanhood and parenthood. Notably, adolescents can have continued fertility distress despite explicit reassurance that their fertility has not been affected. Thus, there is a need for continued assessment of reproductive concerns at all phases of the cancer trajectory from diagnosis to long-term survivorship.

Clinical Pearls and Pitfalls

- Any adolescent or young adult newly diagnosed with cancer should receive an accurate assessment of their risk for compromised fertility following cancer therapy.
- Alkylators are the group of chemotherapeutics most likely to negatively affect ovarian function post cancer treatment. The risk for ovarian compromise is highly correlated with cumulative, lifetime alkylator exposure.
- Any radiation to the uterus or adnexa can negatively affect fertility.
- Standard of care approaches to female fertility preservation include embryo cryopreservation and oocyte cryopreservation. Ovarian tissue cryopreservation is still experimental and should only be undertaken on an IRB-approved trial at a center with appropriate expertise and resources.
- The optimal approach to fertility preservation should be carefully considered, taking into account the patient's age, marital status, and whether she is stable enough to undergo oocyte harvest.
- Fertility preservation techniques are rarely covered by health insurance.
- The biological children born to survivors of childhood or AYA cancer do not have a markedly increased risk for congenital anomalies or cancer.

References

1. Oeffinger KC, et al. Chronic health conditions in adult survivors of childhood cancer. N Engl J Med. 2006;355(15):1572–82.
2. Hudson MM, et al. Clinical ascertainment of health outcomes among adults treated for childhood cancer. JAMA. 2013;309(22):2371–81.

3. Armstrong GT, et al. Late mortality among 5-year survivors of childhood cancer: a summary from the Childhood Cancer Survivor Study. J Clin Oncol. 2009;27(14):2328–38.
4. Benedict C, Shuk E, Ford JS. Fertility issues in adolescent and young adult cancer survivors. J Adolesc Young Adult Oncol. 2016;5(1):48–57.
5. D'Angio GJ. Pediatric cancer in perspective: cure is not enough. Cancer. 1975;35(3 suppl):866–70.
6. Green DM, et al. The cyclophosphamide equivalent dose as an approach for quantifying alkylating agent exposure: a report from the Childhood Cancer Survivor Study. Pediatr Blood Cancer. 2014;61(1):53–67.
7. Fish JD. Fertility preservation for adolescent women with cancer. Adolesc Med State Art Rev. 2012;23(1):111–22, xi.
8. Cardozo ER, et al. Ovarian stimulation and in-vitro fertilization outcomes of cancer patients undergoing fertility preservation compared to age matched controls: a 17-year experience. J Assist Reprod Genet. 2015;32(4):587–96.
9. Loren AW, et al. Fertility preservation for patients with cancer: American Society of Clinical Oncology clinical practice guideline update. J Clin Oncol. 2013;31(19):2500–10.
10. Demeestere I, et al. Live birth after autograft of ovarian tissue cryopreserved during childhood. Hum Reprod. 2015;30(9):2107–9.
11. Raciborska A, et al. Ovarian function in female survivors after multimodal Ewing sarcoma therapy. Pediatr Blood Cancer. 2015;62(2):341–5.
12. Seppanen VI, et al. Risk for congenital anomalies in offspring of childhood, adolescent and young adult cancer survivors. Int J Cancer. 2016;139(8):1721–30.
13. Letourneau JM, et al. The impact of fertility counseling and fertility preservation on long-term psychosocial outcomes in young female cancer survivors. Fertil Steril. 2010;94(4):S65.
14. Fantus S, et al. Addressing fertility preservation for lesbian, gay, and bisexual adolescents and young adults with cancer. J Adolesc Young Adult Oncol. 2015;4(4):152–6.
15. Canada AL, Schover LR. The psychosocial impact of interrupted childbearing in long-term female cancer survivors. Psychooncology. 2012;21(2):134–43.

Suggested Educational Reading

Fish JD. Fertility preservation for adolescent women with cancer. Adolesc Med State Art Rev. 2012;23:111–22, xi.

Loren AW, Mangu PB, Beck LN, et al. Fertility preservation for patients with cancer: American Society of Clinical Oncology clinical practice guideline update. J Clin Oncol. 2013;31:2500–10.

Knight S, Lorenzo A, Maloney AM, et al. An approach to fertility preservation in prepubertal and postpubertal females: a critical review of current literature. Pediatr Blood Cancer. 2015;62:935–9.

Chapter 24
Case of a Girl with Special Needs Seeking Menstrual Management

Erin H. Sieke and Ellen S. Rome

Case

Jessica is a 14-year-old girl who presents to her pediatrician with her parents for her annual well-child check. Her past medical history is significant for birth at 26 weeks gestational age with APGARs of 3/4/7 and birth weight of 780 g. Screening head ultrasound after birth revealed periventricular leukomalacia. She was discharged from the NICU when she reached 40 weeks corrected gestational age but was noted to have hypotonia of the lower limbs at that time. Her gross and fine motor milestones were delayed. She was diagnosed with cerebral palsy at 6 months of age due to poor mobility and significant spasticity in the lower limbs. She continues to have motor and speech delay but enjoys attending school where she is in a classroom for children with multiple disabilities.

Jessica had onset of seizures right after her first birthday. Her seizures were previously well controlled with levetiracetam but have been worsening over the past several months. Jessica's parents report that they have noticed she has a period of increasing seizure frequency around the onset of her menses each month.

Jessica had adrenarche beginning at 9 years of age, followed by thelarche at 10 years of age. Menarche occurred 1 month after her 13th birthday. Her menses were initially irregular but have been coming every month for the past 3 months. She is Tanner 5 for breasts and pubic hair on initial exam. Her parents report that managing her periods have been challenging, as Jessica does not understand what is

E.H. Sieke, B.A.
Cleveland Clinic Lerner College of Medicine at Case, Cleveland, OH, USA

E.S. Rome, M.D., M.P.H. (✉)
Cleveland Clinic Lerner College of Medicine at Case, Cleveland, OH, USA

Center for Adolescent Medicine, Cleveland Clinic Children's Hospital, Cleveland, OH, USA
e-mail: romee@ccf.org

H.J. Talib (ed.), *Adolescent Gynecology*,
https://doi.org/10.1007/978-3-319-66978-6_24

happening and is both afraid and curious, which has led to several "accidents" per her parents.

Jessica's mom has several questions:

1. Are her seizures related to her periods? Why are we having such a problem managing her seizures now when her epilepsy has been so well controlled in the past?
2. Is there anything we can do to better manage her periods and keep her from being afraid?

Background

The onset and progression through puberty can be a difficult period for all adolescents and their families, but girls with mental and physical disabilities may have an even more challenging course. Although studies suggest that the physical changes are similar in patients with disabilities to a normal population (although the tempo and timing of maturation may vary), the concerns of the parent and adolescent may differ, as hygiene, parental/caregiver burden, and menstrual symptoms may be more difficult to manage. Disabilities are common in children and adolescents, with 5.2% of children and adolescents in the United States affected by a disability in 2010 [1].

Causes of Menstrual Irregularities in the Special Needs Population

It is common for adolescent females to have irregular menstrual cycles during the first 2–5 years after menarche. However, adolescents with disabilities may have additional reasons for menstrual irregularity [2]. It is important to screen for other causes of menstrual irregularities in these patients. For example, adolescents with Down's syndrome (trisomy 21) may have alterations in thyroid hormone [3]. Adolescents with disabilities also exhibit increased rates of other common causes of menstrual irregularities. Adolescents with seizure disorders are more likely to have polycystic ovary syndrome (PCOS), and mood-stabilizing medications that are commonly used in this population such as valproate can lead to high prolactin levels [4–8].

Communicating with Patients

When caring for adolescents with disabilities, it is important for providers to start by assessing the patient's knowledge of puberty, menstruation, sexuality, safety, and consent [9]. Gynecologic care for adolescents with special needs should be comprehensive. Communication should be directed to the adolescent and not to a family member or other caregiver. Whenever possible, the clinician should conduct part of the interview in private to allow for confidential discussion between provider and adolescent. Although adolescents with disabilities may not have the same level of understanding about pubertal and sexual development as their peers, clinicians must not assume that they are not sexually active or do not have a sexual drive. In fact, adolescents with disabilities commonly exhibit interest in sex and may express themselves sexually through masturbation.

Clinicians can provide crucial anticipatory guidance to adolescents with disabilities and their parents. Clinicians should tailor education to adolescents with intellectual disability, making sure to provide developmentally appropriate education. Topics should include hygiene, contraception, consent, sexually transmitted infections, and sexual abuse prevention measures. In most cases, adolescents who are capable of toileting without assistance can manage pads or tampons appropriately with proper education.

A complete menstrual history should be taken, assessing age of menarche, frequency and duration of periods, amount of bleeding, dysmenorrhea or associated symptoms, association of menses with headaches, or increased seizure activity. Screening for iron deficiency is important in adolescents with heavy menstrual bleeding.

Communicating with Families

Prior studies have demonstrated that parents of adolescent girls with intellectual disabilities have concerns about pubertal development including menstrual suppression, hygiene, parental burden, and menstrual symptoms [10]. Parents of adolescents with disabilities commonly present to the gynecologist with questions prior to the onset of menses, with one study demonstrating that 31.7% of parents come before their child achieves menarche [10]. The clinician should address any questions that the parents or caregivers may have regarding pubertal development. Clinicians should explain to parents that it is difficult to predict how menses will affect the day-to-day life of a teenager. Thus, it is important to allow pubertal events to advance naturally so that the tolerance and effect of menstrual cycles can be individually evaluated in each patient [11–13]. A discussion of menstrual regulation methods is appropriate after the onset of menses, when goals of promoting hygiene, increasing independence, and reducing discomfort can be tailored to the patient's individual situation. However, anticipatory guidance can be provided at every step to ensure that the parent and adolescent know what options are available to them and have clear expectations about pubertal development. In addition, the clinician should have an open discussion with the family about sexuality, emphasizing that sexual feelings are a normal and expected part of pubertal development [14].

Physical Exam

Pelvic examinations are rarely necessary in adolescents who are not sexually active. However, in the setting of abnormal bleeding, abnormal vaginal discharge, suspected foreign object in the vagina, or evaluation for sexual assault/abuse, a pelvic examination may be indicated.

Providers should utilize current cervical cytology guidelines, which recommend that women younger than 21 years should not be screened for cervical cancer regardless of age of coitarche or the presence of other behavioral risk factors [15, 16]. Providers should never make assumptions about sexual activity in patients with disabilities. Sexually transmitted infections (STIs) are often underdiagnosed in this population because clinicians may assume that the patient is not sexually active. In addition, patients may not be able to detect or report symptoms of sexually transmitted infections, underscoring the importance of careful history taking and physical examination to look for signs of abuse or infection. Screening for STIs should be done using the least invasive method. For example, screening for gonorrhea, chlamydia, and trichomonas can be done using urine tests or vaginal swabs for nucleic acid amplification. Other STI testing such as herpes, human immunodeficiency virus (HIV), hepatitis, and syphilis can be completed with blood samples. In the case of a positive test for a STI, a workup for sexual assault should be considered.

Goals of Menstrual Manipulation

Menstrual suppression or manipulation in adolescents with disabilities can be useful to improve hygiene, diminish or eliminate menstrual flow, reduce dysmenorrhea, decrease catamenial epilepsy or menstrual migraines, improve behavior, and improve quality of life for adolescents with disabilities and their families. In addition, some methods provide pregnancy prevention in the case of consensual sexual activity or sexual assault.

It is important to consider who is requesting menstrual regulation when working with adolescents with special needs and their families. If the patient is requesting menstrual regulation, it is important to identify the reasons behind the request. In addition, this provides an opportunity to conduct a confidential assessment of contraceptive needs and the ability to have a consensual sexual relationship. When family members or caregivers request menstrual regulation, it is important to address the reasons that prompted the request as well as to invite input from the adolescent. The adolescent's wishes and understanding of the topic should be assessed. Important concepts to consider when a parent requests menstrual manipulation include the effect of the cycle (or potential medication to manage the cycle) on the adolescent and the caregivers. Parents should be asked about concerns for abuse or pregnancy, and a thorough safety assessment should be completed. In addition, it is important to consider that adolescents with disabilities may not be able to articulate their concerns about pubertal development or pregnancy. If caregiver discomfort with menstruation is contributing to the request for menstrual regulation, education of the caregivers including school teachers, aides, nurses, and home care providers may help the family to adjust to these developmental changes.

It is important to discuss expectations and priorities with the adolescent and family [9]. For many teenagers, having light but unscheduled menstrual bleeding may be more distressing or inconvenient than heavier but scheduled controlled withdrawal bleeds. This is an especially important consideration in teenagers who rely on others for hygiene assistance. There are multiple options for menstrual manipulation, including regulation of cycles, decreased frequency of cycles, lighter cycles with less associated dysmenorrhea, or no cycles. However, it is important to discuss with families that complete amenorrhea is difficult to achieve. Setting clear goals with both the patient and family or caregivers is necessary, and these goals should be periodically reevaluated based on changing desires or new challenges that may arise.

Side effects must also be considered carefully. Side effects such as weight gain may have substantial consequences in teenagers in wheelchairs, as even a small amount of weight gain could interfere with the patient's ability to transfer herself out of the wheelchair for toileting [2]. In addition, antiepileptic drugs may interact with hormonal methods of contraception, decreasing the contraceptive efficacy. It is important to counsel patients and parents about these side effects and to consider what method may be the best fit to improve symptoms without causing harmful side effects in each patient.

Treatment Options

Nonsteroidal Anti-inflammatory Drugs (NSAIDS)

NSAIDs offer a safe, over-the-counter treatment for dysmenorrhea that can help with pain and reduce bleeding in patients with special needs. Antiprostaglandin drugs have been shown to decrease ovulatory menstrual bleeding by approximately 10–52% [17, 18]. NSAIDs work by reducing the synthesis of prostaglandins (PGE2 and PGF2α) in the endometrium, leading to vasoconstriction and reduced bleeding. Options include aspirin, ibuprofen, and diclofenac, among others. Dosing should be based on weight, with treatment starting on the first day of menses and continuing for 4–5 days or until cessation of menses [17]. Because NSAIDS are ingested for only a few days out of the month, side effects are minimal and the risk of GI upset is low [19].

Estrogen-Containing Methods

There are multiple available hormonal methods that can be used for menstrual regulation. These include combined oral contraceptives (COCs), contraceptive patches, and vaginal rings. Hormonal contraceptives work by suppressing pituitary gonadotropin release, preventing ovulation and leading to endometrial atrophy. Side effects include breast tenderness, nausea, breakthrough bleeding, and possible weight gain. When considering starting hormonal contraception in adolescents with special needs, drug-drug interactions and risk of clotting must be considered. Common interactions include hormonal contraception and antiepileptic agents, which could reduce the efficacy of the antiepileptic drugs while also increasing the risk of pregnancy [4, 20]. In addition, in adolescents with limited mobility, there is a possible increased risk of venous thromboembolism. Family history and other risk factors for clotting should be carefully investigated in this population. Combined oral contraceptives are available in chewable forms for patients who cannot or prefer not to swallow pills or in crushable formulations to be given through a gastrostomy tube [21].

COCs allow for manipulation of the frequency of menstrual cycles. They can be administered continuously or in an extended-cycle manner in order to reduce the frequency and amount of bleeding. However, complete amenorrhea is difficult to obtain even with continuous cycling, with only 58.7% of women reporting amenorrhea after 1 year of continuous dosing [22]. Unscheduled bleeding, commonly known as breakthrough bleeding, is more likely to occur with extended or continuous dosing of COCs and may be more difficult to cope with than scheduled withdrawal bleeds for some adolescents with special needs and their families. Scheduling withdrawal bleeds every 3–4 months can reduce the rates of breakthrough bleeding while still improving dysmenorrhea symptoms and reducing the frequency of menses. Limited data has suggested that there is a higher risk of developing blood clots associated with third-generation progesterones, such as desogestrel, and fourth-generation progesterones, such as drospirenone, when compared with second-generation formulations including levonorgestrel [23]. Thus, a second-generation COC may be preferred for adolescents with decreased mobility who may have increased clotting potential.

The vaginal ring is another method of delivery for combined hormonal contraceptives. However, contraceptive rings are often difficult for adolescents with mobility issues or functional hand limitations to insert. There are clear ethical, physical, and privacy concerns related to having a caregiver insert the ring intravaginally limit the use of the ring in the special needs population. The ring can be used continuously (insert ring, leave in for 28 days, and then remove and replace with a new ring). When used continuously, most patients had no to minimal bleeding with an associated reduction in pelvic pain [24]. However, if breakthrough bleeding does occur, removing the ring for 4 days can help to resolve breakthrough bleeding [24].

The contraceptive patch is administered weekly. It is important to note that the contraceptive patch exposes users to a higher level of estrogen than oral contraceptives or the vaginal ring. It has been postulated that this increased estrogen concentration may increase the risk of deep vein thrombosis, especially in women or adolescents with limited mobility. However, to date no studies have conclusively identified the risk of venous thromboembolism in users of the contraceptive patch. The patch is placed on the abdomen, upper outer arm, upper torso, or buttock for 1 week before being exchanged for a new patch. The patch can be removed every fourth week to have a withdrawal bleed or can be used in an off-label extended or continuous manner. When extended cycling is utilized, similar breakthrough bleeding patterns are observed with the patch as compared to the combined oral contraceptive pills [25].

Progesterone-Only Hormonal Methods

Progesterone-containing methods of contraception work by a negative feedback mechanism on the hypothalamus, preventing follicular maturation and ovulation, which leads to associated endometrial thinning [26]. Similarly to combined hormonal contraceptives, progesterone-containing pills can interact with antiepileptic drugs, leading to decreased efficacy. Another common problem with progesterone-containing agents is breakthrough bleeding, which may be difficult for adolescent with special needs to manage.

Progesterone-containing pills are another method of regulating menses that can be used in adolescents with contraindications to estrogen therapy. However, progesterone-only pills are associated with an increased rate of irregular bleeding and lower rates of amenorrhea than combined oral contraceptives. Of progesterone-only pill users, about 40–50% will have normal menstrual cycles, 40% will have irregular cycles or breakthrough bleeding, and 10% of users will have amenorrhea [27]. Oral progestins, in high doses, can be used to attempt menstrual suppression. However, efficacy is dependent on dosage and adherence to taking the pill at the same time every day, which can be difficult for some adolescents [28].

Depot medroxyprogesterone acetate (DMPA) is a long-acting method of contraception that is effective at achieving menstrual suppression in many adolescents. Although many patients have irregular bleeding initially, high rates of amenorrhea are achieved by 1 year of use (52–64%), with even higher rates of amenorrhea at 2 years of use (71%) [29]. DMPA is available as intramuscular and subcutaneous injections and has a long history of use for both contraception and menstrual suppression. However, there are several important side effects that must be considered carefully before use in teenagers with special needs. DMPA has been shown to be associated with weight gain, averaging 13 pounds in 4 years. In adolescents with mobility challenges, even small amounts of weight gain could have a significant impact on their ability to complete transfers and maintain physical independence. In adolescents who are already obese, even higher rates of weight gain have been observed [30]. The second important consideration is bone health. DMPA carries a black box warning from the FDA recommending limiting dose to 2 years due to its impact on bone mineral density. Some studies have suggested that ever use, long-term use, and current use of DMPA may put adolescents at increased risk of fracture [31]. During adolescence, girls accrue approximately 30–40% of their peak bone mass. In teenagers with limited mobility, bone mineral density is often lower than expected, although it is not clear whether this decrease in BMD is associated with an increased risk of fracture. As DMPA users may have an increased fracture risk, this should be carefully considered with the adolescent and family in order to select a method that meets the needs of the adolescent while minimizing risks.

Contraceptive implants are another long-acting, reversible option for contraception in adolescents. However, due to the unpredictable bleeding patterns associated with implant use, experience with the implant in adolescents with disabilities is limited. Many patients have many days of spotting each month, with 23% of users experiencing normal menstrual patterns and only 13% of users report amenorrhea after 1 year of use [32]. In addition to the irregular bleeding pattern, insertion and removal of the etonogestrel implant requires patient cooperation and may be scary for teenagers with intellectual disabilities, making the procedure difficult to complete. The implant provides contraception for at least 3 years, making it an effective and easy option for adolescents with special needs who are involved in consensual sexual relationships.

Another long-acting, reversible contraceptive (LARC) option for adolescents is intrauterine devices (IUDs). There are two available IUDs currently on the market, with the Mirena IUD approved for 5 years and the Skyla IUD approved for 3 years of contraception. The bleeding profile of the IUDs is more favorable than the implant, with decreased rates of breakthrough bleeding. Many women experience irregular bleeding in the first 6 months after insertion but go on to experience lighter, frequent, or absent periods. Up to 50% of users with have amenorrhea after 1 year of use [33]. Several recent studies have sought to assess the use of a levonorgestrel IUD in adolescents with physical and intellectual disabilities [34, 35]. Both studies found high rates of satisfaction with the levonorgestrel IUD for menstrual suppression. However, it is important to consider that adolescents with disabilities may require anesthesia for insertion and removal of the IUD, with one study finding that 95% of adolescents with disabilities required general anesthesia [35]. However, in many cases, the insertion could be combined with other procedures requiring anesthetic in order to avoid use of anesthesia for solely the IUD insertion. It is recommended that adolescents with IUDs check their IUD strings (palpable against the cervix) at least one time per month to verify that the IUD is still in place. However, adolescents with physical or intellectual disabilities may be incapable of checking the strings. The expulsion rate of the IUD in nulliparous women is approximately 3–4% [36]. Adolescents and caregivers should be observant for a sudden increase in vaginal bleeding, which may indicate expulsion of the IUD.

Surgical Methods

Endometrial ablation seeks to prevent menstrual bleeding by selectively destroying the endometrial lining. However, prior studies have shown that amenorrhea rates are low in an adolescent population. It is not effective as a contraceptive or sterilization procedure, and individuals who do become pregnant after endometrial ablation have a high rate of prenatal complications, including perinatal mortality [37]. Endometrial ablation is not recommended by the American College of Gynecologists or the American Academy of Pediatrics for menstrual regulation in adolescents with special needs, and alternative methods should be preferred [2, 9].

The parents or caregivers of adolescents with disabilities will sometimes request hysterectomy to eliminate menstrual bleeding and prevent pregnancy. It is important to explain to families and patients that performing a hysterectomy represents an irreversible decision with serious risks. As a hysterectomy is a major surgical procedure, it carries significant risk of morbidity and mortality. In addition, a hysterectomy does not protect adolescents with disabilities from sexual abuse or sexually transmitted infections. The risks and costs of the procedure do not outweigh the benefits of menstrual control, and the same standards used in healthy adolescents should be used to determine whether a major surgical procedure is indicated. Thus, hysterectomy should only be considered for menstrual control after other reasonable alternatives have been attempted [2, 9]. The ethical and legal considerations of performing an elective surgery in adolescents with special needs must be carefully considered, and state laws regarding sterilization, hysterectomy, and consent in minors vary [2] (Table 24.1).

Special Considerations

Clot Risk in Adolescents with Limited Mobility

Several studies have sought to determine whether individuals with limited mobility have an increased risk of venous thromboembolism. One study of adult patients with multiple sclerosis found a high rate of deep venous thrombosis (43.9%) of patients, with 24.2% of patients having a history of venous thromboembolism [38]. However, in a sample of para- and tetraparesic patients institutionalized for long durations, no thromboembolisms were observed despite additional risk factors including orthopedic surgery, bone fractures, and hormonal therapy in 60% of participants [39]. Researchers have hypothesized that quadriplegia during childhood may reduce venous lakes, decreasing blood stasis and allowing for a closer to normal risk of venous thromboembolism when compared to patients who acquire quadriplegia later in life [40]. In addition, spasticity may play a role in preventing DVT in patients with limited mobility [39]. No studies to date have examined the risk of venous thromboembolism among adolescents with limited mobility on hormonal

Table 24.1 Available methods for menstrual regulation in adolescents with special needs

Category	Method	Brand names	Mechanism	Frequency of use	Menstrual suppression	Considerations in the special needs population
Estrogen- and progesterone-containing methods	Combined oral contraceptive	Many options available, ranging from first- to fourth-generation COCs	Inhibit ovulation via a negative feedback mechanism on the hypothalamus. Changes in the endometrium occur, reducing the amount of bleeding	Daily dosing	Can space menses out with extended (withdrawal bleed every 3 months) or continuous (no withdrawal bleed) regimens but may have breakthrough bleeding	• Possible drug-drug interactions with antiepileptic agents • Possible increased risk of VTE with limited mobility
	Ring	NuvaRing	Inhibit ovulation via a negative feedback mechanism on the hypothalamus. Changes in the endometrium occur, reducing the amount of bleeding	Monthly	Can space menses out with extended (withdrawal bleed every 3 months) or continuous (no withdrawal bleed) regimens but may have breakthrough bleeding	• Possible drug-drug interactions with antiepileptic agents • Possible increased risk of VTE with limited mobility may require assistance with insertion
	Patch	Ortho Evra, Xulane	Inhibit ovulation via negative feedback on the hypothalamus. Changes in the endometrium occur, reducing the amount of bleeding	Weekly	Can space menses out with extended or continuous cycling, but clot risk may be increased and breakthrough bleeding may occur	• Possible drug-drug interactions with antiepileptic agents • Possible increased risk of VTE with limited mobility • Patients may inadvertently remove patch

Progesterone-only methods	Progesterone-only pill	Micronor, Nor-QD	Negative feedback on the hypothalamus prevents follicular maturation and ovulation and causes endometrial thinning	Daily	May cause irregular bleeding with lighter, delayed, or absent periods. Amenorrhea can occur. Breakthrough bleeding is common	• Possible drug-drug interactions with antiepileptic agents • Irregular bleeding/ breakthrough bleeding
	Depot medroxyprogesterone acetate	Depo-Provera, Depo-SubQ Provera 104, Provera	Negative feedback on the hypothalamus prevents follicular maturation and ovulation and causes endometrial thinning	10–12 weeks	Irregular bleeding initially, high rates of amenorrhea after long-term use (52–64% at 1 year, 71% at 2 year)	• Irregular/ breakthrough bleeding • Bone density • Potential for weight gain
	Implant	Nexplanon	Negative feedback on the hypothalamus prevents follicular maturation and ovulation and causes endometrial thinning	3 years	Irregular	• Irregular bleeding • Insertion may be anxiety-provoking/ painful
	Intrauterine device	Mirena, Skyla	Negative feedback on the hypothalamus leads to thickening of the cervical mucus, alteration of the endometrium preventing implantation, and inhibition of ovulation	Mirena – 5 years Skyla – 3 years	Initial irregular bleeding, but after 6 months most women experience lighter, infrequent, or absent periods. Up to 50% of patients have amenorrhea at 1 year after insertion	• Irregular bleeding in the initial 6 months after insertion • May need anesthesia for insertion and removal • Patients may be unable to check strings

(continued)

Table 24.1 (continued)

Category	Method	Brand names	Mechanism	Frequency of use	Menstrual suppression	Considerations in the special needs population
Surgical	Endometrial ablation		Selectively destroys the endometrial lining to prevent heavy bleeding	Single procedure	Amenorrhea rates are low in an adolescent population	• Ethical and legal considerations • Long-term data needed
	Hysterectomy		Removal of uterus prevents pregnancy and menstrual bleeding	Permanent	Permanent amenorrhea	• Ethical and legal considerations • Not recommended by AAP or ACOG for menstrual suppression unless medically indicated for other reasons • Permanent sterilization
Miscellaneous	Nonsteroidal anti-inflammatory drugs (NSAIDs) such as ibuprofen, naproxen	Aspirin, Advil, Motrin, Voltaren, etc.	Reduces prostaglandin (PGE2 and PGF2 alpha) synthesis in the endometrium, leading to vasoconstriction and reduced bleeding	Frequency depends on medication. Start treatment on the first day of menses and continue for 4–5 days or until menstruation ceases	May improve dysmenorrhea and decrease ovulatory menstrual bleeding by 30–40%	• Nonhormonal does not provide pregnancy prevention • No increase in clotting risk in adolescents

contraception. Thus, the risks and benefits of available methods should be discussed with families prior to initiating a hormonal method of contraception, and a thorough history for patient and familial risk factors should be conducted. If patients and families opt to proceed with combined oral contraceptives, first- and second-generation COCs are optimal given their better clotting profile compared to third- and fourth-generation progestin-containing contraceptives. Further data is necessary to identify whether adolescents with limited mobility are at increased risk of venous thromboembolism when taking hormonal contraceptives.

Sexual Abuse

Adolescents with disabilities are often not viewed as targets for sexual abuse by their family and other members of their community. However, because their intellectual limitations may prevent them from identifying an advance as inappropriate or disclosing the abuse to a caregiver or other adult, some perpetrators may view adolescents with disabilities as an easy target [41]. One study demonstrated that women with severe disability impairments were four times more likely to be sexually assaulted than women with no reported disabilities. Children with disabilities often have limited access to critical information pertaining to personal safety and sexual abuse prevention, and parents of children with disabilities may object to a sexual education curriculum on human sexuality for their adolescents [42]. Pediatricians and pediatric and adolescent gynecologists can help to educate parents about normal sexual development and encourage them to advocate for their children to have appropriate sexual education in the school setting [43]. In the school setting, individualized educational plans (IEPs) can be set up to include human sexuality education geared at an appropriate intellectual level [44]. For example, educational activities can involve parents, teachers, and other care providers and may include role-play, visual aids, and frequent repetition of simple concepts and tasks.

At the University of Michigan, Dr. Elizabeth Quint and colleagues have developed counseling strategies to help prevent abuse. The circle of life helps explain relationships to youth with developmental disabilities. The inner circle involves parents and those closest to the child with the developmental disability, with the explanation that those family members would be appropriate to kiss or hug. The next circle might involve extended family, who it might be appropriate to hug. Next would be peers, teachers, and others in daily life, who it might be appropriate to say hello and give a handshake. Acquaintances might get a wave, while strangers might just be observed but not touched or engaged in conversation. Another example per Dr. Quint and colleagues is the No-Go-Tell strategy, where children with developmental disabilities—and all younger children—are taught their own first line of defense: "say No" to unwanted or unexpected contact, tell the person to "Go away", and then "Tell" someone, no matter what they are told by the perpetrator. This No-Go-Tell strategy can help prevent a cycle of abuse with a developmentally challenged child or adolescent.

Clinical Pearls and Highlights

- Gynecologic care for adolescents with disabilities should incorporate anticipatory guidance regarding pubertal changes and options for menstrual regulation, confidential care with the adolescent, and attention to parental concerns.
- Gynecologic care may be underutilized in adolescents with disabilities as parents and providers may dismiss the possibility that the patient is sexually active.
- If menstrual intervention is warranted, risks, benefits, and alternatives of available options should be discussed with the patient and family. Realistic expectations should be clearly outlined, as complete amenorrhea may be difficult to achieve.
- Options for menstrual regulation include combined hormonal contraceptives (available in pill, patch, and vaginal rings), progesterone-only contraceptives (including pills, injectables, implants, and IUDs), NSAIDs, and, as a last resort, surgical intervention.
- The interaction of hormonal contraceptives and antiepileptic agents must be carefully considered with each individual patient.
- Clot risk may be higher in adolescents with limited mobility. Risk factors for venous thromboembolism should be an important part of an evaluation prior to starting hormonal contraceptives.
- Adolescents with disabilities are at higher risk for sexual abuse and should receive sexual abuse prevention education at an appropriate level for their intellectual abilities. The No-Go-Tell strategy can be a useful construct to help prevent abuse.

References

1. US Census Bureau. Disability characteristics of school age children: 2010 – Children – Newsroom - U.S. Census Bureau. Available at: https://www.census.gov/newsroom/releases/archives/children/cb11-tps49.html. Accessed 1 Sept 2016.
2. Committee Opinion No. 668: Menstrual manipulation for adolescents with physical and developmental disabilities. Obstet Gynecol. 2016;128:e20–25.
3. Prasher VP. Down syndrome and thyroid disorders: a review. Downs Syndr Res Pract. 1999;6:25–42.
4. Hamed SA. The effect of epilepsy and antiepileptic drugs on sexual, reproductive and gonadal health of adults with epilepsy. Expert Rev. Clin. Pharmacol. 2016;9:807–19.
5. Herzog AG, Schachter SC. Valproate and the polycystic ovarian syndrome: final thoughts. Epilepsia. 2001;42:311–5.
6. Reynolds MF, Sisk EC, Rasgon NL. Valproate and neuroendocrine changes in relation to women treated for epilepsy and bipolar disorder: a review. Curr Med Chem. 2007;14:2799–812.
7. Hu X, et al. A meta-analysis of polycystic ovary syndrome in women taking valproate for epilepsy. Epilepsy Res. 2011;97:73–82.
8. Lambert TL, Farmer KC, Brahm NC. Evaluation of serum prolactin levels in intellectually disabled patients using antipsychotic medications. Int J Endocrinol Metab. 2013;11:57–61.
9. Quint EH, O'Brien RF, COMMITTEE ON ADOLESCENCE & North American Society for Pediatric and Adolescent Gynecology. Menstrual management for adolescents with disabilities. Pediatrics. 2016;138. pii: e20160295.

10. Kirkham YA, et al. Trends in menstrual concerns and suppression in adolescents with developmental disabilities. J Adolesc Health. 2013;53:407–12.
11. Quint EH. Menstrual and reproductive issues in adolescents with physical and developmental disabilities. Obstet Gynecol. 2014;124:367–75.
12. Quint EH. Adolescents with special needs: clinical challenges in reproductive health care. J Pediatr Adolesc Gynecol. 2016;29:2–6.
13. Hamilton A, Marshal MP, Sucato GS, Murray PJ. Rett syndrome and menstruation. J Pediatr Adolesc Gynecol. 2012;25:122–6.
14. ACOG Committee Opinion No. 651: menstruation in girls and adolescents: using the menstrual cycle as a vital sign. Obstet Gynecol. 2015;126:e143–6.
15. Moyer VA, U.S. Preventive Services Task Force. Screening for cervical cancer: U.S. Preventive Services Task Force recommendation statement. Ann Intern Med. 2012;156:880–891. , W312.
16. Practice Bulletin No. 157: Cervical cancer screening and prevention. Obstet Gynecol. 2016;127:e1–20.
17. Lethaby A, Augood C, Duckitt K. Nonsteroidal anti-inflammatory drugs for heavy menstrual bleeding. Cochrane Database Syst. Rev. 2000;(2):CD000400. doi:10.1002/14651858.CD000400.
18. Matteson KA, et al. Nonsurgical management of heavy menstrual bleeding: a systematic review. Obstet Gynecol. 2013;121:632–43.
19. Abdel-Tawab M, Zettl H, Schubert-Zsilavecz M. Nonsteroidal anti-inflammatory drugs: a critical review on current concepts applied to reduce gastrointestinal toxicity. Curr Med Chem. 2009;16:2042–63.
20. Reimers A, Brodtkorb E, Sabers A. Interactions between hormonal contraception and antiepileptic drugs: clinical and mechanistic considerations. Seizure. 2015;28:66–70.
21. First chewable oral contraceptive. FDA Consum. 2004;38:4.
22. Benagiano G, Carrara S, Filippi V. Safety, efficacy and patient satisfaction with continuous daily administration of levonorgestrel/ethinylestradiol oral contraceptives. Patient Prefer Adherence. 2009;3:131–43.
23. van Hylckama Vlieg A, Helmerhorst FM, Vandenbroucke JP, Doggen CJM, Rosendaal FR. The venous thrombotic risk of oral contraceptives, effects of oestrogen dose and progestogen type: results of the MEGA case-control study. BMJ. 2009;339:b2921.
24. Sulak PJ, et al. Frequency and management of breakthrough bleeding with continuous use of the transvaginal contraceptive ring: a randomized controlled trial. Obstet Gynecol. 2008;112:563–71.
25. Stewart FH, et al. Extended use of transdermal norelgestromin/ethinyl estradiol: a randomized trial. Obstet Gynecol. 2005;105:1389–96.
26. Emans, Laufer, Goldstein's pediatric & adolescent gynecology. Wolters Kluwer Health/Lippincott Williams & Wilkins Health; 2011.
27. Speroff L, Darney PD. A clinical guide for contraception. Phladelphia: Wolters Kluwer Health/Lippincott Williams & Wilkins; 2011.
28. Altshuler AL, Hillard PJA. Menstrual suppression for adolescents. Curr Opin Obstet Gynecol. 2014;26:323–31.
29. Arias RD, Jain JK, Brucker C, Ross D, Ray A. Changes in bleeding patterns with depot medroxyprogesterone acetate subcutaneous injection 104 mg. Contraception. 2006;74:234–8.
30. Lopez LM, et al. Progestin-only contraceptives: effects on weight. Cochrane Database Syst Rev. 2016;(8):CD008815.
31. Lopez LM, Chen M, Mullins Long S, Curtis KM, Helmerhorst FM. Steroidal contraceptives and bone fractures in women: evidence from observational studies. Cochrane Database Syst Rev. 2015;(7):CD009849. doi:10.1002/14651858.CD009849.pub3.
32. Hubacher D, Lopez L, Steiner MJ, Dorflinger L. Menstrual pattern changes from levonorgestrel subdermal implants and DMPA: systematic review and evidence-based comparisons. Contraception. 2009;80:113–8.
33. Hidalgo M, et al. Bleeding patterns and clinical performance of the levonorgestrel-releasing intrauterine system (Mirena) up to two years. Contraception. 2002;65:129–32.

34. Pillai M, O'Brien K, Hill E. The levonorgestrel intrauterine system (Mirena) for the treatment of menstrual problems in adolescents with medical disorders, or physical or learning disabilities. BJOG Int J Obstet Gynaecol. 2010;117:216–21.
35. Hillard PJA. Menstrual suppression with the levonorgestrel intrauterine system in girls with developmental delay. J Pediatr Adolesc Gynecol. 2012;25:308–13.
36. Alton TM, et al. Retrospective review of intrauterine device in adolescent and young women. J Pediatr Adolesc Gynecol. 2012;25:195–200.
37. Hare AA, Olah KS. Pregnancy following endometrial ablation: a review article. J Obstet Gynaecol. 2005;25:108–14.
38. Arpaia G, et al. Risk of deep venous thrombosis (DVT) in bedridden or wheelchair-bound multiple sclerosis patients: a prospective study. Thromb Res. 2010;125:315–7.
39. Rousseau MC, Guillotel B. Risk factors for deep venous thrombosis in tetraparesic mentally retarded patients. Brain Inj. 2001;15:1041–4.
40. Lohiya G-S, Tan-Figueroa L, Silverman S, Le HV. The wheelchair thrombosis syndrome. J Natl Med Assoc. 2006;98:1188–92.
41. American Academy of Pediatrics: Committee on Child Abuse and Neglect and Committee on Children with Disabilities. Assessment of maltreatment of children with disabilities. Pediatrics. 2001;108:508–12.
42. Murphy GH. Capacity to consent to sexual relationships in adults with learning disabilities. J Fam Plann Reprod Health Care. 2003;29:148–9.
43. Schopp LH, Sanford TC, Hagglund KJ, Gay JW, Coatney MA. Removing service barriers for women with physical disabilities: promoting accessibility in the gynecologic care setting. J. Midwifery Womens Health. 2002;47:74–9.
44. Sweeney L. Human sexuality education for students with special needs. Electron J Hum Sex. 2007;10:1–1.

Suggested Educational Reading, References, and Policies

Altshuler AL, Hillard PJA. Menstrual suppression for adolescents. Curr Opin Obstet Gynecol. 2014;26:323–31.

Committee Opinion No. 668: Menstrual manipulation for adolescents with physical and developmental disabilities. Obstet Gynecol. 2016;128:e20–25.

Quint EH, O'Brien RF, COMMITTEE ON ADOLESCENCE & North American Society for Pediatric and Adolescent Gynecology. Menstrual management for adolescents with disabilities. Pediatrics. 2016;138. pii: e20160295.

Chapter 25
Case of a Girl with Chronic Abdominal Pain, Frequent Emergency Room Visits, and Opioid Abuse

Kanani E. Titchen and Hina J. Talib

A 17-year-old G1P0010 girl was referred to an adolescent medicine specialist by the emergency department (ED) for evaluation of chronic abdominal pain recurring over the past year after she was seen in the ED 2 days ago for cervicitis. She has a history of physical and sexual abuse, extensive psychiatric history, prescription narcotic abuse, gynecologic history of pelvic inflammatory disease, and repeated sexually transmitted infections. Physical exam is significant for multiple tattoos, linear thigh hematoma, diffuse abdominal tenderness to palpation, scant vaginal discharge, and tearfulness on pelvic exam. She seems agitated and uses her cell phone to text throughout the clinic visit. Presentation is concerning for chronic pelvic pain and possible domestic minor sex trafficking (DMST). Because victims of DMST rarely self-identify, it is critical for physicians to recognize the warning signs of sex trafficking and effectively intervene on behalf of these patients to directly affect recovery and outcomes.

Maria is a 17-year-old girl who was referred to an adolescent medicine specialist by the emergency department (ED) for evaluation of chronic abdominal pain recurring over the past year after she was seen in the ED 2 days ago for cervicitis. In the ED, Maria was found to have thick yellow vaginal discharge and severe abdominal pain, but she denied vaginal spotting and dyspareunia. Her gynecologic exam was notable for copious malodorous discharge from her cervical os but no cervical motion or adnexal tenderness. Maria was treated presumptively for cervicitis as per Centers for Disease Control and Prevention's sexually transmitted infection

K.E. Titchen, M.D. (✉)
Division of Adolescent Medicine, Children's Hospital at Montefiore,
The Pediatric Hospital for Albert Einstein College of Medicine, Bronx, NY, USA
e-mail: ktitchen@montefiore.org

H.J. Talib, M.D.
Assistant Professor, Pediatrics, Program Director, Post-doctoral Fellowship in Adolescent Medicine, Division of Adolescent Medicine, Children's Hospital at Montefiore,
The Pediatric Hospital for Albert Einstein College of Medicine, Bronx, NY, USA

H.J. Talib (ed.), *Adolescent Gynecology*,
https://doi.org/10.1007/978-3-319-66978-6_25

2016 treatment guidelines with intramuscular ceftriaxone and a 7-day course of oral doxycycline. She was, additionally, prescribed Percocet for her chronic severe abdominal pain.

Today, she is accompanied by her father and states that her "stomach still hurts." She says the pain is usually lower abdomen and not associated with bowel changes or menses. She appears angry and gives one-word answers while looking at the floor. Her father appears irritated and attempts to answer questions for her. He agrees to step out of the room, looking doubtfully at Maria. Maria continues to text on her cell phone and gives brief answers to your questions.

Maria gives a menarche of 11 years 3 months (gynecologic age of 6 years), her last menstrual period was prior to her most recent DMPA injection 6 weeks ago, and her "daddy always makes sure" she gets her shot on time. On sexual history, Maria discloses coitarche at 12years old and "more than she can remember" number of lifetime sexual male and female partners. Her last sex was yesterday without a condom. She has had one elective pregnancy termination at age 15. With regard to her chronic abdominal pain, she reveals a history of frequent Percocet use following prescriptions given by the ED and admits that sometimes it's just easier to "work something out" on the street for pain medication rather than going to the ED.

On confidential social history, Maria relates that she lives with her father after a history of physical abuse and sexual abuse by her mother's boyfriend when Maria was 12 years old. She says an Administration for Child Services (ACS) caseworker continues to follow up with her. She failed seventh and ninth grades and is currently in ninth grade but with frequent absences. Maria's electronic medical record (EMR) indicates an extensive but nonspecific psychiatric history with diagnoses of bipolar disorder and oppositional defiant disorder and history of non-suicidal self-injurious behaviors. She contracts for safety today, continues texting, and then says she really needs to get going, and is this going to take much longer?

She has been seen in the ED seven times in the past 2 years for pelvic pain, with one episode of gonococcal pelvic inflammatory disease (PID) and an episode of non-gonococcal, non-chlamydial PID. Each time, she received presumptive treatment for STI, was given morphine, prescribed Percocet and/or ibuprofen, referred to adolescent medicine, and sent home. Further, the record shows that pregnancy, HIV, and STI tests done in the ED 2 days ago were negative. This is the first time Maria has followed up with adolescent medicine.

Physical exam reveals a slim, comfortable, but anxious-appearing girl. Vital signs are within normal limits. Exam is significant for diffuse abdominal tenderness to palpation without rebound, guarding, distension, or organomegaly. Pubic hair is shaved but consistent with SMR 5 distribution, and she has a normal external genital exam with no discharge or lesions noted. There is a mild amount of thin, slightly malodorous, white-gray discharge vaginal discharge. On speculum exam, Maria becomes tearful. The cervix is non-friable without lesions, and after some deep breathing and distraction on bimanual exam, there is no cervical motion, uterine, or adnexal tenderness. Her skin is notable for several tattoos of a bow and her boyfriend's initials, a roll of cash, and a nondescript marking at the thenar eminence of her right hand. She has a linear hematoma approximately 6 in. long and 1 cm wide that wraps from the posterior right thigh around to the lateral right thigh.

The nurse knocks on the door and states that Maria's father would like to know if this will take much longer.

Clinical Questions that Might Arise for the Physician

1. *Something feels "off." What are the factors in Maria's history and physical exam that should raise my clinical suspicion for Maria's being a victim of domestic minor sex trafficking (DMST)?*
2. *What are some of the common health and psychological sequelae of DMST?*
3. *How do I approach a patient who I think is a victim of DMST? What do I ask?*
4. *What are some of the resources available to me and to my patient?*

Discussion

Maria's history and current presentation are concerning for possible domestic minor sex trafficking (DMST). With almost 21 million people affected worldwide, human trafficking for sex, labor, or organs is a major public health crisis and an egregious violation of human rights [1]. The US Congress defines DMST as "the recruitment, harboring, transportation, provision, or obtaining of a person for the purpose of a commercial sex act... in which the person induced to perform such act has not attained 18 years of age." [2] Modest estimates suggest that 100,000–300,000 minors in the United States are at risk for DMST annually [3], although data are limited. Most studies indicate that US adolescent females are recruited into sex trafficking in their early to mid-teens [4–6]. Maria exhibited many of the factors that are known to increase risk for DMST, such as female gender, young age, poverty, lack of education, and history of abuse or family instability; in addition, children who are in foster care status or who are marginalized (e.g., racial/ethnic minority, immigrant, or sexual minority status) are at high risk [7].

Something Feels "Off"

Patients who have been victims of human trafficking may present while still being exploited [8, 9]. Maria was accompanied by a man who introduced himself as her father: indeed, many victims are accompanied by an older adult who poses as a father, mother, boyfriend/girlfriend, or spouse but who is actually the trafficker [4]. This person may attempt to speak for the patient and/or rush the appointment along, as Maria's father did. Maria was noted to be texting throughout the clinic visit, which could be construed as typical adolescent behavior. However, this also could be a red flag for trafficking: during the confidential history taking and exam, victims may be required to keep in close cell phone contact with the trafficker through texting [10]. A trafficking victim's failure to reply to the trafficker's texted question(s) in a timely fashion could lead to repercussions such as beatings, starvation, or other punishment later on [10]. Beatings, rape, and torture are not uncommon among trafficking victims, especially younger victims [10].

Although Maria states that she lives with her father, it is possible that she has run away from home, especially in the context of abuse by her mother's boyfriend, her frequent absences from school, and the instability evident in her life. Runaway status and homelessness are other significant risk factors for DMST: more than 10% of US minors living in shelters and 28% of US minors living on the streets report exchanging sex for drugs or money [11].

Victims frequently suffer from post-traumatic stress disorder (PTSD), substance abuse, anxiety, and depression, and these mental health issues can complicate history taking [12, 13]. Maria's history includes vague psychiatric diagnoses and frequent Percocet use, and she admits that the prescriptions she obtains from ED visits are not enough, so she engages in what sounds like transactional sex to obtain drugs on the street. Some traffickers supply their victims with drugs to help patients manage pain so that they can continue working or to control them. Forced substance abuse, in particular, can be a very effective means for traffickers to control their victims, with some victims receiving their "payment" from their trafficker in the form of drugs [14].

Certain physical signs and symptoms serve as red flags for sex trafficking: these include repeated STIs, repeated pregnancy and/or abortion, tattoos, bruises, lacerations, and scars [15–18]. But the physician might detect behaviors associated with abuse and trafficking simply by observing the patient as she enters the room. Maria's angry and agitated affect, her poor eye contact, her impatience for the visit to be over, and her tearfulness during pelvic examination all could be related to DMST, especially in the context of her history and physical exam. While many physicians may dismiss an adolescent patient's poor eye contact as boredom or a lack of respect, it is worth noting that in the world of sex trafficking, victims are taught to respect their pimps by *avoiding* eye contact [10]. The physician who examined Maria might have elicited a clearer picture of abuse and/or trafficking had she or he asked about Maria's tattoos and hematoma, as well as her history of multiple STIs. Her statement that her "daddy always makes sure" she gets her DMPA shot might, upon further questioning, reveal a history of reproductive coercion, which is defined as "behavior intended to maintain power and control in a relationship related to reproductive health by someone who is, was, or wishes to be involved in an intimate or dating relationship with an adult or adolescent." [19] Approximately 9% of women aged 18–49 years old in the United States report history of reproductive coercion [20], and reproductive coercion appears to be more prevalent in women experiencing intimate partner violence than in those who experience more casual relationships [21–25]. Maria's pregnancy and termination of pregnancy might also be related to abuse, and the physician should ask about the circumstances leading to both (Table 25.1).

It is noted on Maria's exam that she has a "linear hematoma" on her thigh, which could be consistent with a mark left from beating with a hanger or extension cord or wire, for example [15]. In one study, women forced or deceived into entering sex

Table 25.1 Potential red flags for human sex trafficking

Repeated STIs
Repeated pregnancy/abortion
Tattoos
Lacerations
Bruises
Scars
Inappropriate clothing
Evidence of controlling relationship or IPV
Is fearful, anxious, depressed, submissive, tense, or nervous/paranoid
Exhibits unusually fearful or anxious behavior after bringing up law enforcement
Avoids eye contact
Has few or no personal possessions
Is not in control of his/her own money, no financial records, or bank account
Is not in control of his/her own identification documents (ID or passport)
Is not allowed to speak (a third party may insist on being present and/or translating)

work before the age of 18 years were at greater risk for physical and sexual violence than those who had entered after the age of 18 years on their own terms, although both groups experienced high levels of violence [15]. Sex-trafficked patients may be hesitant to reveal details of their abuse for fear of trafficker violence, physician judgment, out of embarrassment, or due to their own failure to recognize their treatment as abusive [26].

Maria's case is also significant for lack of follow-up despite multiple referrals to adolescent medicine which is not uncommon in marginalized, including trafficked, youth. Tremendous coordination of care is required for DMST patients when they do present to care, not only to connect them to trafficking specific medical and legal care but also to ensure pediatric or family medicine referral, gynecology referral, and STI screens as indicated [27].

What Are Some of the Common Health and Psychological Sequelae of DMST?

There are several chronic medical and psychiatric health sequelae or presentations of victims of DMST (Table 25.2). One retrospective cohort study of adolescents presenting to a health center for specific evaluation of DMST concerns found that the most common chief complaints of previous medical visits included psychiatric issues (28%), abdominal or back pain (13%), physical injury (9%), gynecologic complaint (8%), and sexual abuse/assault (8%) [28]. Like Maria, victims of physical or sexual abuse may present with chronic pelvic pain (CPP), defined as at least

Table 25.2 Health sequelae of human sex trafficking

Burns, branding, tattoos, and other purposeful and permanent stigmata of "ownership"
Trauma by blunt force, gun, knife, or strangulation
Fractures, dental and oral cavity injuries, traumatic brain injury inconsistent with the history
Neuropathies and other effects of torture
Scarring, especially from unattended prior injuries
Genital trauma
Repeated unwanted pregnancy and/or forced abortion
Sexually transmitted infections (e.g., chlamydia, gonorrhea, human papilloma virus, hepatitis B and C, and HIV)
Infertility, chronic pelvic pain, cervical cancer, liver failure, HIV-AIDS, and chronic disease states resulting from untreated sexually transmitted infections
Impaired social skills
Long-term effects of inadequate treatment of common childhood diseases
Headaches, chronic pain syndromes, abdominal complaints
Fatigue
Substance abuse
Infectious diseases usually prevented through routine immunization
Psychological sequelae: feelings of intense stigma, shame, anxiety, and hopelessness, pathologic fear, panic attacks, sleep disturbances, dissociative disorders, depression, post-traumatic stress disorder, and suicidal ideation and/or attempt

Adapted from http://www.massmed.org/Patient-Care/Health-Topics/Violence-Prevention-and-Intervention/Human-Trafficking-(pdf)/

Table 25.3 Differential diagnosis for chronic pelvic pain in the adolescent female

Outflow tract obstruction (e.g., imperforate hymen, vaginal or cervical agenesis)
Endometriosis
Ovarian cyst
Pelvic inflammatory disease
Urethritis or urinary tract infection
Functional abdominal pain
Chronic constipation
Irritable bowel syndrome
Inflammatory bowel disease
Hernia
Abdominal wall muscle strain
Anxiety/depression
Sexual abuse
Secondary gain

3–6 months of noncyclic pain at or below the umbilicus and interfering with daily activities [29]. The differential diagnosis for CPP in the adolescent female is broad including infectious, such as pelvic inflammatory disease; gynecologic, including dysmenorrhea and endometriosis; and functional abdominal pain (Table 25.3). Depression and anxiety are associated with CPP, and these may be either a cause or result. Finally, the physician should have a high index of suspicion for CPP as sequelae of chronic or acute PID, especially given that adolescents are at increased risk for PID because of cervical ectopy and increased behavioral risk taking [30]. Maria's history included two episodes of PID, which sets her up for CPP.

How Do I Approach a Patient Who I Think Is a Victim of DMST? What Do I Ask?

A 2015 American Academy of Pediatrics clinical report on child sex trafficking recommends asking three pointed questions when the patient exhibits several signs of DMST victimization: (1) Has anyone ever asked you to have sex in exchange for something you wanted or needed (money, food, shelter, or other items)? (2) Has anyone ever asked you to have sex with another person? (3) Has anyone ever taken sexual pictures of you or posted such pictures on the internet? [31] It would have been prudent for the physician to ask Maria if she had ever traded anything for sex and to follow up on Maria's statement that she sometimes would "work something out" on the street to obtain opioid medication: a positive response could alert providers to the possibility that Maria was a victim of DMST. Furthermore, as homelessness is a major risk factor for DMST, Greenbaum and colleagues encourage asking, "Have you ever run away from home? How many times in the last year?" [32], when the clinician has clinical suspicion for DMST. These questions are likely to have been met with positive responses by Maria.

Because sexual abuse may cause or contribute to CPP, it is imperative that the physician obtains a confidential history from the patient without interference by a parent, guardian, or individual accompanying the patient to her appointment, as was done in Maria's case [33]. In addition, it is a good idea to preface questions involving abuse with reassurance that such questions are routine and standard and do not reflect judgmentalism. This is especially relevant when asking about the number of sexual partners: a victim of DMST who discloses his or her situation may report hundreds of sexual encounters. And like Maria, victims of DMST are less likely to have used a condom at last sexual encounter, putting them at high risk for STIs and HIV infection [31].

If an acute history of sexual assault is elicited, a sexual assault evidence kit may be offered within 3–4 days of the trauma as well as pregnancy, STI, HIV, HEP B and C, and syphilis testing. Physicians may refer to CDC guidelines of STI testing in cases of assault [34].

Forced tattoos may also represent physical assault, and many victims of trafficking are branded with symbols that represent a certain pimp or trafficker, or they may be tattooed with dollar signs or profanity [10, 27, 32] (Fig. 25.1). Questions about tattoos may include the open-ended "Tell me about your tattoo," as well as inquiry about use of clean needles and tattoo placement of the patient's own volition versus forced tattooing or branding [35].

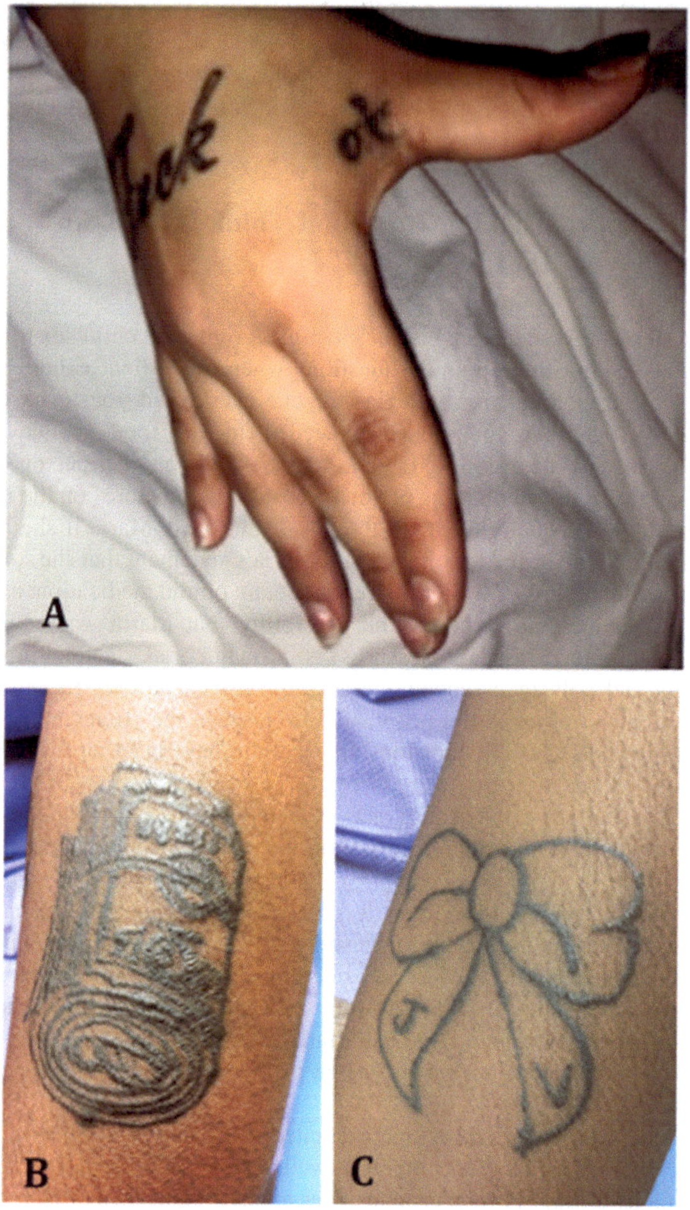

Fig. 25.1 Tattoos found on DMST patients who presented to pediatric clinics. (**a**) Expletive and nondescript pimp's symbol on an 18-year-old DMST victim. (**b**) Roll of cash tattooed on a DMST victim. (**c**) Pimp's initials wrapped up in a bow and tattooed on a DMST victim

Because direct questioning about signs specific to trafficking may elicit anxiety and distress from the patient, a trauma-informed approach is needed. This requires the establishment of rapport and trust by inquiring about the patient's immediate needs, establishing a private and confidential setting, and using sensitive language, with avoidance of terms that confer judgment, such as "prostitute" and "hooker" [10]. Prior to any questioning, limits of confidentiality should be reviewed, and disclosure of trafficking should not be forced [10]. Instead, autonomy should be restored to the patient, and it should be emphasized to the patient that she or he is not required to provide answers to questions and that all questions are being asked for the sole purpose of providing better risk assessment and patient care [36].

What Are Some of the Resources Available to Me and to My Patient?

Unfortunately, in a survey of physicians at all stages of training, researchers found that although a majority of physicians acknowledge the importance of awareness of human sex trafficking, only 40% stated that they knew whom to call if they encountered a DMST victim, and most are not familiar with existing resources [37]. To help guide clinical encounters, the National Human Trafficking Resource Center (NHTRC) created an algorithm to help identify, triage, and refer victims [38]. (Fig. 25.2).

The NHTRC (phone number 888-3737-888) can provide the physician and health-care professional with resources for patients on a state and even local level. The phone number is easily memorized and should be given to patients verbally and privately in the health-care setting. In addition, patients may text "BeFree" if they are in immediate danger. In each case, a volunteer at the NHTRC will return their communication in a safe, private manner and with an ability to provide resources such as housing, medical, and legal help to the patient. For the protection of the patient, no information regarding resources for human trafficking should be printed for the patient in the event that the patient's trafficker finds such materials and is enraged.

In some states, pediatricians are mandated reporters of suspected child abuse and neglect, and as such the provider should be encouraged to report suspected exploitation to law enforcement and Child Protective Services [39].

In summary, this case illustrates common warning signs for sex trafficking in youth who present to the medical setting for routine and/or delayed treatment of acute and chronic disease processes. Because victims of DMST rarely self-identify, recognition of the warning signs of sex trafficking is critical to effectively intervene on behalf of these patients and may directly affect recovery and outcomes. As an increasing number of medical societies acknowledge the impact of sex trafficking on US minors including chronic pain syndromes, substance abuse and dependence, long-term complications from untreated common diseases, unwanted pregnancy, and numerous psychological illnesses (Table 25.3), resources

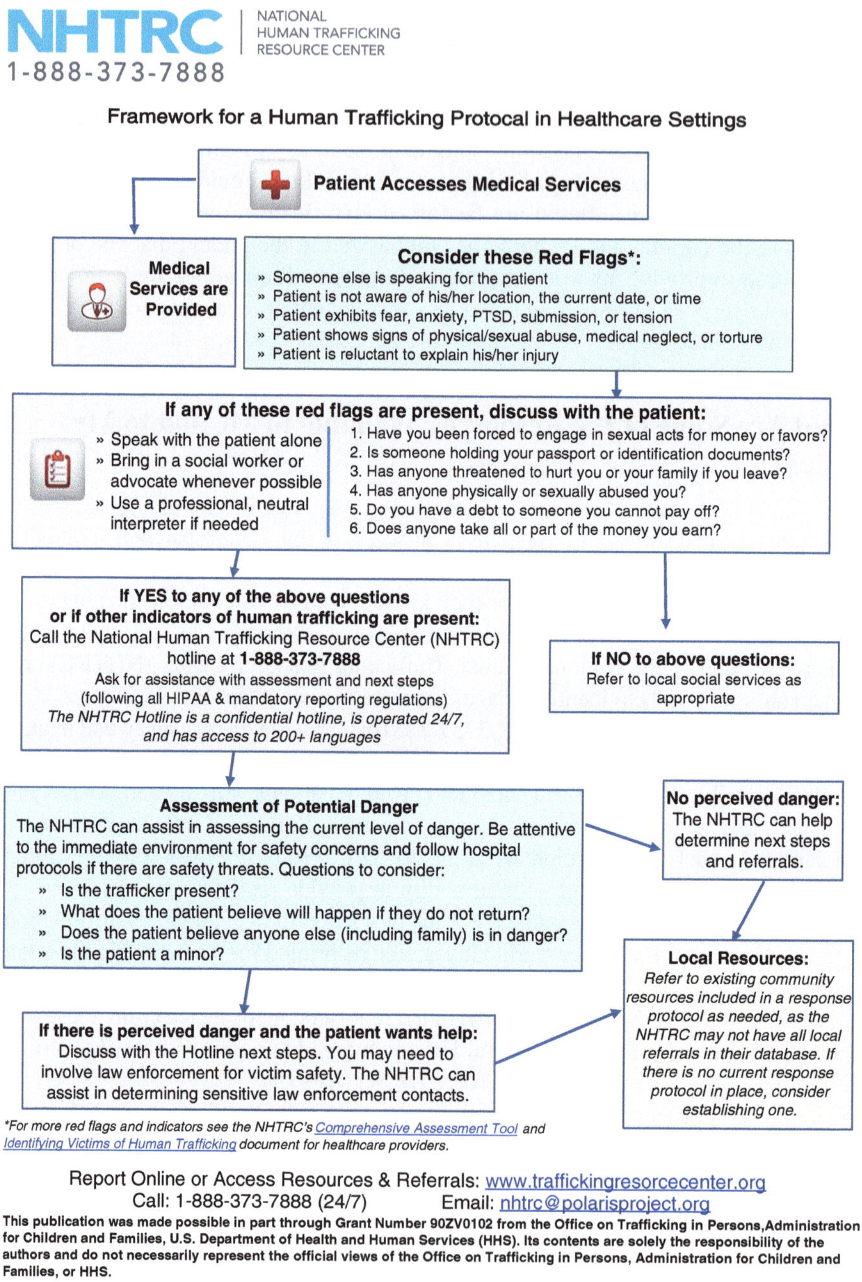

Fig. 25.2 National Human Trafficking Resource Center flowchart for medical professionals when caring for a suspected victim of human trafficking

for screening, identification, and intervention for sex-trafficked patients are growing and should be utilized [7, 10, 32, 40, 41].

Maria did not disclose any history of DMST during this initial visit with her adolescent medicine physician. However, she was provided with the NHTRC hotline number, which she memorized during the visit. Maria did provide her cell phone number to the clinician, and she was given the clinic phone number and a written prescription for follow-up with the same physician for 1 week later.

Clinical Pearls and Pitfalls

- Many domestic US victims of sex trafficking are recruited when they are in their early to mid-teens.
- Sex-trafficked patients may not wish to disclose their situation out of embarrassment, fear, or inability to recognize that they are being abused and exploited.
- Warning signs for sex trafficking include chronic pain syndromes, including chronic pelvic pain, repeated STIs and/or pregnancies and/or abortions, homelessness or unstable housing, transactional sex, frequent texting or the presence of a controlling/dominating person accompanying them to the medical visit, substance abuse, and tattoos/branding.
- Consequences of sex trafficking may be many and severe. They include chronic pain syndromes, depression, anxiety, PTSD, suicide ideation/attempt, infertility, impaired social skills, late presentation of chronic disease, joblessness, and poverty.
- It is the job of the physician or health-care professional to connect the trafficked patient to resources by soliciting the help of a social worker and/or calling the National Human Trafficking Resource Center (NHTRC) for assistance at 1-888-3737-888.
- It is the job of the physician or health-care professional to return a sense of control, well-being, and humanness to the trafficked patient by (1) attending to immediate needs, (2) prescribing/scheduling a follow-up visit, (3) asking if there is a safe person to whom the patient can turn, (4) asking the patient if she would like legal resources, and (5) giving the patient the NHTRC number 888-3737-888 and instructions to text "BeFree" if they are in immediate danger.

American Academy of Pediatrics (AAP)

"Child sex trafficking and commercial sexual exploitation of children (CSEC) are major public health problems in the United States and throughout the world. Despite large numbers of American and foreign youth affected and a plethora of serious physical and mental health problems associated with CSEC, there is limited information available to pediatricians regarding the nature and scope of human trafficking and how pediatricians and other health-care providers may help protect children. Knowledge of risk factors, recruitment practices, possible indicators of CSEC, and common medical and behavioral health problems experienced by victims will help pediatricians recognize potential victims and respond appropriately. As health-care providers, educators, and leaders in child advocacy, pediatricians play an essential role in addressing the public health issues faced by child victims of CSEC. Their roles can include working to increase recognition of CSEC, providing direct care and anticipatory guidance related to CSEC, engaging in collaborative efforts with medical and nonmedical colleagues to provide for the complex needs of youth, and educating child-serving professionals and the public."—Abstract of "Child Sex Trafficking and Commercial Sexual Exploitation: Health Care Needs of Victims," *Pediatrics,* March 2015.

See the full clinical report: http://pediatrics.aappublications.org/content/135/3/566.full.pdf+html.

The American College of Obstetricians and Gynecologists (ACOG)

"Acknowledging the significant interplay of women's human rights with the overall health of women and society, the American College of Obstetricians and Gynecologists and the American Congress of Obstetricians and Gynecologists (ACOG) ardently support efforts to improve the dignity, autonomy, rights and health of women in the United States and globally. ACOG endorses the International Federation of Gynecology and Obstetrics (FIGO) resolutions regarding the rights of women, the relationship of these rights to human rights, and the social responsibility obstetrician-gynecologists have to promote and protect women's health in their individual and professional encounters. To this end, ACOG commits to encourage and uphold policies and action in the United States and across the world to assure that women have:

…The right to decide when and if to have sex, including choosing one's partner, and freedom from coerced marriage and sex trafficking." —Excerpt from Statement of Policy, July 2012.

See the full policy statement: http://www.acog.org/-/media/Statements-of-Policy/Public/2012GlobalWmHlthRights.pdf

American Psychological Association (APA)

"BE IT THEREFORE RESOLVED that the American Psychological Association:

Commits itself to promoting public awareness of the presence of human trafficking consistent with its mission;

Commends individuals, nongovernmental organizations, and governments that are working to create public awareness of human trafficking, to prevent human trafficking and to emancipate trafficked persons, and to assist them in obtaining human services and health care including attention to their psychological needs;

Urges funded research on the social and cultural underpinnings of human trafficking, ways to assist trafficked persons, and research into psychological treatments and educational needs for trafficked persons, consist with their unique circumstances; and.

Urges the United States government, state and local governments, foreign governments, and international non-governmental organizations to work assiduously to end human trafficking and to assist its victims." —Excerpt from "APA Resolution on Emancipating and Assisting Victims of Human Trafficking," 2009.

See the full resolution: https://www.apa.org/pi/women/programs/trafficking/report.pdf.

References

1. International Labor Organization. New ILO Global estimate of forced labour: 20.9 million victims. Available at: http://www.ilo.org/global/about-the-ilo/newsroom/news/WCMS_182109/lang--en/index.htm. Accessed 1 May 2016.
2. Victims of Trafficking and Violence Protection Act of 2000, Pub L No. 106-386, 114 Stat 1464.
3. Richard J, Estes N, Weiner A. The commercial sexual exploitation of children in the U.S., Canada and Mexico. Philadelphia: University of Pennsylvania; 2001. p. 260.
4. Macy RJ, Graham LM. Identifying domestic and international sex-trafficking victims during human service provision. Trauma Violence Abuse. 2012;13(2):59–76.
5. Clarke RJ, Clarke EA, Roe-Sepowitz D, Fey R. Age at entry into prostitution: relationship to drug use, race, suicide, education level, childhood abuse, and family experiences. J Hum Behav Soc Environ. 2012;22(3):270–89. https://doi.org/10.1080/10911359.2012.655583.
6. Spangenberg M. Prostituted youth in New York city: an overview. ECPAT-USA. 2001. Available at: https://d1qkyo3pi1c9bx.cloudfront.net/00028B1B-B0DB-4FCD-A991-219527535DAB/7922f23e-a266-44f4-aae4-0f525f3dbe7d.pdf. Accessed 27 June 2016.
7. Alpert EJ, Ahn R, Albright E, Purcell G, Burke TF, Macias-Konstantopoulos WL. Human trafficking: guidebook on identification, assessment, and response in the health care setting. Boston : MGH Human Trafficking Initiative, Division of Global Health and Human Rights, Department of Emergency Medicine, Massachusetts General Hospital and Waltham: Committee on Violence Intervention and Prevention, Massachusetts Medical Society. Available at: www.massmed.org/Patient-Care/Health-Topics/Violence-Prevention-and-Intervention/Human-Trafficking-(pdf)/. Accessed 27 June 2016.
8. Baldwin SB, Eisenman DP, Sayles JN, Ryan G, Chuang KS. Identification of human trafficking victims in health care settings. Health Hum Rights. 2011;13(1):E36–49.
9. Lederer L, Wetzel CA. The health consequences of sex trafficking and their implications for identifying victims in healthcare facilities. Ann Health Law. 2014;23(1):61–91.
10. Lloyd R, Orman A. Training manual on the Commercial Sexual Exploitation of Children (CSEC). New York: Girls Educational Mentoring Services (GEMS); 2009.
11. Greene JM, Ennett ST, Ringwalt CL. Prevalence and correlates of survival sex among runaway and homeless youth. Am J Public Health. 1999;89(9):1406–9.
12. Oram S, Khondoker M, Abas M, Broadbent M, Howard LM. Characteristics of trafficked adults and children with severe mental illness: a historical cohort study. Lancet Psychiatry. 2015;2:1084–91.

13. Zimmerman C, Hossain M, Yun K, et al. The health of trafficked women: a survey of women entering post-trafficking services in Europe. Am J Public Health. 2008;98:55–9. https://doi.org/10.2105/AJPH.2006.108357.
14. Raphael J, Reichert J, Powers M. Pimp control and violence: domestic sex trafficking of Chicago women and girls. Women Crim Justice. 2010;20:89–104.
15. Oram S, Stöckl H, Busza J, Howard LM, Zimmerman C. Prevalence and risk of violence and the physical, mental, and sexual health problems associated with human trafficking: systematic review. PLoS Med. 2012;9(5):e1001224.
16. Barrows J, Finger R. Human trafficking and the healthcare professional. South Med J. 2008;101(5):521–4.
17. Muftic LR, Finn MA. Health outcomes among women trafficked for sex in the United States: a closer look. J Interpers Violence. 2013;28(9):1859–85.
18. Macias-Konstantopoulos WL, Munroe D, Purcell G, Tester K, Burke TF, Ahn R. The commercial sexual exploitation and sex trafficking of minors in the Boston metropolitan area: experiences and challenges faced by front-line providers and other stakeholders. J Appl Res Child. 2015;6(1):4.
19. ACOG Committee Opinion. http://www.acog.org/Resources-And-Publications/Committee-Opinions/Committee-on-Health-Care-for-Underserved-Women/Reproductive-and-Sexual-Coercion.
20. Black MC, Basile KC, Breiding MJ, et al. National Intimate Partner and Sexual Violence Survey: 2010 summary report; 2011.
21. Bauman LJ, Berman R. Adolescent relationships and condom use: trust, love and commitment. AIDS Behav. 2005;9(2):211–22.
22. Catallozzi M, Bell DL, Short MB, Marcell AV, Ebel SC, Rosenthal SL. Does perception of relationship type impact sexual health risk? Sex Transm Dis. 2013;40(6):473–5.
23. Fortenberry JD, Tu W, Harezlak J, Katz BP, Orr DP. Condom use as a function of time in new and established adolescent sexual relationships. Am J Public Health. 2002;92(2):211–3.
24. Ellen JM, Cahn S, Eyre SL, Boyer CB. Types of adolescent sexual relationships and associated perceptions about condom use. J Adolesc Health. 1996;18(6):417–21.
25. Norris AE, Ford K. Sexual experiences and condom use of heterosexual, low-income African American and Hispanic youth practicing relative monogamy, serial monogamy, and nonmonogamy. Sex Transm Dis. 1999;26(1):17–25.
26. Hom KA, Woods SJ. Trauma and its aftermath for commercially sexually exploited women as told by front-line service providers. Issues Ment Health Nurs. 2013;34(2):75–81.
27. Titchen KE, Katz D, Martinez K, White K. Ovarian cystadenoma in a trafficked patient. Pediatrics. 2016;137(5): pii: e20152201.
28. Goldberg AP, Moore JL, Houck C, Kaplan DM, Barron CE. Domestic minor sex trafficking patients: a retrospective analysis of medical presentation. J Pediatr Adolesc Gynecol. 2017;30(1):109–15.
29. Powell J. The approach to chronic pelvic pain in the adolescent. Obstet Gynecol Clin N Am. 2014;41:343–55.
30. Lee V, Tobin JM, Foley E. Relationship of cervical ectopy to chlamydia infection in young women. J Fam Plann Reprod Health Care. 2006;32:104–6.
31. Greenbaum J, Crawford-Jakubiak J. Child sex trafficking and commercial sexual exploitation: health care needs of victims. Pediatrics. 2015;135(3):566–74.
32. American Professional Society on the Abuse of Children, Greenbaum J, Kellogg N, Isaac R, et al. The commercial sexual exploitation of children: the medical provider's role in identification, assessment and treatment. Available at: www.kyaap.org/wp-content/uploads/APSAC_Guidelines.pdf. Accessed 12 Aug 2015.
33. Lampe A, Sölder D, Ennemoser A, et al. Chronic pelvic pain and previous sexual abuse. Obstet Gynecol. 2000;96:929–33.
34. Centers for Disease Control and Prevention. Sexually transmitted diseases treatment guidelines. 2015. Available at: http://www.cdc.gov/std/tg2015/sexual-assault.htm#table6. Accessed 4 Dec 2016.

35. Shandro J, Chisolm-Straker M, Duber HC, Findlay SL, Munoz J, Schmitz G, Stanzer M, Stoklosa H, Wiener DE, Wingkun N. Human trafficking: a guide to identification and approach for the emergency physician. Ann Emerg Med. 2016;68(4):501–8.e1.
36. Zimmerman C, Watts C. World Health Organization ethical and safety recommendations for interviewing trafficked women. Geneva: World Health Organization; 2003. Available at: http://apps.who.int/iris/bitstream/10665/42765/1/9241546255.pdf. Accessed 4 Dec 2016.
37. Titchen KE, Loo D, Berdan L, Rysavy MB, Ng JJ, Sharif I. Domestic sex trafficking of minors: medical student and physician awareness. J Pediatr Adolesc Gynecol. 2017;30(1):102–8.
38. https://humantraffickinghotline.org/resources/framework-human-trafficking-protocol-health-care-settings. Accessed 5 Dec 2016.
39. Child Welfare Information Gateway. (2016). Mandatory reporters of child abuse and neglect. Washington, DC: U.S. Department of Health and Human Services, Children's Bureau. Available at: https://www.childwelfare.gov/pubPDFs/manda.pdf. Accessed 4 Dec 2016.
40. Baldwin S, Chang K, Chisolm-Straker M, Grace A, Littenberg N, Stoklosa H. Heal trafficking: health professional advocacy, education, & linkage. Available at: http://healtrafficking.org/linkagesresources. Accessed 7 May 2015.
41. American Medical Women's Association. PATH: physicians against the trafficking of humans. Available at: http://www.doc-path.org/path. Accessed 7 May 2016.

Suggested Educational Reading, References, and Policies

https://polarisproject.org/sex-trafficking.
https://healtrafficking.org.
http://www.doc-path.org.

Index

H.J. Talib (ed.), *Adolescent Gynecology*,
https://doi.org/10.1007/978-3-319-66978-6

MIX
Papier aus verantwortungsvollen Quellen
Paper from responsible sources
FSC® C105338

FSC
www.fsc.org

If you have any concerns about our products,
you can contact us on
ProductSafety@springernature.com

In case Publisher is established outside the EU,
the EU authorized representative is:
Springer Nature Customer Service Center GmbH
Europaplatz 3, 69115 Heidelberg, Germany

Printed by Libri Plureos GmbH
in Hamburg, Germany